D1582498

THE YEAR IN
RESPIRATORY MEDICINE
2003

THE YEAR IN RESPIRATORY MEDICINE

2003

**W MACNEE, R FERGUSSON, A HILL
P REID, J SIMPSON**

CLINICAL PUBLISHING SERVICES
OXFORD

Distributed worldwide by
CRC Press
Boca Raton   London   New York   Washington, DC

Clinical Publishing Services Ltd

Oxford Centre for Innovation
Mill Street, Oxford OX2 OJX, UK

Tel: +44 1865 811116
Fax: +44 1865 251550
Web: www.clinicalpublishing.co.uk

Distributed by:

CRC Press LLC
2000 NW Corporate Blvd
Boca Raton, FL 33431, USA
E-mail: orders@crcpress.com

CRC Press UK
23–25 Blades Court
Deodar Road
London SW15 2NU, UK
E-mail: crcpress@itps.co.uk

© Clinical Publishing Services Ltd 2003

First published 2003

A catalogue record for this book is available from the British Library

ISBN 0 9537339 8 X

The publisher makes no representation, express or implied, that the dosages in this book are correct. Readers must therefore always check the product information and clinical procedures with the most up-to-date published product information and data sheets provided by the manufacturers and the most recent codes of conduct and safety regulations. The authors and the publisher do not accept any liability for any errors in the text or for the misuse or misapplication of material in this work

Commissioning editor: Jonathan Gregory
Project managers: Rosemary Osmond and Carolyn Newton
Typeset by Footnote Graphics Limited, Warminster, Wiltshire, UK
Printed in Spain by T G Hostench SA, Barcelona

Contents

Contributors

RON FERGUSSON, MD, FRCPE, Respiratory Medicine Unit, Western General Hospital, Crewe Road, Edinburgh, UK

ADAM HILL, MD, Department of Respiratory Medicine, Royal Infirmary, Lauriston Place, Edinburgh, UK

WILLIAM MACNEE, MB.ChB, MD, FRCP(G), FRCP(E), University of Edinburgh Medical School, Edinburgh, UK

PETER REID, MD, FRCPE, Respiratory Medicine Unit, Western General Hospital, Crewe Road, Edinburgh, UK

JOHN SIMPSON, PhD, FRCPE, Department of Respiratory Medicine, Royal Infirmary, Lauriston Place, Edinburgh, UK

Foreword

Respiratory diseases are a major cause of morbidity and mortality across the world. Lung cancer is now the commonest solid tumour in men, and women are rapidly catching up as the ill-effects of their smoking take their inevitable toll. Equally predictably, the prevalence of chronic obstructive pulmonary disease and its resultant premature death and disability have also been rising steeply. Both these changes are disappointing, given the identification of the principal cause of these disorders (tobacco smoking) many decades ago. Respiratory infections, especially amongst our elderly population, contribute much additional cost and suffering, while tuberculosis has reached the stage of being declared a global emergency by the World Health Organization (WHO). All of this emphasizes the need to keep up to date with the flood of literature published each year in response to the continuing problems posed by respiratory diseases. The practicalities of this are never easy and whilst electronic communication and the increasing availability of full text papers on the Internet have led to greater access to this information, there are still real difficulties in deciding which are the most important papers and evaluating their significance in the wider picture of respiratory medical practice.

This book represents a positive and enjoyable way of dealing with this headache. The editors and their team have conscientiously searched through the literature published in 2001/2002 and have skilfully selected key publications for presentation and analysis. By grouping related topics together, they let the reader understand the themes of the research and, more importantly, how it might apply to the common pulmonary conditions discussed here. Both specialists and generalists would benefit from spending time dipping into this book and are likely to find themselves not just consulting one or two articles but reading on to learn more about the many recent advances that have been made in our understanding of the basis of respiratory diseases and their management.

The team are to be congratulated on the hard work they have undertaken in putting together this extremely useful volume which will certainly help the reader keep up to date, if not ahead, of others in the field! Anyone with an interest in common respiratory diseases will benefit from spending time with this volume.

Professor Peter MA Calverley
Professor of Medicine
(Pulmonary and Rehabilitation Research Group)
University of Liverpool
Liverpool, UK

Preface

The global burden of respiratory diseases continues to increase. Respiratory infections, particularly from tuberculosis and pneumonia, are amongst the commonest presentations of respiratory disease worldwide, but airways disease, from both asthma and chronic obstructive pulmonary disease (COPD), continues to rise and lung cancer is, in most countries, one of the main causes of cancer death. It has been estimated that major respiratory diseases as reasons for mortality will increase over the first few decades of this century. In particular, COPD will rise to become the third commonest cause of death and pneumonia the fourth by the year 2020. Respiratory diseases are often neglected by health-care systems and few countries treat respiratory diseases as a national health priority despite their high prevalence.

There have been considerable advances in respiratory medicine in recent years with the publication of many landmark studies in not only epidemiology, diagnosis and treatment but also in numbers of patients, which have not been previously studied in respiratory diseases. There is also considerable new information on the basic mechanisms of respiratory diseases, particularly relating to inflammatory processes, possibly leading to new treatments for some diseases which have not previously had effective therapies.

The sheer scale of the amount of information published in this field makes it difficult to keep pace with the new developments. *The Year in Respiratory Medicine 2003* is designed to help with this problem as it provides an authoritative review on new clinical and basic research published in the year 2001–2002. It consists of a selection of important journal publications which have a major impact in the field of respiratory medicine and provides the reader with a summary of the key findings from each study. Importantly, there is informed comment from each editor on the topic for readers who wish more detailed analysis of the study. It will therefore provide a rapid update on the year in the field of respiratory medicine for physicians and clinical and basic scientists. This book has been edited by practising clinicians who are working in respiratory medicine in Edinburgh with interests in the specific topics of asthma, COPD, respiratory infection and lung cancer. I am grateful for their efforts in preparing this project and am sure that the reader will benefit from the work that has been devoted to the production of this compilation.

Professor William MacNee
Professor of Respiratory and Environmental Medicine
University of Edinburgh Medical School
Edinburgh, Scotland

Part I

Asthma

Asthma

Introduction

Since it was first recognized as a syndrome characterized by paroxysmal episodes of bronchospasm in 1898, our understanding of asthma has increased enormously. It is now understood that asthma is a chronic inflammatory disorder and this has directed the management of the disease towards anti-inflammatory therapy (principally inhaled corticosteroids) and resulted in major improvements in control for the majority of sufferers.

Asthma is a complex syndrome and it is likely that within this broad heading there are a number of disease phenotypes and consequently multiple genetic and environmental determinants. Consequently, in all but a minority of patients, the causative factor(s) for the emergence of asthma in any individual remain unknown. Alarmingly, the prevalence of the condition has continued to increase in Western society and we are now beginning to observe a similar increase in developing countries. Some answers are beginning to be provided by epidemiological research, but is currently not at a stage where sufficient clarity can be provided to confidently influence lifestyle choices. Many of the key inflammatory and immunomodulatory cells have been identified, including the mediators that co-ordinate the inflammatory response and contribute to the pathophysiological reactions observed in the asthmatic lung. However, our understanding of their precise roles in the initiation and perpetuation of the asthmatic inflammatory response remains rudimentary.

Fortunately, for the majority of patients with asthma, the disease can be effectively managed in primary care by partnerships between doctors, nurses and most importantly patients themselves. However, for a significant minority ongoing morbidity results in absenteeism from education and work and contributes to significant levels of health expenditure. Regrettably, asthma continues to represent an important cause of death, particularly in young people and there is an ongoing need to advise clinicians on how to target and improve the care of these patients. More information is needed on the safe and effective delivery of therapies that are currently available and new drugs that complement these medications and improve asthma control for refractory patients are required.

The following review targets some of the key papers addressing these issues that have been published in 2001 and 2002. Undoubtedly, the choice reflects the bias of the author but greatest attention has been given to those papers published by the leading journals, thus it is hoped that the major themes currently being debated in asthma have been reflected.

1

Incidence and prevalence of asthma

Introduction

Data on incidence and prevalence of asthma is determined from epidemiological studies and the definition of disease is largely based on data obtained from questionnaires reporting wheeze, the diagnosis of asthma, or the prescription of drugs appropriate for asthma. This data is often supplemented by measurement of airway hyper-responsiveness (AHR) and atopy. The different diagnostic criteria used can contribute to differences in reported incidence and prevalence rates and this may confound some of these studies. Thus it is important to understand how different diagnostic criteria may impact on reported figures. It is generally accepted that the incidence and prevalence of asthma have shown a marked increase in the developed countries; however, some authors have suggested that the rapid rise may be beginning to plateau |**1**|. Reports with greatest validity are those performed by the same investigators, employing the same diagnostic criteria, and from a region in which the population base is unlikely to have been influenced by significant demographic swings. Finally, the diagnostic term 'asthma' encompasses several different phenotypes. In some of these diseases, severity and treatment may vary. For example, patients with aspirin-sensitive asthma appear to have a different onset and prognosis than other patients with asthma. There are many other examples, but as these phenotypes become increasingly defined, it will become important to determine the incidence and prevalence of these in any given asthmatic community.

Incidence of asthma and its determinants among adults in Spain.

Basagana X, Sunyer J, Zock JP, *et al. Am J Respir Crit Care Med* 2001; **164**: 1133–7.

BACKGROUND. The aim of this study was to determine the incidence of asthma, and its determinants, in Spain. This study investigated the number of new cases of asthma that arose in a cohort of subjects participating in the European Community Respiratory Health Survey. They employed two different definitions of asthma based on the history and a further definition that required the presence of airway hyper-reactivity.

INTERPRETATION. The incidence of asthma depended on how cases were defined and varied from 5.53 to 1.50 per 1000 person-years. Bronchial hyper-responsiveness and *Immunoglobulin E* (IgE) reactivity to grass (but not house dust mite, cat or any other allergen) appeared to the main determinants of new asthma.

Is the increase in childhood asthma coming to an end? Findings from three surveys of schoolchildren in Rome, Italy.

Ronchetti R, Villa MP, Barreto M, *et al. Eur Respir J* 2001; **17**: 881–6.

BACKGROUND. This is the most recent of a series of studies reporting the prevalence of asthma and atopy by the same team of investigators who have employed identical epidemiological study procedures to schoolchildren (aged 6–14 years) attending two primary schools in Rome with different socio-economic conditions and levels of environmental pollution.

INTERPRETATION. Between 1974 and 1992, the authors reported an increase in the prevalence of asthma and affirmative answers to asthma related questions that have remained stable between 1992 and 1998. They observed lower life asthma prevalence in children of both sexes in older compared to younger children. No further rise in the prevalence of asthma occurred in the last 6 years of the study and this may suggest that the increase in childhood asthma is ending.

The prevalence of aspirin intolerant asthma (AIA) in Australian asthmatic patients.

Vally H, Taylor ML, Thompson PJ. *Thorax* 2002; **57**: 569–74.

BACKGROUND. The aim of this study was to report the prevalence of AIA in a metropolitan area of Perth, Australia.

INTERPRETATION. Aspirin sensitivity is a significant problem with a prevalence of between 10 and 11% in asthmatics and 2.5% in non-asthmatics. AIA was associated with more severe asthma (odds ratio [OR] 2.4, 95% confidence interval [CI] 1.18–4.86), nasal polyposis (OR 3.19, 95% CI 1.52–6.68), atopy (OR 2.96, 95% CI 1.48–5.89), sulphite sensitivity (OR 3.97, 95% CI 1.87–8.41), and sensitivity to wine (OR 3.27, 95% CI 1.65–6.47).

Comment

Thus, variations on the incidence and prevalence of asthma may depend on how the diagnosis was sought and confirmed. This is illustrated by Basagana *et al.* where the incidence rate varied depending on how the at-risk population was defined. When based on a positive answer to the question: 'Have you ever had asthma?' the reported incidence was 5.53 per 1000 person-years (95% CI, 4.28, 7.16) but decreased to 3.28 (95% CI, 2.34, 4.59) following exclusion of individuals who had reported onset of asthma more than 5 years before 1991–1993. The incidence further decreased to 1.97 (95% CI, 1.09, 3.56) when individuals who reported symptoms in 1991–1993 were excluded and to 1.50 (95% CI, 0.78, 2.88) following exclusion of those who had demonstrated airway hyper-responsiveness.

The study by Ronchetti *et al.* provides some grounds for optimism that the increase in asthma may be ending. Technical bias was kept to a minimum by employing the same investigators and the same questionnaire in the same schools over the 24-year period, so it is unlikely that this reflects a change in diagnosis or classification. The authors documented an almost linear increase in asthma of 0.4%/year with each 4-year period for children born between 1962 and 1985, so that the rate of total male and female asthma almost tripled. Asthma rose most prominently in males and those with a family history of atopy.

Valley *et al.* provided information on the prevalence of AIA from three asthmatic populations in Western Australia and found it to be common with a prevalence of 10.7% ($n = 16$, 95% CI 5.8–15.6), and 10.4% ($n = 38$, 95% CI 7.3–13.5) in the hospital and Asthma Foundation cohorts respectively. In addition, 2.5% of non-diagnosed asthmatics in this cohort reported asthma symptoms following aspirin ingestion. It is possible that had they employed oral or inhaled challenge tests, the prevalence of AIA would have been even higher. In keeping with other studies, they reported that AIA was associated with asthma of greater severity, coexistent nasal polyposis, and sensitivity to other food products including wine.

References

1. Burney P. The changing prevalence of asthma. *Thorax* 2002; **57**(Suppl. II): 36–9.

2

Epidemiology

Introduction

The dramatic rise in the incidence and prevalence of asthma in Western society is likely to reflect the impact of the environment. In trying to identify possible candidates, investigators have concentrated on several broad themes. The most popular over the last decade has been the hygiene hypothesis that was originally put forward by the British epidemiologist, David Strachan, in an attempt to explain the observed protective effect of larger family sizes on the incidence of hay fever [1]. Even though less consistently and less strongly demonstrated in asthma, it has emerged as a popular theory to explain the rising prevalence of asthma in European countries. The hygiene hypothesis has been bolstered by an immunological model of asthma suggesting a bias towards T cells that mediate the immunological reactions against parasites, and allergic phenomena with reductions in those that mediate cellular immunity to bacteria and viruses.

T-helper (Th) cells are thought to orchestrate the asthmatic inflammatory response and are believed to differentiate into two relatively distinct subsets: Th1 and Th2. Th2 lymphocytes predominantly secrete cytokines such as interleukin-4 (IL-4), interleukin-5 (IL-5) and interleukin-13 (IL-13) that direct the immune system towards an allergic type of response, whereas Th1 lymphocytes preferentially secrete interferon-gamma and interleukin-2 (IL-2), that are important in fighting viral and bacterial infections. The Th cell polarity of the newborn infant is predominantly skewed to Th2 cell function but as it matures, a shift in polarity of the T cells occurs towards Th1 responses. Thus, if the newborn infant, by remaining in a 'hygienic' environment, fails to be exposed to bacterial and viral infections, the Th cell polarity may remain skewed towards Th2. Thus, the infant is at risk of developing allergic diseases such as asthma. However, although this model has been widely recognized and will be referred to below, it is beginning to be questioned and viewed as an oversimplification [2].

Other investigators have examined the role of the diet, either with regard to its impact on the gut microflora or the intake of foods that may influence the immune response. Furthermore, as the increase in asthma has occurred in line with the increase in obesity in Western society, so some investigators have focused on possible links between the two. Lastly, an awareness of the possible contribution of environmental pollutants accompanying the industrialization of societies has been examined.

Asthma and infection

Early childhood infectious disease and the development of asthma up to school age: a birth cohort study.

Illi S, von Muitus E, Lau S, *et al*. *Br Med J* 2001; **322**: 390–5.

BACKGROUND. The aim of this study was to prospectively investigate the association between different types of early childhood infections and the subsequent development of asthma, atopic sensitization (Immunoglobulin E [IgE] to various allergens) and airway hyper-responsiveness (AHR) (histamine challenge), in a cohort of newborn infants at risk of atopy defined as the presence of ≥2 atopic family members or elevated cord blood IgE. Patients were recruited from the ongoing multi-centre allergy study (MAS).

INTERPRETATION. Children who experienced two or more episodes of runny nose before the age of 1 year, were less likely to have physician-diagnosed asthma at the age of 7 years (odds ratio [OR] 0.52, 95% confidence interval [CI] 0.29–0.92) or to have wheeze (OR 0.60, 95% CI 0.38–0.94). They were also less likely to be atopic before the age of 5 years. Reporting ≥1 viral infection of the herpes type during the first 3 years of life was inversely associated with asthma at the age of 7 years (OR 0.48, 95% CI 0.26–0.89). By contrast, repeated lower respiratory tract infections during the first 3 years of life were positively associated with wheeze up to the age of 7 years (OR 3.37, 95% CI 1.92–5.92) for ≥4 infections vs ≤3.

Independent effects of intestinal parasite infection and domestic allergen exposure on risk of wheeze in Ethiopia: a nested case–control study.

Scrivener S, Yemaneberhan H, Zebenigus M, *et al*. *Lancet* 2002; **358**: 1493–9.

BACKGROUND. The authors of this study had previously noted that the prevalence of self-reported wheeze in Jimma, an urban area of Ethiopia, was related to skin sensitization to *Dermatophagoides pteronyssinus*. However, although the prevalence of skin sensitization to *D. pteronyssinus* was more common in rural areas, self-reported wheeze was less common |3|. The aim of this study was to determine whether an interaction between parasites and house dust mites, protection from previous infection with hepatitis A, or the level of exposure to organophosphorus insecticides might explain this discrepancy.

INTERPRETATION. Hookworm (predominantly *Necator americanus*) was present in 24% of participants and was associated with a significant reduction in the risk of wheeze (adjusted OR 0.48, 95% CI 0.29–0.82, *P* = 0.03), with some relation to intensity of infection. Increased levels of Der p 1 were associated with an increased risk of wheeze (adjusted OR 1.26, 95% CI 1.00–1.59, $P = 0.05$) but this was unrelated to hepatitis A seropositivity or cholinesterase concentration. *D. pteronyssinus* skin sensitization was more strongly related to wheeze (OR 9.45, 95% CI 5.03–17.75) in the urban than the rural population, where although high levels were observed, the risk of wheeze decreased with increasing intensity of parasitic infection. Thus, high degrees of parasite infection appeared to prevent asthma symptoms in atopic individuals.

Comment

The study by Illi *et al.* is consistent with other studies suggesting that the exposure to infection in early life appears to protect the infant from the subsequent development of atopy and asthma |4–6|. They suggest that both the total burden of infection and the type of infection are relevant. The fact that lower respiratory tract infections were associated with the development of asthma can probably be explained by reverse causation, where children already predisposed to develop asthma may be more likely to develop symptoms of a lower respiratory tract infection when exposed to respiratory viruses. Although the increases in asthma observed in Africa have occurred under conditions that cannot be described as clean, Scrivener *et al.* suggest that the increased occurrence of wheeze in Urban Ethiopia (and the dissociation between the usual relationships between Der p 1 sensitization) may be associated with a loss of a protective effect from hookworm infection.

These papers and the observations of others raise the possibility that it may be possible to exploit the protective effects of these infections and intervene in the development of asthma. This has led to speculation regarding the use of vaccines that would induce a Th1 response such as Mycobacterium vaccae or Bacillus Calmette-Guerin (BCG) |7|. Parasitic infections are classically associated with a Th2 cell response and the production of IgE antibodies and have been postulated to prevent IgE-mediated allergic disease by blocking effector-cell IgE receptors with parasite induced specific and polyclonal IgE |8,9|. Scrivener *et al.* suggest that any protection in their population was not due to an IgE-receptor blocking mechanism. An alternative mechanism that was not tested is the induction of the anti-inflammatory cytokine interleukin-10 |10|.

Asthma and outdoor allergens

Does living on a farm during childhood protect against asthma, allergic rhinitis and atopy in childhood?

Leynaert B, Neukirch C, Jarvis D, Chinn S, Burney P, Neukirch F.
Am J Respir Dis Crit Care Med 2001; **164**: 1829–34.

BACKGROUND. The aim of this study was to determine whether the timing of exposure to a farm environment affects the protection against asthma, hay fever and

allergic sensitization and reports data from the European Community Respiratory
Health Survey recruiting from 48 study centres.

INTERPRETATION. After adjusting for potential confounders, living on a farm during
childhood was associated with a decrease in the risk of atopic sensitization as an adult
(OR 0.76, 95% CI 0.60–0.97). When specific allergens were considered there was
reduced risk of sensitization to cats (OR 0.63, 95% CI 0.41–0.96), and timothy grass
(OR 0.68, 95% CI 0.50–0.94). Nasal symptoms in the presence of pollen were less
common (OR 0.80, 95% CI 0.64–1.02). No protection was observed against asthma,
wheeze or nasal symptoms in the presence of animals or dust in adulthood.

Exposure to farming in early life and development of asthma and allergy: a cross-sectional study.

Reidler J, Braun-Fahrländer C, Eder W, *et al.*, and the ALEX study team.
Lancet 2001; **358**: 1129–33.

BACKGROUND. In this study, the authors performed a cross-sectional survey in rural
areas of Austria, Germany and Switzerland to determine whether increased microbial
pressure is associated with a reduced risk of development of allergic diseases.

INTERPRETATION. The prevalence of asthma and hay fever symptoms was
significantly lower in farmers' children than in those from a non-farming environment.
Children living on farms were also less likely to be atopic. The difference between
farming and non-farming groups was most pronounced for grass pollen. The greatest
protection against the development of asthma, hay fever and allergic sensitization was
observed in children exposed to stables and farm milk in the first year of life and the
effect of these variables appeared to be additive. Prenatal exposure (assessed by the
activity of the mother on farm during pregnancy) also appeared to provide a substantial
protective effect.

Environmental exposure to endotoxin and its relation to asthma in school-age children.

Braun-Fahrländer C, Riedler J, Herz U, *et al.*, for the Allergy and Endotoxin
Study team. *N Engl J Med* 2002; **347**: 869–77.

BACKGROUND. The aim of this cross-sectional study was to investigate whether the
early life innate immune system can recognize viable and non-viable parts of
microorganisms and to determine if this could lead to the development of tolerance to
allergens implicated in the development of atopy and asthma.

INTERPRETATION. Endotoxin exposure displayed a strong inverse association with hay
fever, hay-fever symptoms, and atopic sensitization. Control for covariates showed a
largely monotonic decrease in prevalence with an increasing endotoxin load (Fig. 2.1). An

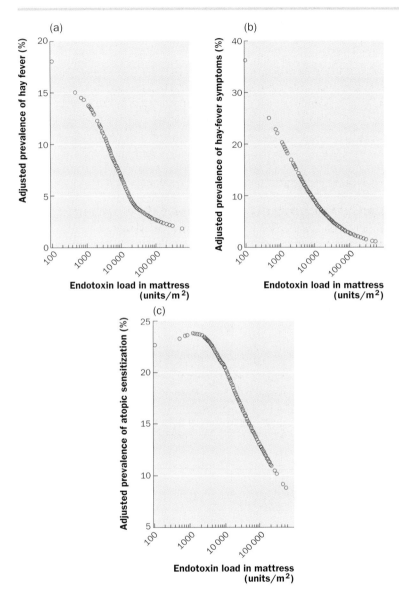

Fig. 2.1 Smoothed plots of the prevalence of hay fever (a), hay-fever symptoms (b) and atopic sensitization (c) in relation to the log-transformed endotoxin-load values. The analyses controlled for age, sex, study area, family history of asthma and hay fever, educational level of the parents, and number of siblings. For each outcome, there was a monotonic decrease with increasing endotoxin load. A smoothing span of 0.9 was used for all three graphs. Source: Braun-Fahrländer et al. (2002).

inverse relation was also found between the level of endotoxin exposure and the capacity of peripheral-blood leukocytes to produce inflammatory and regulatory cytokines after lipopolysaccharide (LPS) stimulation. There was also a strong negative association between the current level of endotoxin exposure and the occurrence of atopic wheeze and asthma (Fig. 2.2). However, there was a non-significant trend toward increasing prevalence for cases of non-atopic wheeze and asthma. The level of cytokine production by leukocytes (tumour necrosis factor α, interferon-γ, interleukin-10 and interluekin-12) was inversely related to the endotoxin level in the bedding, suggesting that down-regulation of immune responses had occurred in exposed children. Thus, environmental exposure to microbial products appears to be associated with a significant decrease in the risk of childhood hay fever, atopic sensitization, atopic asthma and atopic wheeze in children from farming and non-farming households and this may be due to the development of tolerance to allergens encountered in this environment.

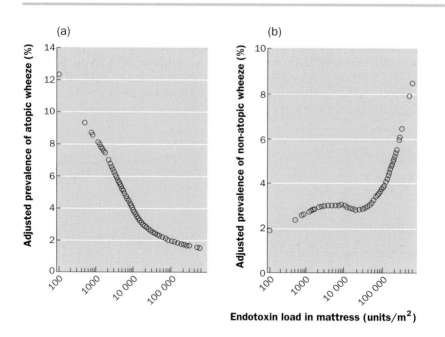

Endotoxin load in mattress (units/m^2)

Fig. 2.2 Smoothed plots of the prevalence of atopic wheeze (a) and non-atopic wheeze (b) in relation to the log-transformed endotoxin-load values. The analyses were controlled for age, sex, study area, family history of asthma and hay fever, educational level of the parents, and number of siblings. There was a negative association for atopic wheeze, whereas for non-atopic wheeze there was a non-significant positive trend with increasing levels of current endotoxin exposure. For Panel (a), a smoothing span of 0.9 was used; for Panel (b), a span of 0.5 was used. Source: Braun-Fahrländer *et al.* (2002).

Comment

Farming environments have been shown to provide more consistent protection from hay fever and allergic sensitization than from asthma |**11–15**|. The study by Leynaert *et al.* demonstrates that protection against atopic sensitization and hay fever persists even when the child no longer lives on the farm. The study by Reidler extends previous observations by demonstrating that protection appears to occur independently of the state of allergic sensitization and may even begin *in utero*. Furthermore, both the amount and duration of exposure appeared to be important with long-term and early life exposure to stables and farm milk protecting from the development of asthma, hay fever and allergic sensitization. Protection against asthma was independent of the state of allergic sensitization. Although short exposure times to stables conferred protection, the lowest levels of asthma in those with continuing exposure from the first year of life. The authors suggest that exposure to stables may provide a surrogate for markers of the microbial environment such as endotoxin, other bacterial-wall components, or bacterial DNA that is rich in CpG dinucleotides that modulate innate immune responses. However, they did not test this and did not provide information on T-helper cell status.

Braun-Fahrländer *et al.* extend our knowledge by demonstrating that apparent protection afforded by the farm environment may be mediated through endotoxin exposure and they show a functional change in the cytokine profile of inflammatory cells following stimulation by LPS. They also demonstrate that the effect of endotoxin exposure is independent of, and additional to, the protective effect of exposure to stables within the first year of life and protects following exposure at school age. This protective effect was also observed in children who had not grown up on a farm. Whereas exposure to farming in the first year of life was associated with a protective effect against non-atopic wheeze, exposure at school age was related to an increased risk.

Asthma and pet ownership

Decreased prevalence of sensitization to cats with high exposure to cat allergen.

Custovic A, Hallam CL, Simpson BM, Craven M, Simpson A, Woodcock A.
J Allergy Clin Immunol 2001; **108**: 537–9.

BACKGROUND. The authors devised this study in response to the conflicting reports on the relationship between early life exposure to cats and the later development of respiratory allergy. They were able to gain information from parents and children currently participating in a prospective study on atopy and asthma in children.

INTERPRETATION. Dividing the levels of the cat allergen Fel d 1 into deciles, the authors observed that although cat ownership was associated with higher Fel d 1 levels,

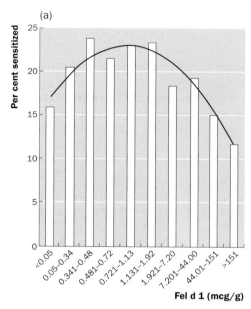

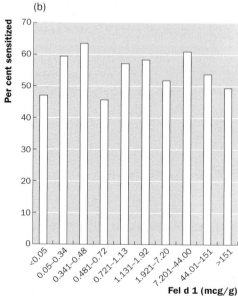

Fig. 2.3 (a) Prevalence of sensitization to cat in 10 cat allergen exposure groups. (b) No significant differences were seen in the proportion of subjects sensitized to mite, dog and mixed grasses between different cat allergen exposure groups.
Source: Custovic *et al.* (2001).

the risk of sensitization to cats was greatest in those with medium exposure to Fel d 1. By contrast, the prevalence of sensitization to cat was significantly decreased in the lowest and the highest cat allergen exposure groups (Fig. 2.3).

Sensitization, asthma and a modified Th2 response in children exposed to cat allergen: a population-based cross-sectional study.

Platts-Mills T, Vaughan J, Squillace S, Woodfolk J, Sporik R. *Lancet* 2001; **357**: 752–6.

BACKGROUND. Platts-Mills *et al*. had previously observed that increasing concentrations of cat allergen (by contrast with mite allergen) did not increase the risk of sensitization to cat allergen |16–18|. Further interrogation of their data showed that a large number of these patients were in fact atopic but exposure to high concentrations of cat allergen was associated with a decreased risk of sensitization. In this paper, they performed a population-based cross-sectional study in children aged 12–14 years to investigate the immune response to cat and mite allergens with a wide range of allergen exposure.

INTERPRETATION. Sensitization to mite or cat allergens was the strongest independent risk factor for asthma. However, there was a different dose–response between cat exposure and mite exposure. Increasing exposure to mite was associated with increased prevalence of sensitization and IgG antibody to Der f 1, but although higher exposures to cat were associated with a higher prevalence of IgG antibody to Fel d 1, reported rates of sensitization were lower. The authors were also able to demonstrate that individuals who were not sensitized despite high levels of Fel d 1 had high levels of IgG antibody to Fel d 1. Furthermore, antibodies to Fel d 1 of the IgG4 isotype were strongly correlated with IgG antibody in both allergic and non-allergic children ($r = 0.84$ and $r = 0.66$, respectively). This suggested that exposure to cat allergen can result in the development of an IgG and IgG4 antibody response that is not associated with sensitization or the development of asthma.

Exposure to cat allergen, and wheezing in first 5 years of life.

Celedón JC, Litonjua AA, Ryan L, Platts-Mills T, Weiss ST, Gold DR. *Lancet* 2002; **360**: 78–2.

BACKGROUND. The aim of this short report was to provide further insight into the link between pet ownership in early life and asthma.

INTERPRETATION. The risk of wheezing associated with exposure to cat appeared to be determined by the presence of a history of allergy in the mother but not the father. In the absence of a maternal history of asthma, exposure to cat appeared to protect against wheezing up to 5 years of age (RR [relative risk] 0.7, 95% CI 0.5–1.0). If the mother had asthma, the risk of wheezing associated with exposure to cat increased with age and by the age of 3 years, exposures to cat and a Fel d 1 concentration of at least 8 μg/g in early life were significantly associated with asthma (RR 2.4 95%, CI 1.3–4.5). There was no association between wheezing and exposure to dog or dog allergen.

Comment

The evidence for a causal relationship between allergen and asthma is based on the epidemiological observation of a strong association between specific IgE antibodies, total IgE and asthma |19|. For many of the allergens commonly implicated in the development of asthma such as house dust-mite, this relationship between exposure and the development of atopy and asthma appears to be linear |20|. However, the relationship between exposure to pet animals and the development of asthma appears to be more complicated, particularly with relation to cats.

There is good evidence from adult studies that ownership and exposure to cats is associated with the onset and worsening of asthma |21–23|. However, several studies have observed that cat ownership is associated with a decreased rate of sensitization and can exert a protective effect on the development of asthma. In a Swedish 5-year cohort study of 402 school children, the cumulative incidence of asthma was lower among those who had a pet in the home during the first year of life: adjusted OR 0.34 (95% CI 0.07–0.77). In a Norwegian cohort study of 2531 children followed for 4 years from birth, the risk of asthma was lower in children with any pet at birth: adjusted OR 0.7 (95% CI 0.5–1.1) |24,25|. This may simply reflect avoidance of pet ownership in allergic and asthmatic families but it is possible that exposure to cats may protect against the development of allergy.

The above papers use current exposure as a surrogate for the measurement of cumulative or lifetime exposure. However, the results are consistent and suggest that for cats, the maximum prevalence of sensitization appears to occur with moderate exposure and higher exposure appears to confer protection against the development of atopy and asthma. The work by Celedón *et al.* extends this observation by reporting that although cat ownership in early life protects against asthma this only appears to be operative in the absence of a maternal history of asthma. If the child's mother has a history of asthma, then exposure to cat allergen is associated with an increased risk of wheeze.

Platts-Mills *et al.* suggest a possible mechanism to explain protection by high cat allergen exposure in some individuals. High levels of exposure may preferentially direct the immune system towards a modified Th2 response, were instead of manufacturing IgE antibodies (associated with atopy), IgG4 antibodies are made. Interestingly, this does not support the widely held theory that tolerance is induced by a shift towards a Th1 response. It is also interesting that cat allergen appears to behave differently from mite allergen. Possible suggestions include differences in the physical characteristics of the allergen, differences in biological potency or biochemical activity. Why these two behave differently could be of great importance in understanding the genesis of allergy.

Asthma and diet

Long-term relation between breast-feeding and development of atopy and asthma in young adults.

Sears MR, Greene JM, Willan AR, *et al. Lancet* 2002; **360**: 901–7.

BACKGROUND. The aim of this study was to test the claims that breast-feeding is protective against atopy and asthma. The authors examined 1037 of the 1139 children born at a Dunedin Hospital between April 1972 and March 1973, and residing in Otago province at the age of 3 years.

INTERPRETATION. At age 13 and 21 years, children who had been breast-fed were more likely to test positive for skin test allergen (except aspergillus) and by the age of 9 years they were more likely to report asthma and this effect persisted at all ages to 26 years. The relationship remained strong even when AHR was used to confirm the diagnosis of asthma. Allowing for repeated measures children who were breast-fed were more than twice as likely as those who were not to develop wheeze with AHR or current asthma with AHR. No duration of breast-feeding had a protective effect. In conclusion, breast-feeding does not protect children against atopy and asthma and may even increase the risk.

Probiotics in primary prevention of atopic disease: a randomized placebo controlled trial.

Kalliomäki M, Salminen S, Arvilommi H, Kero P, Koskinen P, Isolauri E. *Lancet* 2001; **357**: 1076–9.

BACKGROUND. It has been suggested that promotion of *Lactobacillus* and other potentially beneficial gut microorganisms may protect against the development of atopic disease. The aim of this study was to prospectively test whether lactobacillus rhamnosus (Lactobacillus GG) administered to pregnant mothers before delivery and then for up to 6 months while breast-feeding and to babies who were not breast-fed would protect against the development of atopic disease.

INTERPRETATION. The frequency of atopic eczema in the probiotic group was half that of the placebo group (RR 0.51, 95% CI 0.32–0.84) and the number needed to treat was 4.5 (95% CI 2.6–15.6). There was no reduction in positive skin prick tests or specific IgE by 2 years of age, and no reduction in severity of disease in children who developed atopic eczema. In conclusion, in children at high risk of atopic disease, Lactobacillus GG was effective in preventing early symptoms.

Dietary antioxidants and asthma in adults: population based case–control study.

Shaheen SO, Sterne JAC, Thompson RL, Songhurst CE, Margetts BM, Burney PGJ. *Am J Respir Crit Care* 2001; **164**: 1823–8.

BACKGROUND. **Epidemiological studies have suggested that diets rich in antioxidants such as vitamin E and selenium appeared to exert a protective effect against the development of asthma and wheezing syndromes. This population-based, case–control study was designed to determine whether a higher intake of dietary antioxidants protected against asthma and if, in addition, it was associated with asthma of lesser severity.**

INTERPRETATION. After controlling for potential confounders, the dietary intake of foods rich in flavonoids appeared to provide a protective effect against both the development of asthma and the severity of asthma in patients suffering from the condition. This was shown by a negative association between the development of asthma and the consumption of apples (OR 0.89, 95% CI 0.82–0.97) and selenium (OR 0.85, 95% CI 0.76–0.95). There was no evidence for an association between the development of asthma and dietary intake of tea, onions, red wine, vitamin C and vitamin E. There was evidence of a weak association with carotene intake. For subjects with asthma, the amount of red wine consumed was negatively associated with asthma severity.

Comment

Dietary intake has the potential, either directly or indirectly, to modify the immune system |26|. The plasticity of the immune system in early life suggests that it will be dietary influences at this stage that will have the greatest impact. Indeed, early exposure to cows' milk protein has been linked to the development of atopy and asthma |27|. Evidence that the gut microflora may be associated with the development of atopy comes from studies comparing Estonian infants with Swedish infants. Estonian infants have a low prevalence of atopy and display greater gut colonization with *Lactobacilli* and *Eubacteria*, whereas Swedish infants, who have a higher prevalence of atopy, display greater levels of *Clostridium difficile* |28|. Furthermore, iso-caproic acid, a compound associated with *C. difficile*, has been detected almost exclusively in allergic infants, and the levels of other compounds associated with a *Lactobacillus* flora were higher in non-atopic infants |29|. Thus, it has been suggested that promotion of *Lactobacillus* and other potentially beneficial gut microorganisms may protect against the development of atopic disease. By inference, breast-feeding, which promotes gut colonization with bifidobacterium, ought to be associated with a reduction of atopy and/or asthma |30|. Thus, the finding by Sears *et al.* that breast-feeding is associated with an increased risk is surprising. Nevertheless, the authors have performed a careful prospective study, taking care to minimize confounding factors, and although breast-feeding has many advantages, protection against atopy and asthma does not appear to be one of them.

Another method with potential to enhance the numbers of potentially beneficial organisms in the gut is the use of probiotics. These agents have produced beneficial results in the management of atopic eczema and food allergy |**31,32**|. The study by Kalliomäki *et al.* provides prospective confirmation that probiotics can prevent atopic disease and may provide a natural means of beneficially modulating the immune system. However, the mechanism remains unclear and more data needs to be available before conclusions can be made on their ability to impact on the development of other allergic diseases including asthma.

Epidemiological studies have suggested that diets rich in antioxidants such as vitamin E and selenium appeared to exert a protective effect against the development of asthma and wheezing syndromes. Thus it has been proposed that diets lacking antioxidants may predispose to asthma |**33,34**|. Shaheen *et al.* report that diets rich in flavonoids and selenium appeared to protect against asthma. The study utilized a detailed questionnaire that probably contributed to the low response rates but the authors managed to survey a large group that included a range of socioeconomic conditions. The protective effects of a higher intake of apples or higher consumption of red wine on asthma have not been previously reported. However, there is some evidence that apples and other hard fruits are associated with improved lung function and protection from chronic obstructive pulmonary disease |**35,36**|. Selenium may protect against asthma through modulating glutathione and enhancing antioxidant levels. More information is needed on the role of selenium, as it is known that selenium levels are declining in the UK population |**37**|.

Asthma and obesity

Body mass index and asthma in adults in families of subjects with asthma in Anqing, China.
Celedón JC, Palmer LJ, Litonjua AA, *et al. Am J Respir Crit Care Med* 2001; **164**: 1835–40.

BACKGROUND. The authors undertook a cross-sectional study of 7109 adults from 2544 families with asthma in the eight rural counties of the Anhui Province to determine the relation between body mass index (BMI) and asthma. The authors employed two separate definitions of asthma. The first depended on the combination of physician-diagnosed asthma, AHR to methacholine at ≤25 mg/ml and ≥2 respiratory symptoms or attacks was taken as confirmation of asthma. The second definition (symptomatic AHR) required a combination of AHR (≤8 mg/ml) and ≥2 respiratory symptoms or attacks of asthma. Generalized estimating equations were used to study the association between BMI and asthma in study participants while adjusting for familial correlations and potential confounders.

INTERPRETATION. Multivariate analysis demonstrated that both being underweight and overweight were associated with asthma in women and that being underweight was

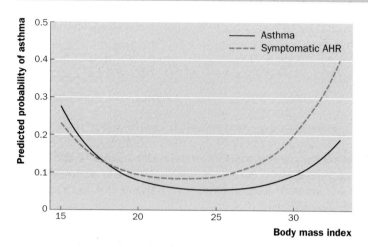

Fig. 2.4 Relation between body mass index (kg/m²) and risk of asthma and symptomatic airway hyper-responsiveness in 3386 men in Anqing, adjusting for age, intensity of cigarette smoking, skin test reactivity to one or more allergens, and familial correlations. Source: Celedón *et al.* (2001).

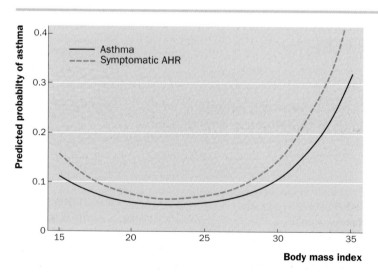

Fig. 2.5 Relation between body mass index (kg/m²) and risk of asthma and symptomatic airway hyper-responsiveness in 3723 women in Anqing, adjusting for age, intensity of cigarette smoking, skin test reactivity to one or more allergens, and familial correlations. Source: Celedón *et al.* (2001).

associated with physician diagnosed asthma in men. Among men, those with a BMI of 16 and 30 kg/m^2 had a 2.5 and 2.3 times greater odds of symptomatic AHR, respectively, than those whose BMI was 21 kg/m^2. Among women, those with a BMI of 16 and 30 kg/m^2 had 2.0 and 2.3 times higher odds of symptomatic AHR than those whose BMI was 21 kg/m^2. The associations were unchanged following exclusion of former and current smokers and excluding subjects over 45 years of age (Figs 2.4 and 2.5).

Increased incidence of asthma-like symptoms in girls who become overweight or obese during the school years.

Castro-Rodriguez JA, Holberg CJ, Morgan WJ, Wright AL, Martinez FD.
AJRCCM 2001; **163**: 1344–9.

BACKGROUND. Rather than the existence of a truly causal link between obesity and asthma, the apparent association between the two may be explained by the hypothesis that asthmatic individuals refrain from exercise (a recognized precipitant of their disease) and thus become obese. Such conundrums cannot be addressed by cross-sectional studies, hence the authors of this study from Tucson, Arizona, utilized a longitudinal design to determine whether a new diagnosis of asthma or chronic asthma are associated with weight gain or reduced physical activity.

INTERPRETATION. At the age of 11 years, females who were overweight or obese were more likely to have experienced wheezing compared to females who were not overweight. Similar but non-significant trends were observed for males. Females who became overweight or obese at 6 and 11 years of age were between 5.5 and 6.8 times more likely to develop new asthma symptoms at 11 or year 13 years of age, compared with those who did not. New weight gain between the ages of 6 and 11 years was associated with new asthma symptoms (infrequent wheeze), at 13 years of age, with an OR of 8.7 (95% CI 1.8–42.4, $P = 0.0002$). Females who become overweight or obese between 6 and 11 years of age had a significantly higher prevalence of peak expiratory flow record (PEFR) variability, and were more likely to demonstrate positive responses to albuterol, compared with those who did not.

Comment

Obesity has increased in the West and may be associated with the development of asthma. In some individuals, the link may be mechanical and associated with the higher incidence of gastro-oesophageal reflux or alterations that may occur in airway smooth muscle operating at low lung volumes. However, interesting theories have been developed exploring the relevance of shared genetic traits, immune modification by diet, or modification of airway responsiveness by changes in hormonal levels. Others have speculated whether the development of obesity favours an indoor lifestyle with a resultant increased exposure to indoor allergens |**38**|. Obesity is best described in terms of the BMI, which links height and weight: BMI = weight (kg) divided by height (m^2). Overweight, or grade 1 obesity, is defined by a BMI of

25.0–29.9, grade 2 obesity by a BMI of 30.0–39.0 and a BMI >40 represents grade 3 obesity.

Celedón *et al.* studied a group at risk of developing asthma and demonstrated that both being underweight (particularly in men) and overweight were associated with asthma. This study is particularly commendable as the authors took great care to clarify the diagnosis of asthma, employing two different definitions and used AHR. However, the study is cross-sectional in design and it is inappropriate to speculate regarding causation. Thus, it cannot be determined whether weight loss preceded the development of asthma or whether asthma led to failure to thrive and malnutrition in childhood that persisted into adult life. Equally, it is not possible to determine if the association between obesity and asthma reflects a lack of physical exercise due to asthma or that weight gain precedes the development of asthma. Castro-Rodriguez *et al.* performed a prospective study that allowed the issue of obesity to be addressed and suggest that asthma is associated with weight gain, particularly in females. These results were consistent with a further study published in 2001 following a cohort of 4547 African American and white adults (aged 18–30 years) participating in the Coronary Artery Risk Development in Young Adults Study |**39**|.

The importance of obesity lies in the fact that it is a modifiable risk factor. Weight loss is difficult, but if achieved may be associated with beneficial outcomes for lung function, asthma symptoms, morbidity and health status |**40**|. The association between being underweight and asthma needs to be addressed by prospective studies. Possible explanations may lie in the association between malnutrition and abnormal lung growth and reduced lung function |**41,42**|.

Asthma and outdoor pollutants (ozone)

Asthma in exercising children exposed to ozone: a cohort study.

McConnell R, Berhane K, Gilliland F, *et al. Lancet* 2002; **359**: 386–91.

BACKGROUND. In an attempt to answer whether the amount of ozone exposure is related to the development of asthma in children, the authors examined the relationship between playing team sports with the subsequent development of asthma in 3535 children during a 5-year follow-up of participants in the Southern California Children's Health Study. Children were categorized into those who played no team sports, and those who played 1, 2 and ≥3 team sports. Sporting activities were further classified according to their likely metabolic index. Each cohort was split into children playing more than the median time outdoors and those playing less. The concentrations of ozone, PM_{10} and NO_2 measured by air pollution monitoring stations and communities were categorized as either high or low pollution.

INTERPRETATION. The incidence of new diagnosis of asthma is associated with heavy exercise in communities with high concentrations of ozone (Tables 2.1 and 2.2).

Comment

Air quality is an important public health issue and health professionals have become increasingly aware of the potential for numerous pollutants including ozone to contribute to respiratory illness |43|. This paper suggests that playing sport, particularly if it involves high levels of activity, in an environment with high ozone concentration is associated with the development of physician-diagnosed asthma. As asthma also appeared in children with a previous history of wheeze, the results may also suggest that exercise in high ozone environments is associated with exacerbation of previously undiagnosed asthma. The greater effect observed according to the number of outdoor sports played and time spent outdoors strengthens the biological

Table 2.1 Effect of sports on incidence of asthma diagnoses

	n (incidence)*	RR (95% CI)
Number of sports played		
0	104 (0.022)	1.0
1	90 (0.026)	1.3 (1.0−1.7)
2	36 (0.021)	1.1 (0.7−1.6)
⩾3	29 (0.033)	1.8 (1.2−2.8)

n = number of cases of asthma; RR = relative risk (hazard ratio), adjusted for ethnic origin, and for stratified baseline hazards by sex and age group.
* Denominator = person-years of follow-up.

Source: McConnell et al. (2002).

Table 2.2 Effect of number of team sports played on the risk of new asthma diagnosis in high and low ozone communities

	Low ozone communities		High ozone communities	
	n (incidence)*	RR (95% CI)	n (incidence)*	RR (95% CI)
Number of sports played				
0	58 (0.027)	1.0	46 (0.018)	1.0
1	50 (0.033)	1.3 (0.9−1.9)	40 (0.021)	1.3 (0.8−2.0)
2	20 (0.023)	0.8 (0.5−1.4)	16 (0.020)	1.3 (0.7−2.3)
⩾3	9 (0.019)	0.8 (0.4−1.6)	20 (0.050)	3.3 (1.9−5.8)

n = number of cases of asthma; RR = relative risk, adjusted for ethnic origin, and for stratified baseline hazards by sex and age group. * Denominator = person-years of follow-up.

Source: McConnell et al. (2002).

plausibility of the results. Ozone has been shown to enhance AHR in response to house dust mite allergen challenge in children undertaking exercise, thus it is possible that ozone acts by increasing the potency of other aeroallergens encountered when exercising outdoors |44|. The study was underpowered to exclude an independent association of other pollutants with the development of newly diagnosed asthma, or to identify interaction between sports, ozone, and other pollutants, so it is possible that pollutants other than ozone could have explained the association. However, no effect of sports was seen in communities with high concentrations of pollutants other than ozone.

References

1. Strachan DP. Hay fever, hygiene and household size. *Br Med J* 1989; **299**: 1259–60.
2. Salvi S, Babu KS, Holgate ST. Is asthma really due to a polarized T cell response toward a helper T cell type 2 phenotype? *Am J Respir Crit Care Med* 2001; **164**: 1343–6.
3. Yemaneberhan H, Bekele Z, Venn A, Lewis S, Perry E, Britton J. Prevalence of wheeze and asthma and relation to atopy in urban and rural Ethiopia. *Lancet* 1997; **350**: 85–90.
4. Ball TM, Castro-Rodriguez JA, Griffith KA, Holberg CJ, Martinez FD, Wright AL. Siblings day-care attendance, and the risk of asthma and wheezing during childhood. *N Engl J Med* 2000; **343**: 538–43.
5. Shaheen SO, Aaby P, Hall AJ, Barker DJ, Hayes CB, Shiell AW *et al.* Measles and atopy in Guinea-Bissau. *Lancet* 1996; **347**: 1792–6.
6. Matricardi PM, Rosmini F, Riondino S, Fortini M, Ferrigno L, Raicetta M *et al.* Exposure to foodborne and orofecal microbes versus airborne viruses in relation to atopy and allergic asthma: epidemiological study. *Br Med J* 2000; **320**: 412–17.
7. Shirtcliffe PM, Easthope SE, Cheng S, Weatherall M, Tan PL, Le Gros G, Beasley R. The effect of delipidated deglycolipidated (DDMV) and heat-killed Mycobacterium vaccae in asthma. *Am J Respir Crit Care Med* 2001; **163**: 1410–14.
8. Godfrey RC, Gradidge CF. Allergic sensitization of human lung fragments prevented by saturation of IgE binding sites. *Nature* 1976; **259**: 484–6.
9. Weiss ST. Parasites and asthma/allergy: what is the relationship? *J Allerg Clin Immunol* 2000; **105**: 205–10.
10. van den Biggelar AHJ, van Ree R, Rodrigues LC *et al.* Decreased atopy in children infected with Schistosoma haematobium: a role for parasite-induced IL-10. *Lancet* 2000; **356**: 1723–7.
11. Braun-Fahrländer C, Gassner M, Grize L, *et al.* Prevalence of hay fever and allergic sensitization in farmers' children and their peers living in the same rural community. SCARPOL team—Swiss Study on Childhood Allergy and Respiratory Symptoms with Respect to Air Pollution. *Clin Exp Allergy* 1999; **29**: 28–34.
12. Reidler J, Eder W, Oberfeld G, Schreuer M. Austrian children living on a farm have less hay fever, asthma, and allergic sensitization. *Clin Exp Allergy* 2000; **30**: 194–200.

13. Von Ehrnestien OS, von-Mutius E, Illi S, Hachmeister A, von Kries R. Reduced risk of hay fever and asthma among children of farmers. *Clin Exp Allergy* 2000; **30**: 187–93.

14. Kilpelainen M, Terho EO, Helenius H, Koskenvuo M. Farm environment in childhood prevents the development of allergies. *Clin Exp Allergy* 2000; **30**: 201–8.

15. Ernst P, Cormier Y. Relative scarcity of asthma and atopy among adolescents raised on a farm. *Am J Respir Crit Care Med* 2000; **161**: 1563–6.

16. Sporik R, Ingram JM, Price W, Sussman JH, Honsinger RW, Platts-Mills TAE. Association of asthma with serum IgE and skin test reactivity to allergens among children living at high altitude. *Am J Respir Crit Care Med* 1995; **151**: 1388–92.

17. Sporik R, Squillace SP, Ingram JM, Rakes G, Honsinger RW, Platts-Mills TAE. Mite, cat and cockroach exposure, allergen sensitization, and asthma in children: a nested case–control study of three schools. *Thorax* 1999; **54**: 675–80.

18. Squillace SP, Sporik R Rakes G, *et al.* Sensitization to dust mites as a dominant risk factor for adolescent asthma. Multiple regression analysis of a population-based study. *Am J Respir Crit Care Med* 1997; **156**: 176–4.

19. Burrows B, Martinez FD, Halonen M, Barbee RA, Cline MG. Association of asthma with serum IgE levels and skin-test reactivity to allergens. *N Engl J Med* 1989; **320**: 271–7.

20. Sporik R, Holgate ST, Platts-Mills TAE, Cogswell JJ. Exposure to house-dust mite allergen (Der p 1) and the development of asthma in childhood: a prospective study. *N Engl J Med* 1990; **323**: 502–7.

21. Augusto A, Litonjua A, Sparrow D, Weiss ST, O'Connor GT, Long AA, Ohman JL. Sensitization to cat allergen is associated with asthma in older men and predicts new-onset airway hyperresponsiveness. *Am J Respir Crit Care Med* 1997; **156**: 23–7.

22. Siracusa A, Marabini A, Sensi L, Bacoccoli R, Ripandelli A, Anulli R, Pettinan L. Prevalence of asthma and rhinitis in Perugia, Italy. *Monaldi Arch Chest Dis* 1997; **52**: 434–9.

23. Noretjojo K, Dimich-Ward H, Obata H, Manfreda J, Chan-Yeung M. Exposure and sensitization to cat dander: asthma and asthma-like symptoms among adults. *J Allergy Clin Immunol* 1999; **104**: 941–7.

24. Hasslemar B, Åberg N, Åberg B, Eriksson B, Björkstén B. Does early exposure to cat or dog protect against later allergy development? *Clin Exp Allergy* 1999; **29**: 611–17.

25. Roost HP, Künzli N, Schindler C, Jarvis D, Chinn S, Peruchoud AP, Ackermann-Liebrich U, Burney P, Wüthrich B, for the European Community Respiratory Health Survey. Role of current and childhood exposure to cat and atopic sensitization. *J Allergy Clin Immunol* 1999; **104**: 941–7.

26. Sudo N, Sawamura S, Tanaka K, Aiba Y, Kubo C, Koga Y. The requirement of intestinal microflora for the development of an IgE production system fully susceptible to oral tolerance induction. *J Immunol* 1997; **159**: 1739–45.

27. Hide DW, Guyer BM. Clinical manifestations of allergy related to breast and cows' milk feeding. *Pediatrics* 1985; **76**: 973 5.

28. Björkstén B, Naaber P, Seep E, Mikelsaar M. The intestinal microflora in allergic Estonian and Swedish 2-year old children. *Clin Exp Allergy* 1999; **29**: 342–6.

29. Böttcher M, Nordin EK, Sandin A, Midtvedt T, Bjorksten B. Microflora associated characteristics in faeces from allergic and non-allergic children. *Clin Exp Allergy* 2000; **30**: 1590–6.

30. Rubaltelli FF, Biadaioli R, Pecile P, Nicoletti P. Intestinal flora in breast- and bottle-fed infants. *J Perinat Med* 1998; **26**: 186–91.

31. Isolauri E, Arvola T, Sütas Y, Salminen S. Probiotics in the management of atopic eczema. *Clin Exp Allergy* 2000; **105**: 61–70.

32. Majamaa H, Isolauri E. Probiotics: a novel approach in the management of food allergy. *J Allergy Clin Immunol* 1997; **99**: 179–85.

33. Seaton A, Godden DJ, Brown KM. Increase in asthma: a more toxic environment or a more susceptible population. *Thorax* 1994; **49**: 171–4.

34. Devereux G, Seaton A. Why don't we give chest patients dietary advice. *Thorax* 2001; **56**(Suppl. ii); ii15–1122.

35. Butland BK, Fehily AM, Elwood PC. Diet, lung function and lung function decline in a cohort of 2512 middle-aged men. *Thorax* 2000; **55**: 102–8.

36. Tabak C, Arts IC, Smit HA, Heederik D, Kromhout D. Chronic obstructive pulmonary disease and intake of catechins, flavonols and flavones: the MORGAN Study. *Am J Respir Crit Care Med* 2001; **164**: 61–4.

37. Rayman MP. Dietary selenium: time to act. *Br Med J* 1997; **314**: 387–8.

38. Tantisira KG, Weiss ST. Complex interactions in complex traits: Obesity and asthma. *Thorax* 2001; (Suppl II): ii64–ii74.

39. Beckett WS, Jacobs DR Jr, Yu X, Iribarren C, Williams OD. Asthma is associated with weight gain in females but not males, independent of physical activity. *Am J Respir Crit Care Med* 2001; **164**: 2045–50.

40. Stenius-Aarniaia B, Poussa T, Kvarnstrom J, Gronlund EL, Ylikahri M, Mustajoki P. Immediate and long term effects of weight reduction in obese people with asthma: randomized controlled study. *Br Med J* 2000; **320**: 827–32.

41. Kelly YJ, Brabin BJ, Milligan P, Heaf DP, Reid J, Pearson MG. Maternal asthma, premature birth, and the risk of respiratory morbidity in schoolchildren in Merseyside. *Thorax* 1995; **50**: 525–30.

42. Ong TJ, Mehta A, Ogston S, Mukhopadhyay S. Prediction of lung function in the inadequately nourished. *Arch Dis Child* 1998; **79**: 18–21.

43. Koren HS. Associations between criteria air pollutants and asthma. *Environ Health Perspect* 1995; **103**(Suppl.): 235–42.

44. Kehrl HR, Peden DB, Ball B, Folinsbee LJ, Horsman D. Increased specific airway reactivity of persons with mild allergic asthma after 7.6 hours of exposure to 0.16 ppm ozone. *J Allergy Clin Immunol* 1999; **104**: 1198–204.

3

Genetics of asthma

Introduction

The development of asthma, the course of the disease and the response to treatment appear to be under genetic as well as environmental control and the recent
publication of the human genome project is likely to generate a substantial amount
of interest in this area. In common with other complex disease phenotypes, it is
unlikely that a single asthma gene will emerge. However, the identification of one
or more genes that appear to exert a moderate influence has the potential to provide insight into the pathological processes that determine the perpetuation of the
inflammatory state or govern response to treatment.

Association of *IL12B* promoter polymorphism with severity of atopic and non-atopic asthma in children.
Morahan G, Huang D, Wu M, *et al. Lancet* 2002; **360**: 455–9.

BACKGROUND. The association between atopy and asthma has led investigators to
target genetic markers in chromosome 5q31-33. This region includes genes important
in the control of T-helper cell differentiation including interleukin 12 (IL-12). The IL-12
glycoprotein consists of two subunits: *IL12A* and *IL12B*. The *IL12B* gene encodes the
p40 subunit of IL-12. The aim of this study was to assess the relationship between
IL12B promoter polymorphism and the development of asthma in both atopic and
non-atopic individuals.

INTERPRETATION. There was no relationship between individual *IL12B* polymorphisms
and asthma susceptibility. However, the presence of *IL12B* heterozygosity was more
common in those with severe asthma. Among all asthmatic children the relative risk for
IL12B promoter heterozygotes developing severe asthma was 4.6 (95% confidence
interval [CI] 2.1–11.1). The *IL12B* polymorphisms appeared to have a functional
consequence as heterozygotes produced significantly less IL12 gene products.

Association of the ADAM33 gene with asthma and bronchial hyper-responsiveness.

Van Eerdwegh P, Little RD, Dupuis J, *et al. Nature* 2002; **418**: 426–30.

BACKGROUND. **The authors identified 460 Caucasian families in which there were at least two siblings with physician-diagnosed asthma and on therapy for asthma. Performing linkage analysis, they identified a specific DNA 'signature' on chromosome 20p13 that was linked to asthma (Log$_{10}$ of the likelihood ratio [LOD], 2.94) and bronchial hyper-responsiveness (LOD 3.93). The region spanned 4.28 centimorgans and the investigators characterized a potential of 40 genes. A survey of 135 polymorphisms in 23 genes identified the ADAM33 gene as being significantly associated with asthma as demonstrated by linkage disequilibrium in both the UK and USA populations. As multiple single nucleotide polymorphisms (SNPs) may act in combination to increase the risk of asthma, haplotype pairs were constructed and their frequencies compared in cases and controls, again only ADAM33 was significantly associated with asthma. The association was further strengthened by use of the transmission disequilibrium test in which the observed frequency of gene variants transmitted from healthy parents to children with asthma was compared to the frequency that would be observed if the gene distribution occurred by chance.**

INTERPRETATION. As ADAM33 encodes a protein-processing enzyme known as a metalloproteinase expressed in lung fibroblasts and airway smooth muscle, the authors speculate that altered expression of ADAM33 in these tissues may be linked to the development of bronchial hyper-responsiveness and airway remodelling characteristic of the asthmatic phenotype.

Comment

Given the current immunological views on asthma development, the association between a polymorphism in the *IL12B* promoter and the severity of asthma, explored by Morahan *et al.* appears logical. IL-12 is important in determining the balance between Th1 and Th2 cells, and mice deficient in IL-12 are unable to generate a Th1 immune response |1|. In keeping with their hypothesis, these authors report that heterozygosity for the *IL12B* promoter polymorphism is associated with increased severity of both atopic and non-atopic asthma. They bolster their finding by demonstrating that this polymorphism is associated with reduced expression of the *IL12B* gene and reduced production of the interleukin 12 p70 protein. This abnormality could lead to attenuated Th1 function in response to viral infection, a known trigger of asthma. Additionally, animal models have demonstrated that reduced levels of IL12 contribute to the development of enhanced AHR |2|. However, it is not clear why heterozygosity is associated with a reduced functional response but homozygosity is not.

This paper by Eerdewegh *et al.* provides an elegant model for the investigation of genetic traits in complex diseases. In this study, the authors identify ADAM33 as being significantly associated with asthma. The finding that the association was not influenced by serum IgE, a marker of atopy, suggests that ADAM33 is linked to the asthmatic phenotype *per se*. Its expression in key target tissues will provide a basis to extend research to the mechanisms that may be operative in defining the asthmatic phenotype. The ADAM genes encode metalloproteinases and this paper will direct further work towards understanding the role of these enzymes in the regulation of the pathological processes observed in the asthmatic lung [3].

References

1. Magram J, Connaughton SE, Warrier RR, *et al.* IL-12 deficient mice are defective in IFN gamma production and type 1 cytokine responses. *Immunity* 1996; **4**: 471–81.

2. Gavett SH, O'Hearn DJ, Li X, Huang S-K, Finkelman FD, Wills-Karp M. Interleukin 12 inhibits antigen-induced airway hyperresponsiveness, inflammation, and Th2 cytokine expression in mice. *J Exp Med* 1995; **182**: 1527–36.

3. Yoshinaka T, Nishii K, Yamada K, *et al.* Identification and characterization of novel mouse and human ADAM33s with potential metalloproteinase activity. *Gene* 2002; **282**: 227–36.

4

Clinical course of asthma

Introduction

It is widely held that most children will 'out-grow' asthma, but many will continue to experience ongoing symptoms and asthma will return in some of those who have experienced remission |1–4|. Furthermore, it is recognized that asthma may present as a new diagnosis at any age. In the past two years, several papers have been published reporting the results from cohort studies that provide further insight into the factors associated with remission, persistence and new-onset asthma. When assessing patients with persistent asthma it is pertinent to identify whether the patient is exposed to factors known to perpetuate the disease such as allergens. A further possibility, often of concern to patients, is the possible role of stressful situations or life-events. Finally, some patients with asthma experience exacerbations that necessitate hospital admission. This group accounts for a significant proportion of the morbidity and mortality associated with asthma and the factors associated with this group require clarification in order to identify possible factors for intervention. The risk of death appears to be highest in those who suffer rapid and severe deterioration in lung function |5,6|.

Risk factors for onset and remission of atopy, wheeze and airway hyper-responsiveness.
Xuan W, Marks GB, Toelle BG, *et al. Thorax* 2002; **57**: 104–9.

BACKGROUND. This study reports on a cohort of 8–10 year old children who were enrolled in 1984 and surveyed at 2-yearly intervals, and provides information from the seventh survey conducted between 1997 and 1999 of 401 subjects (age range 23–27 years). Atopy, airway hyper-responsiveness (AHR), wheeze in the last 12 months, and lung function had been recorded at each survey. Late onset, remission, and persistence were defined based on characteristics in the initial survey and changes in these at follow-up surveys. The aim of this study was to investigate characteristics associated with onset and progression of atopy and asthma during adolescence and young adulthood.

INTERPRETATION. The prevalence of atopy increased, as both persistence and late-onset were more common than remission. A similar pattern was observed regarding a history of recent wheeze. The development of late-onset wheeze was independently associated with atopy (odds ratio [OR] 2.8; 95% confidence interval [CI] 1.5–2.10) and the presence of a parental history of asthma (OR 2.1, 95% CI 1.02–4.13), but not AHR following adjustment for atopy. Being female was associated with a trend towards late-onset wheeze (OR 1.7, 95% CI 0.95–2.97), but this did not attain statistical significance. Persistence of wheeze from childhood was associated with the presence of AHR (OR 4.3, 95% CI 1.3–5.0). Neither the presence of a family history of asthma, nor atopy was associated with persistent wheeze. Late-onset AHR was more likely with a history of atopy aged 8–12 years (OR 2.9, 95% CI 1.5–5.4) and being female (OR 1.9, 95% CI 1.01–3.60). Being male was associated with the development of late-onset atopy (Table 4.1, Fig. 4.1).

Table 4.1 Prognosis and development of recent wheeze, airway hyper-responsiveness (AHR), and atopy in the study sample (*n* = 498)

	Never	Intermittent	Late onset	Remission	Persistent
Recent wheeze	60.4%	13.1%	12.4%	5.6%	8.4%
AHR	78.7%	7.8%	1.8%	7.2%	4.4%
Atopy	43.4%	11.2%	13.7%	3.2%	28.5%

Source: Xuan *et al.* (2002).

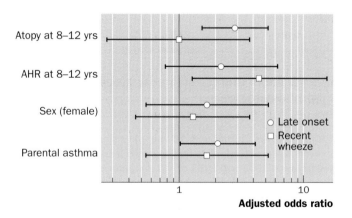

Fig. 4.1 Risk factors for late onset and persistence of recent wheeze.
Source: Xuan *et al.* (2002).

Incidence and remission of asthma: a retrospective study on the natural history of asthma.

de Marco R, Locatelli F, Cerveri I, Bugiani M, Marinoni A, Giammanco G.
J Allergy Clin Immunol 2002; **110**: 228–35.

BACKGROUND. **This multi-centre, cross-sectional survey on a young adult Italian population reported the incidence, persistence and remission of asthma from birth to the age of 44 years during the period between 1953 and 2000. The onset of asthma was defined as the age of the first attack and remission when a subject was neither under treatment nor had experienced an asthma attack in the last 24 months. Person years and survival techniques were used for analysis and efforts were made to minimize recall and selection bias.**

INTERPRETATION. There appear to be two different forms of asthma: early onset asthma, which is more common in boys and carries a good prognosis; and late-onset asthma, occurring during or after puberty, which is more common in women and less favourable in prognosis.

Comment

Although the diagnosis of asthma differs in these (and indeed many epidemiological papers), some consistent messages emerge. Xuan *et al.* reiterate the presence of atopy as one of the strongest risk factors for the development of asthma, and highlight the importance of the family history. Both of these factors are consistent with previous reports |**7,8**|. However, this paper reassures us that neither of these factors conveys an adverse prognostic impact on the disease, with asthma being as equally likely to remit whether these factors are present or not.

Also consistent with previous reports is the observation by Xuan *et al.* that the persistence of asthma is more likely in the presence of AHR |**9,10**|. It is often not possible to measure AHR and so the observations of de Marco *et al.* are helpful as they provide information on remission from more easily accessible clinical parameters. In their paper, asthma was more likely to remit if the onset of the condition occurred early, the patient was male and the duration of asthma had not been longer than 5 years.

Both papers confirm that asthma can occur in adolescence even in the absence of a history of atopy or family history of asthma. Indeed, the rate of onset is greater than the rate of remission, which accounts for the generational increase in the observed incidence of asthma. That this appears to be more common in women may reflect the greater female prevalence of AHR. Unfortunately, when acquired post-puberty, asthma is less likely to remit.

Sensitization to airborne moulds and severity of asthma: cross-sectional study from European Community respiratory health survey.

Zureik M, Neukirch C, Leynaert B, Liard R, Bousquet J, Neukirch F. *Br Med J* 2002; **325**: 411–14.

BACKGROUND. The European Community Respiratory Health Survey is an international multi-centre epidemiological study on asthma, collecting standard information on asthma prevalence and known or suspected risk factors for atopy and asthma. This study analysed data from 1132 patients (20–44 years) with the aim of determining whether the severity of asthma is associated with sensitization to airborne moulds rather than to other seasonal or perennial allergens.

INTERPRETATION. In this study, sensitization to moulds was rare but multivariate logistic regression demonstrated that the odds ratios for sensitization to moulds was 1.48 (95% CI 0.97–2.26) for moderate vs mild asthma and 2.16 (95% CI 1.37–3.35) for severe vs mild asthma (P <0.001 for trend). Thus, it appeared that sensitization to moulds may be associated with severe asthma and should be taken into account in the management of these patients.

Housing characteristics, reported mold exposure, and asthma in European Community Respiratory Health Survey.

Zock J-P, Jarvis D, Luczynska C, Sunyer J, Burney P. *J Allergy Clin Immunol* 2002; **110**: 285–92.

BACKGROUND. This study also reported data from the European Community Respiratory Health Survey but herein the authors report information regarding house dampness, type of heating and ventilation systems, presence of double glazing, type of floor cover in the bedroom and living room, water damage, water collection or mould/mildew on any surface inside the house and house dust mite levels. The aim of the study was to determine the relationship between these factors and the level of adult asthma.

INTERPRETATION. A significant ecological association between asthma and mould exposure (Spearman $r_s = 0.55$, P <0.001) was observed across all study centres. Water damage and the presence of mould in the home were related to asthma symptoms, and mould exposure was also related to AHR but in models with mutual adjustment, the effect of recent water damage was explained by exposure to moulds. Individuals with sensitization to *C. herbarum* were at a significantly increased risk of current asthma if they reported mould exposure (OR 2.41, 95% CI 1.32–4.39), compared with those who did not (OR 1.17, 95% CI 1.02–1.36). Findings for wheezing and bronchial hyper-responsiveness were less consistent.

School examinations enhance airway inflammation to antigen challenge.

Liu LY, Coe CL, Swenson CA, Kelly EA, Kita H, Busse W. *Am J Respir Crit Care Med* 2002; **165**: 1062–7.

BACKGROUND. It is widely held that stressful life-events are associated with exacerbations of asthma. The aim of this study was to suggest a possible mechanism by investigating whether chronic stressful life events could enhance airway inflammation.

INTERPRETATION. Compared to the relatively less stressful period of mid semester or the period post final examination, the level of eosinophilic airway inflammation was higher when college students were assessed during a period of high stress: final examination week.

Comment

Several case–control studies have suggested that patients with asthma are more likely to live in homes with evidence of dampness, particularly in the bedroom |**11–13**|. One possible mechanism is that growth of house dust mite is favoured by damp conditions |**14**|. However, a further possibility is that dampness favours growth of moulds that initiate or perpetuate asthma. Moulds have been associated with asthma severity as judged by asthma death, near fatal episodes, emergency room attendance and hospital admission |**15,16**|. The large population-based studies over wide geographical regions by Zoch *et al.* and Zureik *et al.* extend these observations. Zoch *et al.* demonstrate that mould exposure in the home is associated with current asthma symptoms and AHR. Zureik *et al.* employed a symptom score to demonstrate that mould exposure is associated with asthma of greater day-to-day severity. The cross-sectional design of these studies means that it is inappropriate to speculate on causation and prospective studies would be needed to distinguish between new-onset asthma and aggravation of asthma. A possible mechanism may lie in the ability of polymers in the fungal cell wall to promote airway inflammation |**17**|.

Patients are often interested in the role of stress and the severity of asthma. The paper by Liu *et al.* provides an interesting observation on the changes in airway inflammation that appear to accompany a stressful situation. They suggest that during stress, there is a shift towards a Th2 response. The authors accept that other confounding factors may be operative that accompany the lifestyle changes students may make approaching exams and note that none of their patients experienced a significant decline in lung function.

Risk factors for hospital admission for asthma from childhood to young adulthood: a longitudinal population study.

Rasmussen F, Taylor RD, Flannery EM, *et al*. *J Allergy Clin Immunol* 2002; **110**: 220–7.

B A C K G R O U N D . In order to determine factors associated with single or multiple hospital admissions from asthma, the authors examined a birth cohort of 1037 New Zealand children followed to the age of 26 years. The participants were characterized according to respiratory questionnaires, lung function, AHR and atopic status on seven occasions over the course of the study.

I N T E R P R E T A T I O N . Hospitalization was reported in 62 individuals (8.3% of those at risk and 6.2% of the unselected cohort). Admission to hospital was associated with being male, an earlier age of onset of symptoms, a history of atopy, and a greater degree of AHR. Fifty-five admissions occurred in children <9 years, 40 admissions between the ages of 9 and 18 years, and 41 admissions >18 years. Frequent symptoms and low lung function were evident among the 45 study members with single admissions and even more evident among the 17 study members with multiple admissions.

Frequency and clinical characteristics of rapid-onset fatal and near-fatal asthma.

Plaza V, Serrano J, Picado C, Sanchis J. *Eur Respir J* 2002; **19**: 846–52.

B A C K G R O U N D . The aim of this prospective, descriptive, hospital-based, multi-centre study was to provide information on the frequency and clinical characteristics of rapid-onset asthma (ROA) in patients experiencing a fatal or near-fatal attack. ROA was defined as deterioration over 2 hours from a previously stable state.

I N T E R P R E T A T I O N . ROA was not rare accounting for 20% of attacks. The clinical characteristics for ROA differed from those of slow-onset asthma (SOA). The ROA group had significantly fewer episodes of suspected respiratory tract infection (7 vs 38%), higher rates of fume/irritant inhalation (9 vs 1%), and a higher intake of non-steroidal anti-inflammatory drugs (14 vs 3%). The ROA group exhibited significantly higher rates of impaired consciousness (63 vs 42%), absence of lung sounds on admission (68 vs 42%), fewer hours of mechanical ventilation (13 vs 28 hours), and fewer days of hospitalization (8 vs 9.5 days) than the SOA group.

Comment

Ramussen *et al*. detail that during the first 26 years hospitalization occurs in approximately 6% of an unselected asthmatic population. Although more common in childhood, hospitalization is also a feature of adolescent and adult asthma and is more common in males and those with severe asthma (characterized by frequent symptoms, AHR and atopy). Under-treatment was recognized in patients prone to hospitalization but the reasons why this occurred were not possible to be determined using this study design.

ROA is a particularly distressing form of asthma attack characterized by a precipitous onset and the rapid progression to severe features. This form of asthma is associated with death. Plaza *et al.* highlight some of the features associated with these individuals. They identify that patients with ROA more frequently reported sensitivity to non-steroidal anti-inflammatory drugs. This is consistent with observations made in two other studies, although others have failed to identify this link |18–20|. This study failed to implicate strongly, respiratory infections or certain allergens as major factors but did note a seasonal variation with more cases presenting in spring and winter. The identification of under-treatment is consistent with other studies |21–22|. Although, many reasons may be operative, it is an important reminder that clinicians must emphasize compliance, particularly with inhaled corticosteroids, to this patient group |23|.

References

1. Jenkins MA, Hopper JL, Bowes G, Carlin JB, Flander LB, Giles GG. Factors in childhood as predictors of asthma in adult life. *Br Med J* 1994; **309**: 90–3.

2. Oswald H, Phelan PD, Lanigan A, Hibbert M, Bowes G, Olinsky A. Outcome of childhood asthma in mid-adult life. *BMJ* 1994; **309**: 95–6.

3. Blair H. Natural history of childhood asthma. *Arch Dis Child* 1977; **52**: 613–19.

4. Godden DJ, Ross S, Abdalla M, McMurray D, Douglas A, Oldman D, Friend JAR, Legge JS, Douglas JG. Outcome of wheeze in childhood: symptoms and pulmonary function 25 years later. *Am J Respir Crit Care Med* 1994; **149**: 106–12.

5. Wasserfallen JB, Schaller MD, Feihl F, Perret CH. Sudden asphyxic asthma: a distinct clinical entity. *Am Rev Respir Dis* 1990; **142**: 108–11.

6. Sur S, Crotty TB, Kephart GM, Hyma BA, Colby TV, Reed CE, Hunt LW, Gleich GJ. Sudden-onset fatal asthma. A distinct entity with few eosinophils and relatively more neutrophils in the airway submucosal. *Am Rev Respir Dis* 1993; **148**: 713–19.

7. Burrows B, Martinez FD, Halonen M, Barbee RA, Cline MG. Association of asthma with serum IgE levels and skin-test reactivity to allergens. *N Engl J Med* 1989; **320**: 271–7.

8. Dodge R, Burrows B, Lebowitz MD, Cline MG. Antecedent features of children in whom asthma develops during the second decade of life. *J Allergy Clin Immunol* 1993; **92**: 744–9.

9. Xu X, Rijcken B, Schouten JP. Airway hyperresponsiveness and development and remission of chronic respiratory symptoms in adults. *Lancet* 1997; **350**: 1431–4.

10. Toelle BG, Peat JK, Salome CM, Mellis CM, Woolcock AJ. Toward a definition of asthma for epidemiology. *Am Rev Respir Dis* 1992; **146**: 633–7.

11. Mohamed N, Ng'ang'a L, Odhiambo J, Menzies R. Home environment and asthma in Kenyan school-children: a case–control study. *Thorax* 1995; **50**: 74–8.

12. Verhoeff AP, van Strien RT, van Wijnen JH, Brunekreef B. Damp housing and childhood respiratory symptoms: the role of sensitization to dust mites and moulds. *Am J Epidemiol* 1995; **141**: 103–10.

13. Williamson IJ, Martin CJ, McGill G, Monie RDH, Fennerty AG. Damp housing and asthma: a case–control study. *Thorax* 1997; **52**: 229–34.

14. Kuehr J, Frischer T, Karmaus W, Meinert R, Barth R, Schraub S *et al.* Natural variation in mite antigen density in house dust and relationship to residential factors. *Clin Exp Allergy* 1994; **24**: 229–37.

15. O'Hollaren M, Yunginger JW, Offord KP, Sommers MJ, O'Connell EJ, Ballard DJ *et al.* Exposure to aeroallergen as a possible precipitating factor in respiratory arrest in young patients with asthma. *N Engl J Med* 1991; **324**: 359–63.

16. Black PN, Udy AA, Brodie SM. Sensitivity to fungal allergens is a risk factor for lifethreatening asthma. *Allergy* 2000; **55**: 501–4.

17. Douwes J, Zuidhof A, Doekes G, van der Zee SC, Wouters I, Boezen MH, *et al.* (1→3)-β-D-glucan and endotoxin in house dust and peak flow variability in children. *Am J Respir Crit Care Med* 2000; **162**: 1348–54.

18. Picardo C, Castillo JA, Montserrat JM, Agusti Vidal A. Aspirin-intolerance as a precipitating factor of life-threatening attacks of asthma requiring mechanical ventilation. *Eur Respir J* 1989; **2**: 127–9.

19. Matsuse H, Shimoda T, Matsuo N, *et al.* Aspirin-induced asthma as a risk factor for asthma mortality. *J Asthma* 1997; **34**: 413–17.

20. Woodruff PG, Emond SD, Singh AK, Camargo CA Jr. Sudden-onset severe acute asthma: clinical features and response to therapy. *Acad Emerg Med* 1998; **5**: 695–701.

21. Hartert TV, Windom HH, Peebles RS, *et al.* Inadequate out-patient medical therapy for patients with asthma admitted to two urban hospitals. *Am J Med* 1996; **100**: 386–94.

22. Rabe KF, Vermeire PA, Soriano JB, *et al.* Clinical management in asthma in 1999: the Asthma Insights and Reality in Europe (AIRE) study. *Eur Respir J* 2000; **16**: 802–7.

23. Suissa S, Ernst P, Benayoun S, Baltzan, Cai B. Low-dose inhaled corticosteroids and the prevention of death from asthma. *N Engl J Med* 2000; **343**: 332–6.

5

Airway wall remodelling

Introduction

Airway wall remodelling refers to a dynamic process that is thought to be characterized by the gradual alteration in airway wall structure that occurs in a subset of asthmatic patients. Over time this is thought to lead to the development of airflow obstruction that no-longer responds fully to bronchodilator or corticosteroid therapy and contributes to the loss of lung function reported in these individuals.

Factors associated with persistent airflow limitation in severe asthma.
ten Brinke A, Zwinderman AH, Sterk PJ, Rabe KF, Bel EH. *Am J Respir Crit Care Med* 2001; **164**: 744–8.

BACKGROUND. The aim of this study was to determine the prevalence of persistent airflow limitation in patients with severe asthma and to determine the associated clinical and pathophysiological characteristics.

INTERPRETATION. Factors associated with persistent airflow limitation included a significantly older age (mean: 49 vs 42 years) and a longer duration of asthma (median: 26.5 vs 15 years). It was also associated with sputum eosinophils $\geq$2%, (OR 7.7, 95% CI 2.4–25), PC_{20} histamine $\leq$1 mg/ml (OR 3.9, 95% CI 1.2–13) and adult onset ($\geq$18 years) of asthma (OR 3.3, 95% CI 1.2–9.0). Only sputum eosinophilia was independently associated with persistent airflow limitation (OR 8.9, CI 1.3–59). Thus, persistent airflow limitation is common in severe asthma and may be the result of uncontrolled eosinophilic airway inflammation.

Risk factors for airway remodelling in asthma manifested by a low post-bronchodilator FEV_1/vital capacity ratio.
Rasmussen F, Taylor R, Flannery EM, *et al. Am J Respir Crit Care Med* 2002; **165**: 1480–8.

BACKGROUND. The changes associated with low lung function or an accelerated decline of lung function may begin in childhood. Using the post-bronchodilator forced expiratory volume$_1$/vital capacity (FEV_1/VC) ratio as a functional marker of remodelling, Rasmussen *et al.* performed a longitudinal population-based epidemiological study on a birth cohort of 1037 New Zealand children to determine the prevalence of airway remodelling in relation to childhood asthma, airway hyper-responsiveness (AHR), atopy, sex, pulmonary function and smoking.

INTERPRETATION. Airway remodelling (as defined by a low FEV_1/VC ratio) is detectable in childhood and continues into adulthood. A low post-bronchodilator FEV_1/VC ratio was found in 62 of 839 (7.4%) and 58 of 913 (6.4%) study members aged 18 and 26 years, respectively and was more common in males. AHR (even when asymptomatic) was more common in those with a low post-bronchodilator FEV_1/VC ratio. It was possible to classify the subjects into three groups: a consistently low FEV_1/VC ratio, a variable ratio and a consistently normal ratio. Those with consistently low ratios more often had

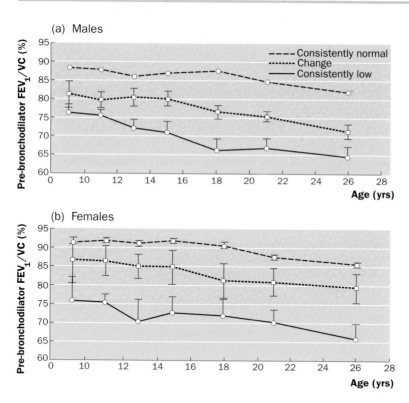

Fig. 5.1 Mean (95% confidence interval) FEV_1/VC ratio (%) before bronchodilator from age 9 to age 26 by sex. Study members with a consistently normal post-bronchodilator FEV_1/VC ratio at both ages 18 and 26. Study members with a change in FEV_1/VC ratio from age 18 to age 26. Study members with a consistently low post-bronchodilator FEV^1/VC ratio at both age 18 and 26. Source: Rasmussen *et al.* (2002).

asthma, AHR and symptomatic AHR and demonstrated a greater decline in the pre-bronchodilator FEV_1/VC ratio from 9 to 26 years of age. Asthma, male sex, AHR, and low lung function in childhood were each independently associated with a low post-bronchodilator FEV_1/VC ratio, which in turn was associated with an accelerated decline in lung function and diminished reversibility (Fig. 5.1.).

Comment

Until recently, asthma has been considered as a fully reversible disorder. However, several studies have identified a subgroup of patients that display an accelerated loss of lung function and develop a degree of fixed airflow obstruction |**1,2**|. This is thought to reflect structural remodelling of the airway with proliferation of smooth muscle, blood vessels, an increase in bronchial glands and deposition of collagen. The study by ten Brinke *et al.* suggests that persistent airflow limitation is very common in patients with severe asthma and may be associated with uncontrolled eosinophilic inflammation. The cross-sectional design means that any temporal relationship between these two findings is blurred and causality cannot be determined but this is an interesting observation in the light of other papers suggesting that control of asthma may be improved by targeting the level of airway eosinophilia |**3**|.

Ramussen *et al.* have performed a very detailed and thorough cohort study. They tackled the problem of describing lung function during growth, and have used this as a surrogate for remodelling. The study suggests that being male is associated with a worse outcome as 1 in 4 in males compared with 1 in 10 in females with asthma developed a consistently low ratio. Male subjects also demonstrated an accelerated decline in FEV_1 predicted and FEV_1/VC ratio from the age of 9 to the age of 26 years and displayed more reversibility to β2-agonist in terms of both absolute FEV_1 and FEV_1/VC ratio. The observation that AHR is associated with accelerated decline in lung function is consistent with previous work and has been associated with remodelling in asymptomatic individuals |**4,5**|.

References

1. Strachan DP, Griffiths JM, Johnston ID, Anderson HR. Ventilatory function in British adults after asthma or wheezing illness at ages 0–35. *Am J Respir Crit Care Med* 1996; **154**: 1629–35.

2. Lange P, Parner J, Vestbo J, Schnohr P, Jensen G. A 15-year follow-up study of ventilatory function in adults with asthma. *N Engl J Med* 1998; **339**: 1194–200.

3. Green RH, Brightling CE, McKenna S, Hargadon B, Parker D, Bradding P, Wardlaw AJ, Pavord ID. Asthma exacerbations and sputum eosinophil counts: a randomized controlled trial. *Lancet* 2002; **360**: 1715–21.

4. Sherrill D, Sears MR, Lebowitz MD, Holdaway MD, Hewitt CJ, Flannery EM, Herbison GP, Silva PA. The effects of airway hyperresponsiveness, wheezing, and atopy on longitudinal pulmonary function in children: a 6 year follow-up study. *Pediatr Pulmonol* 1992; **13**: 78–85.

5. Laprise C, Laviolette M, Boutet M, Boulet LP. Asymptomatic airway hyperresponsiveness: relationships with airway inflammation and remodelling. *Eur Respir J* 1999; **14**: 63–73.

6

Investigations

Airway hyper-responsiveness

Enhanced bronchoconstriction to a variety of direct and indirect stimuli such as exercise, cold air, dusts, smoke and chemicals such as histamine and methacholine is an integral part of the definition of asthma. It is believed (although remains unproven) that this reflects underlying airway inflammation. The level of airway hyper-responsiveness (AHR) appears to correlate with the severity of asthma symptoms and the need for treatment [1,2]. Worsening of asthma following viral infection or antigen exposure is associated with an increase in AHR [3]. AHR has traditionally been demonstrated by bronchial challenge tests. These are based on the administration of sequentially increasing concentrations of either histamine or methacholine. The responsiveness of the airways is expressed as the concentration or dose of either chemical required to produce a certain decrease (usually 20%) in the FEV_1 (PC_{20} or PD_{20}).

PC_{20} adenosine 5′-monophosphate is more closely associated with airway inflammation in asthma than PC_{20} methacholine.

Van den Berge M, Meijer RJ, Kerstjens HA, *et al. Am J Respir Crit Care Med* 2001; **163**: 1546–50.

BACKGROUND. The aim of this study was to determine if AHR to adenosine monophosphate (AMP) provided a better marker of airway inflammation that AHR to methacholine in patients with atopic asthma of mild to moderate severity. In order to model loss of asthma control the authors tapered, or if possible discontinued, the dose of inhaled corticosteroids.

INTERPRETATION. Although the levels of PC_{20} methacholine and PC_{20} AMP are both related to the baseline level of FFV1, PC_{20} AMP provides a better reflection of airway inflammation than PC_{20} to methacholine (Fig. 6.1).

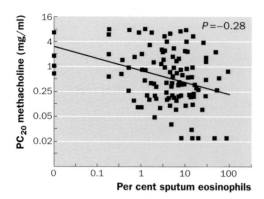

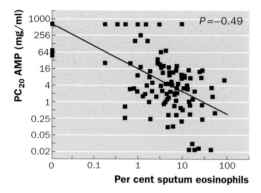

Fig. 6.1 Unadjusted relationship between PC_{20} methacholine and PC_{20} AMP with the percentage of sputum eosinophils. Source: Van den Berge *et al.* (2001).

Corticosteroid-induced improvement in the PC_{20} of adenosine 5′-monophosphate is more closely associated with airway inflammation in asthma than PC_{20} methacholine.

Van den Berge M, Kerstjens HA, Meijer RJ, *et al. Am J Respir Crit Care Med* 2001; **164**: 1127–32.

BACKGROUND. In an extension of the above study, patients in whom inhaled corticosteroids were either discontinued or tapered to the lowest dose possible until symptoms consistent with an impending asthma exacerbation were experienced, were then randomized to receive treatment for 2 weeks with prednisolone (30 mg/day), fluticasone (2000 µg/day), or fluticasone (500 µg/day). **The aim of this study was to determine if improvement in airway inflammation was more closely associated with the PC_{20} AMP than PC_{20} methacholine.**

INTERPRETATION. Both the PC_{20} methacholine and the PC_{20} AMP improved significantly with steroid therapy but the total explained variance of the improvement in bronchial hyper-responsiveness was greater for AMP as compared to methacholine (36 vs 22% respectively), thus PC_{20} AMP appears to be more sensitive to changes in airway inflammation than PC_{20} methacholine (Table 6.1).

Comment

Both histamine and methacholine act directly on airway smooth muscle (ASM) and stimulate contraction. However, many of the stimuli known to induce broncho-constriction, such as adenosine, have no direct effect on ASM and probably act by indirect pathways mediated through inflammatory cells. Testing AHR with these chemicals may provide a more clinically relevant measure of airway inflammation. As AMP is soluble in aqueous solution and is rapidly metabolized to adenosine, it has been employed as a novel indirect method of testing AHR [4]. Evidence of its clinical relevance has emerged from a study demonstrating dose-related broncho-constriction in asthmatic but not normal individuals [5]. More severe AMP respons-iveness has been shown to be associated with enhanced peak flow variability and higher symptom scores whereas anti-inflammatory therapy reduces AHR to AMP in patients with asthma to a greater extent than AHR to methacholine. Further-more, in contrast to methacholine, AMP responsiveness is associated with indirect

Table 6.1 Individual correlations of corticosteroid-induced changes in clinical and inflammatory parameters with improvement in the provocative concentrations of methacholine and adenosine monophosphate causing a 20% decrease in forced expiratory volume in 1 second

	ΔPC_{20} methacholine†		ΔPC_{20} AMP†	
ΔFEV_1 %predicted	$r = 0.31$	$P = 0.001$	$r = 036$	$P = 0.0001$
Sputum differential				
ΔEosinophils†, 10^3/ml	$r = -0.28$	$P = 0.004$	$r = -0.43$	$P = 0.000005$
ΔLymphocytes†, 10^3/ml	$r = 0.27$	$P = 0.052$	$r = 0.15$	$P = 0.132$
ΔMacrophages†, 10^3/ml	$r = 0.25$	$P = 0.01$	$r = 0.01$	$P = 0.901$
ΔNeutrophils†, 10^3/ml	$r = 0.14$	$P = 0.15$	$r = -0.08$	$P = 0.441$
ΔBronchial epithelial cells†, 10^3/ml	$r = 0.05$	$P = 0.59$	$r = -0.14$	$P = 0.17$
ΔSputum ECP†, ng/ml	$r = -0.07$	$P = 0.483$	$r = -0.24$	$P = 0.015$
ΔNO exhaled breath, ppb	$r = -0.128$	$P = 0.065$	$r = -0.38$	$P = 0.0001$

Δ = change; ECP = eosinophil cationic protein; PC_{20} AMP = provocative concentration of adenosine monophosphate causing a 20% decrease in FEV_1.
† Value is log transformed.

Source: Van den Berge *et al.* (2001).

parameters of airway inflammation such as exhaled nitric oxide (eNO), and eosinophilia in peripheral blood and sputum.

AHR measures both a fixed component of airway wall remodelling and a variable component that probably relates to airway inflammation. The two studies by van den Berge *et al.* provide further evidence that AHR measured by AMP provides a better assessment of airway inflammation than methacholine. In the first study they report that PC_{20} methacholine was predominantly predicted by the FEV_1 % predicted (explained variance [ev] = 18%). Interestingly, the percentage of peripheral blood monocytes provided a weak additional independent predictor (total ev = 23%). By contrast PC_{20} AMP was predominantly predicted by the percentage of eosinophils in sputum (ev = 25%) while FEV_1 % predicted was only an additional independent predictor (total ev = 36%). In the second study, they also demonstrate that the PC_{20} AMP may also provide a better assessment of improvement in airway inflammation following treatment. Here, the improvement of PC_{20} AMP was solely related to a reduction in airway inflammation. In contrast, the improvement in PC_{20} methacholine was related to both a reduction in airway inflammation (change in number of sputum eosinophils and lymphocytes) and an increase in the FEV_1 % predicted. The authors propose that more information is required including studies of longer duration and it will also be interesting to determine how AHR to AMP reflects other parameters of airway inflammation that are relevant to asthma.

Induced sputum and exhaled breath

Safety and reproducibility of sputum induction in asthmatic subjects in a multicentre study.

Fahy JV, Boushey HA, Lazarus SC, *et al.*, for the National Heart Lung, and Blood Institute's Asthma Clinical Research Network. *Am J Respir Crit Care Med* 2001; **163**: 1470–5.

BACKGROUND. There have been no published studies on the safety and reproducibility of induced sputum in the setting of multi-centre trials. A trial co-ordinated through the Asthma Clinical Network, investigating airway inflammation as an outcome indicator of treatment provided an opportunity to report the safety and repeatability of induced sputum in this setting and compare it to the reproducibility of the FEV_1 and methacholine PC_{20}.

INTERPRETATION. Induced sputum may be safely performed in patients with moderate-to-severe asthma. Although eleven out of 79 patients experienced a fall in FEV_1 of at least 20% from the post-albuterol baseline, all responded promptly to β2 agonist, and none developed refractory bronchospasm, required emergency room treatment or hospitalization. Induced sputum markers of inflammation were as reproducible as a methacholine PC_{20} (Table 6.2).

Table 6.2 Reproducibility of sputum markers, PC_{20} methacholine and FEV_1

Variable	n	Concordance correlation coefficient and 95% CI
Sputum eosinophil %*	59	0.74 (0.59, 0.84)
Sputum ECP*	54	0.81 (0.68, 0.88)
Sputum tryptase	56	0.79 (0.67, 0.87)
PC_{20} methacholine*	52	0.74 (0.58, 0.84)
FEV_1	59	0.93 (0.88, 0.96)

* The concordance correlation estimates are based on log transformed data (log base 2 for PC_{20}).
Source: Fahy et al. (2001).

The predictive value of exhaled nitric oxide measurements in assessing changes in asthma control.
Jones SL, Kiielson J, Cowan JA, et al. Am J Respir Crit Care Med 2001; **164**: 738–43.

BACKGROUND. The aim of this study was to assess the usefulness of eNO in detecting and predicting loss of control of asthma and to correlate this with sputum eosinophils and AHR to hypertonic saline.

INTERPRETATION. The authors reported highly significant correlations between changes in eNO and symptoms ($P < 0.0001$), FEV_1 (0.002), sputum eosinophils ($P < 0.0002$), and saline PD_{15} ($P < 0.0002$). There were significant differences between the loss of control (LOC) and no LOC groups. These values were similar to these obtained using sputum eosinophils and saline PD_{15} measurements. An absolute value of eNO of ≥ 15 ppb, or an increase of ≥ 10 ppb or 60% over baseline, provided a useful threshold for the detection of ongoing airway inflammation and predicts breakthrough symptoms. However, the absence of these changes did not preclude the possibility of deteriorating asthma.

Comment
Although airway inflammation is central to our understanding of asthma, the diagnosis and assessment of asthma on clinical grounds are made with reference to symptoms and lung function rather than measures of airway inflammation. Reliable, reproducible and safe methods to assess the extent of airway inflammation are clearly needed. The technique of sputum induction has been utilized as a research tool for some time and an increasing body of evidence supports its potential utility. However, it is usually performed by research centres with established expertise in the technique. The paper by Fahy et al. adds to the body of evidence suggesting that sputum induction is safe but also demonstrates that it can produce reliable

information within the context of many centres participating in clinical trials. The authors acknowledge that their results will only refer to this technique and that similar data should be obtained from methods that employ lower doses of $\beta 2$ agonist, higher concentrations of hypertonic saline for longer periods or use nebulisers with a higher output. A higher incidence of bronchoconstriction may be anticipated in patients not taking inhaled corticosteroids.

Exhaled nitric oxide is also becoming recognized as a non-invasive marker of airway inflammation. Increased levels have been reported in patients with newly diagnosed asthma. Levels increase following allergen exposure and during exacerbations and improve following administration of inhaled corticosteroids. Thus, eNO may be a useful marker in the longitudinal assessment of asthma control. Jones *et al.* tested this hypothesis by inducing LOC by withdrawal of inhaled corticosteroids (ICS). The best positive predictive value (PPV), sensitivity and specificity for anticipating and diagnosing LOC were observed by recording changes in eNO over time. A doubling dose increase in saline PD_{15} was marginally better than the other measurements for diagnosing LOC, with a PPV of 95% and a 4% change in eosinophils was associated with a PPV of 84%. However, as a method of making frequent recordings in patients exhaled breath may be more user-friendly than either measurement of AHR or induced sputum, although comparative studies will be required. Furthermore, the authors point out that they used an exhalation flow rate 250 ml/sec that is significantly greater than currently recommended 50 ml/sec. Had they used a slower flow rate, their observations may have been improved.

References

1. Gustafsson PM, Kjellman B. Asthma from childhood: course and outcome of lung function. *Respir Med* 2000; **94**: 466–74.

2. Gray L, Peat JK, Belousova E *et al.* Family patterns of asthma, atopy and airway hyperresponsiveness: an epidemiological study. *Clin Exp Allergy* 2000; **30**: 393–9.

3. Cockcroft DW, Ruffin RE, Dolovitch J, Hargreave FE. Allergen-induced increase in nonallergic bronchial reactivity. *Clin Allergy* 1977; **7**: 503–13.

4. Polosa R, Rorke S, Holgate ST. Evolving concepts on the value of adenosine hyperresponsiveness in asthma and chronic obstructive pulmonary disease. *Thorax* 2002; **57**: 649–54.

5. Cushley MJ, Tattersfield AE, Holgate ST. Inhaled adenosine and guanosine on airway resistance in normal and asthmatic subjects. *Br J Clinical Pharmacol* 1983; **15**: 161–5.

7

Pathology of asthma

Introduction

The appreciation that even mild asthma was associated with airway inflammation has led to the central recognition that asthma is a chronic inflammatory disorder of the airways. Numerous inflammatory cells including eosinophils, CD4+ T-lymphocytes, macrophages and mast cells infiltrate the airways. In addition, the structural cells of the airway undergo changes with fragmentation of the delicate respiratory epithelium, thickening of the sub-epithelial collagen layer, hypertrophy and hyperplasia of the airway smooth muscle (ASM) and a marked increase in bronchial capillary bed. At a molecular level, numerous inflammatory genes are up-regulated including those encoding cytokines, chemokines, growth factors, adhesion molecules and their receptors.

Eosinophil

Asthma exacerbations and sputum eosinophil counts: a randomized controlled trial.
Green RH, Brightling CE, McKenna S, *et al. Lancet* 2002; **360**: 1715–21.

BACKGROUND. The aim of this study was to determine whether a management strategy directed towards maintaining the sputum eosinophil count below 3% would provide better asthma control that one following the current British Thoracic Society (BTS) guidelines (based on symptoms and lung function). The primary end-point was the prevention of an asthma exacerbation and the control of eosinophilic inflammation as assessed by induced sputum.

INTERPRETATION. Compared to those patients managed in accordance with BTS principles, the sputum management group experienced significantly fewer severe exacerbations and required fewer rescue courses of oral corticosteroids. This was achieved without the need for additional anti-inflammatory treatment (Fig. 7.1).

Comment

An influx of eosinophils is characteristic of the inflammatory response in asthma and although their precise role remains to be clarified, their appearance in the

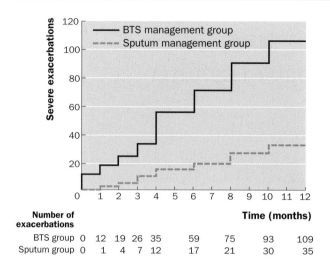

Number of exacerbations	0	1	2	3	4		5		6		7		8	
BTS group	0	12	19	26	35		59		75		93		109	
Sputum group	0	1	4	7	12		17		21		30		35	

Fig. 7.1 Cumulative asthma exacerbations in the BTS management group and the sputum management group. Source: Green *et al.* (2002).

sputum appears to predate and predict the onset of an exacerbation |1|. The study by Green *et al.* provides further evidence for the utility of the airway eosinophil in predicting asthma exacerbations and suggests that therapy directed towards maintaining sputum eosinophils within a defined target provides superior asthma control to more traditional methods recommended in the BTS guidelines. The general applicability of this data requires to be more thoroughly tested but it points the way toward improving asthma control through targeting the underlying inflammatory response.

Neutrophil

Association of forced expiratory volume with disease duration and sputum neutrophils in chronic asthma.
Little SA, MacLeod KJ, Chalmers GW, Love JG, McSharry C, Thomson NC. *Am J Med* 2002; **112**: 446–52.

B A C K G R O U N D . The aim of this study was to investigate whether induced sputum cell counts and soluble mediator components were associated with pulmonary function in non-smoking asthmatic subjects.

INTERPRETATION. The duration of asthma and sputum neutrophil counts were negatively associated with maximal forced expiratory volume$_1$ (FEV_1).

Comment

The neutrophil has classically been thought of as the first line in defence against bacterial infections and is not typically associated with asthma. However, there is evidence that neutrophils are present in the airways of asthmatic individuals, particularly in those with more severe disease, and those prone to near-fatal attacks [2–4]. The paper by Little *et al.* adds further weight to the evidence that neutrophils participate in the asthmatic inflammatory response and suggests that they may play a role in the process of airway wall remodelling and the accelerated decline in lung function seen in some asthmatic individuals. Certainly, neutrophils have the potential to secrete proteases and reactive oxygen species that could initiate injury and repair processes within the airway.

Mast cell

Mast cell infiltration of airway smooth muscle in asthma.

Brightling CE, Bradding P, Syman FA, Holgate ST, Wardlaw AJ, Pavord I.
N Engl J Med 2002; **346**: 1699–705.

BACKGROUND. To test whether the absence of airway hyper-reactivity (AHR) in eosinophilic bronchitis was due to differences in the relationship between mast cells and airway smooth muscle, the authors performed a comparative immunohistochemical analysis of bronchial-mucosa-biopsy specimens obtained from symptomatic individuals with each condition.

INTERPRETATION. The infiltration of airway smooth muscle by mast cells appears to be associated with the disordered airway function in asthma. The number of mast cells per square millimetre of smooth muscle was significantly higher in the subjects with asthma than in subjects with eosinophilic bronchitis or in normal controls. There was a significant inverse correlation between the number of mast cells infiltrating the bronchial smooth muscle and the PC_{20} for methacholine in the subjects with asthma ($r = -0.5$, $P = 0.03$) (Fig. 7.2).

Comment

AHR is consistently observed in asthma, yet also exists in many normal non-asthmatic and individuals, patients with allergic rhinitis who do not have asthma [5]. Interestingly, AHR is not observed in patients with eosinophilic bronchitis [6]. By virtues of its ability to secrete an array of mediators known to induce broncho-constriction, the mast cell is believed to be a major effector of AHR. However, a greater number of mast cells and higher concentration of their mediators can be recovered from subjects with eosinophilic bronchitis than asthma |7|. A possible explanation for this may relate to differences in the relationship between the mast cells and ASM in the two disorders. Thus, the paper by Brightling *et al.* represents a potentially exciting breakthrough in understanding the relationship between AHR

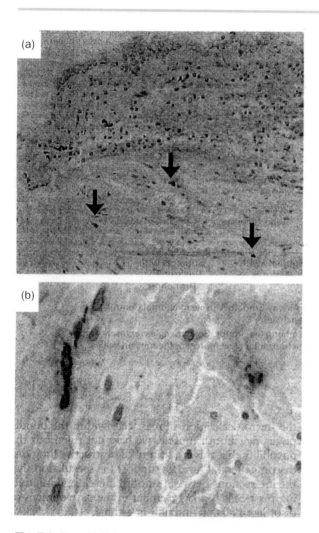

Fig. 7.2 Bronchial-biopsy specimens from subjects with asthma. Panel (a) shows epithelium, submucosa and smooth muscle with mast cells (arrows) infiltrating the airway smooth muscle (×100). Panel (b) shows mast cells within the airway smooth muscle (hematoxylin, ×400). Source: Brightling *et al.* (2002).

and inflammation reporting that mast cells infiltrate the ASM in asthma but not in eosinophilic bronchitis. It is not clear whether this localization is a feature of other obstructive lung diseases such as chronic obstructive pulmonary disease and further reports will be awaited.

Airway smooth muscle

Airway smooth muscle proliferation is increased in asthma.

Johnson PRA, Roth M, Tamm M, Hughes M, Ge Q, King G, burgess JK, Black JL. *Am J Respir Crit Care Med* 2001; **164**: 474–7.

BACKGROUND. In this study the authors were able to isolate and culture ASM from asthmatic and normal individuals to determine if ASM from patients with asthma exhibit a different pattern of proliferation from those obtained from non-asthmatic patients.

INTERPRETATION. The proliferation of ASM isolated from patients with asthma was significantly increased compared to control. Flow cytometric analysis of DNA content on days 1 and 2 demonstrated that a significantly greater percentage of asthmatic ASM cells were on the $G_2 + M$ phase than controls at 24 and 48 h (Table 7.1, Fig. 7.3).

Comment

One of the characteristic features of the asthmatic airway is an increased bulk of ASM due to both hypertrophy and hyperplasia |**8**|. In addition to acting as an effector cell, ASM is known to participate in the inflammatory response and probably contributes to persistent airway narrowing |**9**|. The report by Johnson *et al.* is the first report of the growth of human ASM cells obtained from endobronchial biopsies and the first study to demonstrate that ASM from asthmatic patients proliferate faster than those obtained from non-asthmatic individuals. Although care must be exercised in extrapolating these *in vitro* findings to *in vivo* conditions, the authors speculate that increased proliferation probably does occur *in vivo* and contribute to the increased muscle bulk observed.

Table 7.1 Details of asthmatic and non-asthmatic patients

Patient No.	Age	Sex	Disease	Treatments	Type of Sample	Sensitization
1	33	M	Asthma and primary pulmonary hypertension	Corticosteroids, bronchodilators	Explanted lung	Yes
2	15	M	Asthma (status asthmaticus)	Corticosteroids, bronchodilators	Autopsy	Yes
3	44	M	Asthma with emphysema	Bronchodilators	Explanted lung	Yes
4	44	F	Asthma	Corticosteroids, bronchodilators	Endobronchial biopsy	Yes*
5	46	M	Asthma	Corticosteroids, bronchodilators	Endobronchial biopsy	Yes*
6	78	M	Asthma	Corticosteroids, bronchodilators	Endobronchial biopsy	Yes*
7	25	M	Asthma	Corticosteroids, bronchodilators	Endobronchial biopsy	Yes*
8	55	F	Asthma	Corticosteroids, bronchodilators	Endobronchial biopsy	Yes*
9	49	F	Asthma	Corticosteroids, bronchodilators	Endobronchial biopsy	Yes*
10	34	F	Asthma	Corticosteroids, bronchodilators	Endobronchial biopsy	Yes*
11	42	F	Asthma	Corticosteroids, bronchodilators	Endobronchial biopsy	Yes*
12	50	M	Asthma	Corticosteroids, bronchodilators	Endobronchial biopsy	Yes*
13	59	M	Carcinoma	No treatment	Lobectomy	No
14	47	F	Carcinoma	Corticosteroids, bronchodilators	Lobectomy	No
15	52	F	Emphysema	Corticosteroids, bronchodilators	Explanted lung	No
16	51	M	Emphysema	Corticosteroids, bronchodilators	Explanted lung	No
17	49	M	Emphysema	Bronchodilators	Explanted lung	No
18	56	M	Cryptogenic fibrosing alveolitis	Corticosteroids, cyclophosphamide	Explanted lung	Yes
19	50	F	No lung disease	No treatment	Whole lung	No
20	55	F	Emphysema	Corticosteroids, bronchodilators	Explanted lung	No
21	40	M	No lung disease	No treatment	Whole lung	No
22	16	F	Carcinoma	Corticosteroids, bronchodilators	Lobectomy	No

* Sensitization assessed by skin prick test.

Source: Johnson et al. (2001).

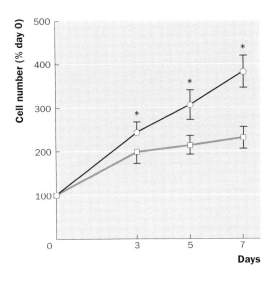

Fig. 7.3 Cell number in response to exposure to 5% FBS in DMEM for Days 0, 3, 5 and 7. Results are expressed as a percentage of the cell number in the presence of 1% FBS in DMEM on Day 0. *Significant differences from non-asthmatic ($P < 0.05$, $n = 12$ asthmatic and 10 non-asthmatic). Source: Johnson *et al.* (2001).

Inflammation and remission of asthma

Airway inflammation is present during clinical remission of atopic asthma.

van den Toorn LM, Overbeek SE, de Johgste JC, Leman K, Hoogsteden HC, Prins J-B. *Am J Respir Crit Care Med* 2001; **164**: 2107–13.

B A C K G R O U N D . **To establish whether subjects in clinical remission of atopic asthma suffer from ongoing active airway inflammation and/or remodelling, the authors compared bronchial biopsy specimens of subjects with a long-standing clinical remission of atopic asthma with subjects currently symptomatic with asthma and healthy controls.**

I N T E R P R E T A T I O N . Compared to healthy control subjects, subjects in clinical remission of atopic asthma have evidence of persistent airway inflammation and airway wall remodelling.

Comment

Remission will occur in many patients with asthma. However, it has been demonstrated that it is possible to demonstrate abnormalities of lung function including AHR during remission and that for some individuals the disease will return |**10–12**|. The study by van den Toorn *et al.* is the first study to demonstrate persistent inflammation despite clinical remission of asthma. The cross-sectional design of the study does not permit causative links to be drawn, but it is tempting to speculate that it is the ongoing inflammatory process that later leads to relapse of the disease. This would require to be addressed by further prospective studies.

References

1. Jatakanon A, Lim S, Barnes PJ. Changes in sputum eosinophils predict loss of asthma control. *Am J Respir Crit Care Med* 2000; **161**: 64–72.

2. Sur S, Crotty TB, Kephart GM, Hyma BA, Colby TV, Reed CE, Hunt LW, Gleich GJ. Sudden onset fatal asthma: a distinct entity with few eosinophils and relatively more neutrophils in the airway submucosal. *Am Rev Respir Dis* 1993; **148**: 713–19.

3. Jatakanon A, Uasuf C, Maziak W, Lim S, Chung KF, Barnes PJ. Neutrophilic inflammation in severe persistent asthma. *Am J Respir Crit Care Med* 1999; **160**: 1001–8.

4. Ordonez CL, Shaughnessy TE, Matthay MA, Fahy JV. Increased neutrophil numbers and IL-8 levels in airway secretions in acute severe asthma—clinical and biological significance. *Am J Respir Crit Care Med* 2000; **161**: 1185–90.

5. Brucsasco V, Crimi E, Pellegrino R. Airway hyperresponsiveness in asthma: not just a matter of airway inflammation. *Thorax* 1998; **53**: 992–8.

6. Gibson PG, Dolovich J, Denburg J, Ramsdale EH, Hargreave FE. Chronic cough: eosinophilic bronchitis without asthma. *Lancet* 1989; **i**: 1346–8.

7. Brightling CE, Ward R, Woltmann G, Bradding P, Sheller JR, Dworski R, Pavord ID. Induced sputum inflammatory mediator concentrations in eosinophilic bronchitis and asthma. *Am J Respir Crit Care Med* 2000; **162**: 878–82.

8. Ebina M, Takahashi T, Chiba T, Motomiya M. Cellular hypertrophy and hyperplasia of airway smooth muscles underlying bronchial asthma. A 3-D morphometric study. *Am Rev Respir Dis* 1993; **148**: 720–6.

9. Fredburg JJ. Airway smooth muscle in asthma. Perturbed equilibrium of myosin binding. *Am J Respir Crit Care Med* 2000; **161**: S158–60.

10. Kerrebijn KF, Fioole AC, van Bentveld RD. Lung function in asthmatic children after a year or more without symptoms or treatment. *Br Med J* 1978; **1**: 886–8.

11. Gruber W, Eber E, Steinbrugger B, Modl M, Weinhandl E, Zach MS. Atopy, lung function and bronchial hyperresponsiveness in symptom-free paediatric asthma patients. *Eur Respir J* 1997; **10**: 1041–5.

12. Panhuysen CIM, Vonk JM, Koëter GH, Schouten JP, van Altena R, Bleeker ER, Postma DS. Adult patients may outgrow their asthma: a 25-year follow-up study. *Am J Respir Crit Care* 1997; **155**: 1267–72.

8

Treatment

Introduction

The treatment of asthma should embrace a search for the underlying cause of the condition and the presence of aggravating factors in the patients' lifestyle that could be addressed to either abolish the condition (e.g. occupational asthma) or reduce its severity. Nevertheless, the majority of patients presenting to their physician with symptomatic asthma will require pharmacological therapy. The appreciation of the inflammatory nature of asthma has shifted the emphasis of treatment onto the central role of regularly administered inhaled corticosteroids, with the use of short-acting β-2 agonists for predominantly symptomatic (rescue) purposes. Long acting β-2 agonists have emerged as a useful add-on therapy for those not controlled on moderate doses of inhaled corticosteroids. More information is available on the role of the leukotriene receptor antagonists that were the first new treatment to be released for the management of asthma in over twenty years but newer therapies such as a monoclonal antibody directed against IgE may soon become available. Finally, although they remain underused, most guidelines encourage the use of management plans to empower patients to manage their own disease.

Allergen avoidance

Clinical evaluation of the effect of anti-allergic mattress covers in patients with moderate to severe asthma and house dust mite allergy: a randomized double-blind placebo-controlled study.
Rijssenbeek-Nouwens LHM, Oosting AJ, de Bruin-Weller MS, Bregman I, de Monchy JGR, Postma DS. *Thorax* 2002; **57**: 784–90.

B A C K G R O U N D. Thirty-eight patients with moderate to severe clinically stable asthma and allergy to house dust mite underwent a one-year, randomized, double-blind, placebo-controlled, parallel-group study comparing the effect of allergen impermeable encasings on the mattresses, pillows and bedcovers to determine if reduction in house dust mite (HDM) levels in bedding would improve asthma control in adult patients.

INTERPRETATION. The use of allergen impermeable bedding resulted in a significant reduction in Der p 1 mattress concentrations (decreasing from 26.19 [8.58] to 2.79 [0.88] µg/g fine dust). However, it was not possible to demonstrate any significant difference from placebo in terms of airway hyper-responsiveness (AHR), quality of life, symptoms scores, morning and evening peak expiratory flow record (PEFR), peak flow variability, or the use of rescue medication over the study period. Although there was a significant decrease in nasal symptoms in the active group, there was no difference between groups.

Comment

Sensitization to a range of allergens followed by subsequent and continued exposure has been implicated in the initiation and perpetuation of the asthmatic response. The number of potential allergens is extensive and varies with climatic conditions. In the UK and other European countries, HDMs are a major source of allergens and significant exposure in sensitized individuals is recognized in the development of asthma, with those exposed to the highest levels reporting more severe disease [1–3]. The principle allergenic component is the protease, Der p 1, found in the faeces. The improvement of asthma in mite free environments such as hospitals and the dry air of high altitude Alpine sanatoria suggest that avoidance of allergen may lead to a reduction in airway inflammation, AHR and symptoms [4–6]. However, it has proven difficult to achieve significant and sustained reductions in levels of exposure. This has been reflected by a recent Cochrane review on the topic including 23 studies and 686 subjects. However, most of the studies were small in number and in the majority (n = 17), no reported reduction in HDM allergen levels was observed. Allergen levels were reduced in six studies but only two of these were double-blind [7]. Better studies are needed to provide good quality information on allergen avoidance.

The paper adds to the volume of disappointing studies but, as with other studies, the authors were only able to recruit small numbers and the time course may still be relatively short. Confounding this study, and many of the others, is the possibility that the patients were continually exposed to other relevant allergens which may continue to drive the disease. Furthermore, it is possible that other end-points would provide more specific information on airway inflammation and these may be more useful as a marker to demonstrate effectiveness from allergen avoidance studies.

Short acting β-2 agonists

β-2 agonist tolerance and exercise-induced bronchospasm.
Hancox RJ, Subbarao P, Kamada D, Watson PM, Hargreave FE, Inman MD.
Am J Respir Crit Care Med 2002; **165**: 1068–70.

BACKGROUND. Eight subjects who demonstrated a ≥15% fall in forced expiratory volume$_1$(FEV$_1$), sustained at ≥10% for 5 minutes were entered into a randomized double-blind cross-over study receiving either regular salbutamol 200 μg qid or placebo, to determine if clinically relevant loss of bronchodilator response could be observed in response to a natural stimulus (exercise) following regular administration of β-agonist.

INTERPRETATION. Regular β-2 agonist treatment leads to enhanced exercise-induced bronchoconstriction and a sub-optimal bronchodilator response to rescue β-2 administration.

Comment

Short acting β-2 agonists are currently recommended as rescue medication, targeted towards the relief of symptoms, and therefore, administered on as required rather than regular basis. Used in this manner they also act as a barometer of control allowing the patient to judge how often they require rescue medication and how effective it is when administered. In patients with exercise-induced asthma, they may also be administered as bronchoprotective agents, offsetting an anticipated bronchoconstriction |8|. Although not currently recommended, the regular use of the short acting β-2 agonist, salbutamol, has been shown to be safe |9|. However, the aim of this study was to investigate whether clinically relevant tolerance may develop. Regular salbutamol treatment has been shown to increase in post-exercise bronchoconstriction, but the finding that the FEV$_1$ remains low despite salbutamol is a new observation |10|. This raises the possibility that regular administration of β-2 agonists may result in these agents being less effective in the setting of an acute severe asthma attack. These studies need to be repeated using long acting β-2 agonists.

Long acting β-2 agonists

Comparison of formoterol and terbutaline for as-needed treatment of asthma: a randomized trial.

Tattersfield AE, Löftdahl C-G, Postma DS, *et al. Lancet* 2001; **357**: 257–61.

BACKGROUND. **The onset of action of formoterol is equivalent to short acting β-2 agonists and could potentially be used as a rescue medication. The authors performed a double-blind, randomized, parallel-group study 362 patients (157 men) from 35 European centres, to assess the safety and efficacy of use of 4.5 μg inhaled formoterol with 0.5 mg terbutaline, each as needed, in moderate to severe asthma requiring as-needed medication despite taking inhaled corticosteroids (ICS).**

INTERPRETATION. Patients randomized to terbutaline experienced more exacerbations than those randomized to formoterol (48 exacerbations in 43 patients compared with 29 exacerbations in 26 patients). The time to first severe exacerbation was longer in the formoterol group than the terbutaline group ($P = 0.013$), and the relative risk ratio for having a first exacerbation in the formoterol group compared to the terbutaline group was 0.55 (95% confidence interval [CI] 0.34–0.89). However, the relative risk ratio for having an exacerbation defined by a need for oral corticosteroids was not significantly different 0.61 (0.35–1.06). Formoterol was also associated with improvements in PEFR, pre-bronchodilator FEV_1 and a reduction in rescue inhaler requirement compared to terbutaline. Both treatments were well tolerated and no safety issues were identified (Figs 8.1 and 8.2).

Comment

Both formoterol and salmeterol have become established in the management of asthma that is not adequately controlled by inhaled corticosteroids. Both drugs are highly potent and selective β-2 receptor agonists and act over at least 12 hours. When used regularly, and in combination with inhaled corticosteroids, they reduce symptoms, reduce exacerbations, and improve quality of life. Thus, current guide-lines recommend that they be administered as regular therapy. Whereas salmeterol has a relatively slow-onset of action, formoterol is believed to enter the plasmalemma and interacts immediately with the β-2 receptor, thus the onset of action is similar to short-acting β-2 agonists which suggests it may also be used on demand as a rescue medication. In this study, Tattersfield *et al.* demonstrate that formoterol may be used safely as an alternative to terbutaline and that it is associated with improved asthma control. The authors recognize that in comparing these two drugs at these doses, that they cannot be certain they have compared like-with-like (relative dose equivalence), but speculate that they have probably compared formoterol at lower equivalent dose to terbutaline.

Given that the authors selected a group of patients with demonstrable reversibil-ity, it might be anticipated that a long acting bronchodilator would reduce the

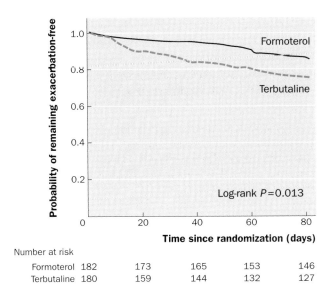

Fig. 8.1 Kaplan–Meier plot showing estimated probability of remaining without a severe asthma exacerbation. Source: Tattersfield *et al.* (2001).

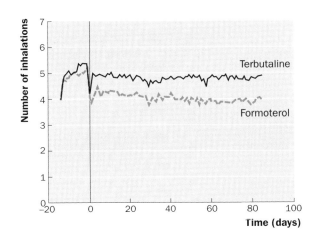

Fig. 8.2 Mean number of inhalations of relief medication in patients. 0 = day of randomization. Source: Tattersfield *et al.* (2001).

number of exacerbations defined on PEFR criteria (28% of exacerbations in ter-butaline group defined on PEFR criteria compared with 19% in the formoterol group). It is not clear whether these results can be extrapolated to other asthmatics with less reversibility. The authors suggest that the lack of significance reported with exacerbations defined by requirement for oral corticosteroids reflected the small numbers in this arm of the trial. This paper confirms that formoterol may be used as required instead of a shorter acting agent but this should not divert the emphasis on asthma management away from the importance of using optimal doses of ICS.

Corticosteroids

Significant variability in response to inhaled corticosteroids for persistent asthma.
Szefler SJ, Martin RJ, Sharp King T, *et al.*, for the Asthma Clinical Research Network of the National Heart, Lung and Blood Institute. *J Allergy Clin Immunol* 2002; **109**: 410–18.

BACKGROUND. This investigation was designed as a feasibility study (rather than a comparative trial), to establish a clinical model in which it would be possible to compare the relative beneficial and systemic effects in a dose–response relationship for two ICSs: beclomethasone dipropionate (BDP) and fluticasone propionate (FP), administered via a pressurized metered dose inhaler (MDI) with the OptiChamber spacer. The doses were chosen to achieve <5%, 20–30%, and 40–60% adrenal suppression.

INTERPRETATION. Responsiveness to ICS treatment varied markedly among subjects but the maximum FEV_1 response and the near-maximum methacholine PC_{20} improvement were observed with low dose FP–MDI and medium dose BDP–MDI produced the maximum. Higher doses were not associated with further efficacy but it was possible to demonstrated a greater systemic effect including dose-dependent cortisol suppression.

Dose–response relation of inhaled fluticasone propionate in adolescents and adults with asthma: meta-analysis.
Holt S, Suder A, Weatherall M, Cheng S, Shirtcliffe P, Beasley R. *Br Med J* 2001; **323**: 1–8.

BACKGROUND. The authors performed a meta-analysis of double-blind, randomized, placebo-controlled trails of adolescents (≥12 years of age) or adults with asthma reporting measures of clinical efficacy from fluticasone to determine the dose–response relation of inhaled FP in adolescents and adults with asthma.

INTERPRETATION. Eight studies fulfilled inclusion criteria and included a total of 2324 adolescents and adults with asthma (mostly moderate to severe) The majority of the therapeutic benefit from inhaled fluticasone is achieved with a total daily dose of 100–250 µg/day, and the maximum effect is achieved at a dose of 500 µg/day.

Comment

Inhaled corticosteroids are the most effective anti-inflammatory drugs in the treatment of asthma and are recommended for most adults with symptomatic chronic asthma. They rapidly improve symptoms, airway inflammation, reduce the frequency and severity of exacerbations, attenuate AHR and improve quality of life |11,12|. More recently they have been shown to reduce hospitalizations (including admissions to intensive care) and protect against asthma death |13–15|. The optimal dose of ICSs has been difficult to study but for beclometasone and budesonide, maximum efficacy has been suggested with doses of 400–800 µg/day |16,17|.

In line with other published studies, the data provided by Szefler *et al.* demonstrate that measures of pulmonary function improve rapidly on low doses of ICS |18–20|. Increasing the dose failed to deliver any greater efficacy but resulted in greater systemic effects. The results for FP are consistent with the meta-analysis by Holt *et al.* which suggests that, when delivered by MDI or Diskhaler the beneficial effects as regards lung function, nocturnal awakenings, β-agonist use, and major exacerbations, begins to plateau at 100–200 µg/day and the maximum achievable benefit occurs by a dose of around 500 µg/day. The authors, therefore, suggest that guidelines be modified to suggest that the recommended dosage of fluticasone for chronic asthma should be 200–500 µg/day, increasing to >500 µg/day in oral corticosteroid dependent patients.

The study by Szefler *et al.* demonstrates that considerable variability exists between individual patients. Good (>15%) FEV_1 response, in contrast to poor (<5%) response was found to be associated with high exhaled NO, high bronchodilator reversibility, and a low FEV_1/FVC ratio before treatment. Excellent compared to poor improvement in methacholine PC_{20}, was associated with high sputum eosinophil levels and older age of onset of asthma. This was also consistent with data from a further study by the Asthma Clinical Research Network where a poor FEV_1 response was observed in approximately 40% of a study population testing six ICS delivery devices and is consistent with the meta-analysis of Holt in which wide confidence intervals are seen with regard to the data using higher doses of FP |21|. Although some predictive features emerged from Szefler's study, larger studies will be required to define the characteristics of the most steroid-responsive patients. Furthermore, there may be clinical circumstances in which higher doses may be appropriate: management of exacerbations, weaning from oral corticosteroids, and the management of the relatively steroid resistant patient.

Corticosteroid safety issues

Symptomatic adrenal insufficiency presenting with hypoglycaemia in asthmatic children receiving high dose inhaled fluticasone propionate.

Drake AJ, Howells RJ, Shield JPH, Prendiville A, Ward PS, Crowne EC.
Br Med J 2002; **324**: 1081–2.

BACKGROUND. **The maximum licensed dose for children is 200 μg daily. The use of higher doses has been associated with growth retardation and adrenal suppression in children. However hypoglycaemia has not been a feature of previous reports.**

INTERPRETATION. In this paper, the authors report four cases of children with asthma presenting with acute hypoglycaemia secondary to adrenal suppression caused by inhaled fluticasone propionate. In all of the cases, a thorough investigation failed to identify any other underlying cause and all cases were managed with oral hydrocortisone and reducing the dose of ICS. The authors recommended that long acting β-2 agonists or leukotriene receptor antagonists should be considered in children whose asthma is not controlled on 200 μg fluticasone daily, and that the hypothalamic-pituitary-adrenal axis should be assessed in all children taking high dose inhaled steroids (greater than 400 μg daily) long-term. These children should also carry a steroid card.

Effect of inhaled glucocorticoids on bone density in pre-menopausal women.

Israel E, Banerjee TR, Fitzmaurice GM, Kotlov TV, LaHive K, LeBoff MS.
N Eng J Med 2001; **345**: 941–7.

BACKGROUND. **In this study, the authors performed a prospective cohort study over 3 years to investigate the relationship between the dose of ICS and the rate of bone loss in pre-menopausal women with asthma. They also wished to determine if serum or urinary markers of bone turnover could provide a surrogate measure for the assessment of bone mineral density measured by dual-photon absorptiometry. ICS were standardized by switching all patients to triamcinalone acetonide (100 μg/puff) and women were categorized as those taking no ICS ($n = 28$), those taking between 4–8 puffs/day ($n = 39$) and those taking >8 puffs/day ($n = 42$).**

INTERPRETATION. It was possible to demonstrate a negative linear association between the average number of puffs per day of ICS and the yearly change in bone density at both the total hip and the trochanter with each additional puff of ICS being associated with a decline in bone density of 0.00044 g per square centimetre ($P = 0.01$ and $P = 0.005$ respectively). No dose-related effect was noted at the femoral neck or spine. The association persisted after exclusion of all women who received oral or parenteral glucocorticoids at any time during the study. Biochemical and urinary markers of bone turnover do not provide a surrogate marker for the measurement of BMD (Table 8.1).

Comment

Since their introduction in the early 1960s, doses of ICS prescribed to patients with asthma have progressively increased. British Thoracic Society (BTS) guidelines for steps 3–5 recommend that patients with chronic asthma should take beclometha-sone or budesonide in doses of 800–2000 µg/day through a large volume spacer. Because of its greater potency, fluticasone propionate is recommended in doses of 400–1000 µg/day |22|. The maximum licensed dose of fluticasone for children is 200 µg/day, but a series of reports is raising concern that many children are prescribed higher doses and that this is associated with adrenal suppression and growth retardation |23|. The series of reports by Drake *et al.* alerts clinicians that the use of high dose fluticasone can lead to adrenal insufficiency presenting as hypo-glycaemia. They recommend that the hypothalamic-pituitary-adrenal axis should be assessed in all children taking long-term high-dose ICSs and suggest these children should carry a steroid card. In assessing this paper, it should be remem-bered that these children had been prescribed doses of fluticasone in excess of the licensed dose and that inhaled corticosteroids administered in appropriate doses remain the most safe and effective for the majority of patients |24,25|.

One of the greatest concerns regarding long-term treatment with ICSs is their effect on bone. In health, bone is in a constant state of turnover with up to 10% of the skeleton being replaced each year. Osteoporosis (a progressive skeletal disease characterized by low bone mass and micro-architectural deterioration of bone tissue) leads to increased bone fragility and predisposes to low trauma fractures. Bone mass is assessed by measurement of bone mineral density (BMD) and osteo-porosis is defined as a BMD that is 2.5 SD below the mean peak value in young adults.

Bone mass is determined by a complex interplay of factors including peak bone mass achieved, age, sex, ethnic background, body habitus, diet, physical activity, use of alcohol, smoking, thyroid hormone and sex hormone status, use of medi-cations including oral corticosteroids. These act as confounding factors when investigating the possible relationship between abnormal bone loss and inhaled corticosteroids, contributing to the difficulties involved in designing and interpret-ing these studies. Corticosteroids affect bone formation and resorption at a number of direct and indirect interactions with bone metabolism. Oral glucocorticoids are known to decrease bone mineral density and have their greatest effect at skeletal sites with a higher proportion of trabecular rather than cortical bone. The study by Israel *et al.* highlights concern that ICS are associated with a measurable dose-related loss of bone at the hip in pre-menopausal women with asthma. There was considerable inter-patient scatter, so it is likely that not all patients are equally susceptible to the bone mineral loss.

Table 8.1 Mean yearly change in bone density associated with inhaled glucocorticoid therapy*

Site	All women (n = 109)				Women who received no oral or parenteral glucocorticoid therapy (n = 83)			
	Unadjusted yearly change (g/cm²/puff)	P value	Adjusted yearly change (g/cm²/puff)†	P value	Unadjusted yearly change (g/cm²/puff)	P value	Adjusted yearly change (g/cm²/puff)‡	P value
Total hip	−0.00044 ± 0.00017	0.01	−0.00048 ± 0.00018	0.008	−0.00041 ± 0.00019	0.03	−0.00041 ± 0.00020	0.047
Trochanter	−0.00044 ± 0.00016	0.005	−0.00042 ± 0.00017	0.01	−0.00048 ± 0.00019	0.01	−0.00047 ± 0.00019	0.02
Femoral neck	−0.00005 ± 0.00028	0.85	−0.00017 ± 0.00028	0.54	0.00015 ± 0.00030	0.61	0.00015 ± 0.00031	0.63
Spine (L1–L4)	−0.00008 ± 0.00019	0.68	0.00012 ± 0.00018	0.51	0.00001 ± 0.00020	0.95	0.00015 ± 0.00019	0.41

* Plus–minus values are means ± SE. P values are for the test of whether the change in bone density differs from zero.
† The results have been adjusted for age, the use of inhaled and oral glucocorticoids, and the use of oral contraceptives.
‡ The results have been adjusted for age, the use of inhaled glucocorticoids, and the use of oral contraceptives.

Source: Israel et al. (2001).

The strengths of the study were that it was large, prospective in design and verification of dose was achieved. Nevertheless, it is unclear why cortical bone was affected rather than trabecular bone as would be expected from studies using oral corticosteroids. This has led some to question whether the demineralizing effect in cortical bone is associated with asthma *per se* rather than its treatment |**26**|. As such the greatest bone loss in those taking the largest doses of ICS would reflect the fact that these patients had the greatest disease activity. The authors did not measure levels of oestrogen, which may have been confounding. The women in the high-dose group were slightly older and a higher percentage of women who were using ICS had used oral glucocorticoids in the past but this is unlikely to be important.

Long acting β-2 agonists and inhaled corticosteroids

Long-acting β-2 agonist monotherapy vs continued therapy with inhaled corticosteroids in patients with severe asthma: a randomized controlled trial.

Lazarus SC, Boushey HA, Fahy JV, *et al.*; Asthma Clinical Research Network for the National Heart, Lung, and Blood Institute. *JAMA* 2001; **285**: 2583–93.

B A C K G R O U N D . The aim of this study was to determine whether asthma control would be maintained if salmeterol xinafoate was substituted for triamcinolone acetonide in patients with persistent asthma who had achieved good control with the combination of ICS and long acting β-2 agonists (LABA).

I N T E R P R E T A T I O N . Patients who stepped down therapy to salmeterol alone experienced more exacerbations, a greater increase in sputum eosinophils, and a worsening of AHR. Patients with persistent asthma that is well controlled by low dose triamcinolone cannot be switched to salmeterol monotherapy without the risk of clinically significant loss of asthma control (Fig. 8.3a,b).

Inhaled corticosteroid reduction and elimination in patients with persistent asthma receiving salmeterol.

Lemanske RF, Sorkness CA, Mauger EA, *et al.*, for the Asthma Clinical Research Network for the National Heart, Lung, and Blood Institute. *JAMA* 2001; **285**: 2594–603.

B A C K G R O U N D . Lemanske *et al.* performed a randomized, controlled, double-dummy, parallel-group study to determine whether ICS therapy can be reduced or eliminated in patients with persistent asthma following the addition of a LABA to their treatment.

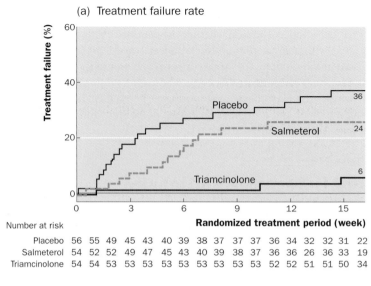

(a) Treatment failure rate

Number at risk

Placebo	56	55	49	45	43	40	39	38	37	37	37	36	34	32	32	31	22
Salmeterol	54	52	52	49	47	45	43	40	39	38	37	36	36	26	36	33	19
Triamcinolone	54	54	53	53	53	53	53	53	53	53	53	52	52	51	51	50	34

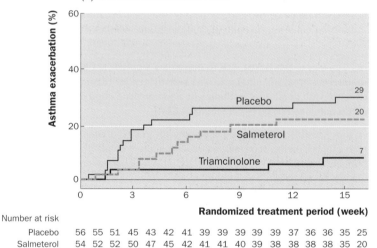

(b) Asthma exacerbation rate

Number at risk

Placebo	56	55	51	45	43	42	41	39	39	39	39	39	37	36	36	35	25
Salmeterol	54	52	52	50	47	45	42	41	41	40	39	38	38	38	38	35	20
Triamcinolone	54	54	52	52	52	52	52	52	52	52	52	51	51	50	49	48	33

Fig. 8.3 Kaplan–Meier survival curves for treatment failure and asthma exacerbation during the randomized treatment period. (a) For placebo vs triamcinolone, $P = 0.001$; for salmeterol vs triamcinolone, $P = 0.004$; and for placebo vs salmeterol, $P = 0.18$. (b) For placebo vs triamcinolone, $P = 0.003$; for salmeterol vs triamcinolone, $P = 0.04$; and for placebo vs salmeterol, $P = 0.29$. Statistical comparisons are based on the log-rank test. Source: Lazarus et al. (2001).

INTERPRETATION. For the majority of patients in whom the control of asthma improves following the addition of salmeterol, it is possible to make a reduction in ICS dosages by as much as 50%. However, total elimination of ICS results in significant deterioration in asthma control.

Low dose inhaled budesonide and formoterol in mild persistent asthma.

O'Byrne PM, Barnes PJ, Rodriguez-Roisin R, *et al. Am J Respir Crit Care Med* 2001; **164**: 1392–7.

BACKGROUND. **The aim of this study was to determine whether regular treatment with low doses of inhaled budesonide, with or without low doses of inhaled formoterol, would reduce severe asthma exacerbations and improve control in patients with mild asthma. Two groups of patients were included: Group A consisted of 698 patients with mild asthma who had not used corticosteroids for ≥3 months, Group B consisted of 1272 mild asthmatics taking ≤400 µg/day of inhaled budesonide, or its equivalent, for ≥3 months.**

INTERPRETATION. Patients with mild asthma who are not taking inhaled corticosteroids (Group A) will experience fewer exacerbations and less poorly controlled days when managed with regular inhaled budesonide. The addition of formoterol to this group improves lung function but provides no further clinical benefit. In patients with mild asthma who are already taking an ICS (Group B), the addition of regular formoterol was better than doubling the dose of ICS for all outcome variables (Figs 8.4 and 8.5).

Comment

The clinical effectiveness of the addition of LABA to inhaled corticosteroids has been established by numerous clinical studies and some new data suggests that this may be attributed to important interactions between β-2 agonists and cortico-steroids that promote the efficacy of each drug |**27–30**|. The beneficial effects of LABA and the suggestion that these agents may have some anti-inflammatory therapy have led some to speculate that they may be used as monotherapy in place of maintenance ICS. Concern that such was occurring in clinical practice led Lazarus *et al.* to undertake a study investigating whether asthma control would be maintained if salmeterol was substituted for triamcinalone. Although the salmeterol group had fewer symptoms, less need for rescue medication and better airway function than patients who received placebo, they experienced treatment failures and asthma exacerbations at a rate similar to the placebo group. Thus, ICS remains preferable to LABA monotherapy in patients with persistent asthma. However, the study by Lemanskc *et al.* demonstrates that LABA may safely facilitate a dose-reduction in ICS by as much as 50% in patients with persistent asthma. Long-term studies would be required to demonstrate that these patients remain protected

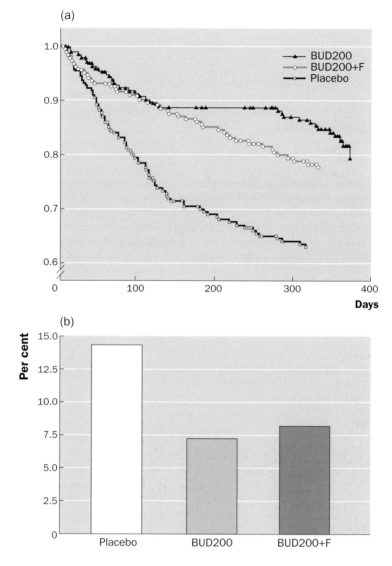

Fig. 8.4 (a) Kaplan–Meier survival curve for the time to the first severe asthma exacerbation. (b) Proportion (%) of poorly controlled asthma days in Group A (corticosteroid-free patients). BUD 200 = budesonide 100 μg twice daily; F = formoterol 4.5 μg twice daily. Source: O'Byrne *et al.* (2001).

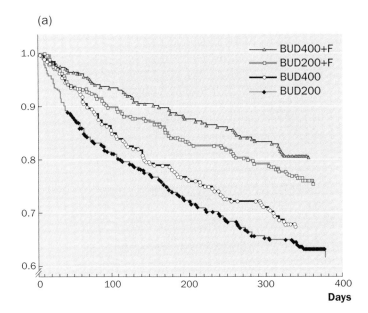

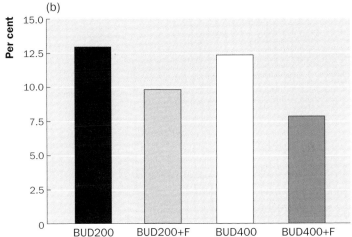

Fig. 8.5 (a) Kaplan–Meier survival curve for the time to the first severe asthma exacerbation. (b) Proportion (%) of poorly controlled asthma days in Group B (corticosteroid-treated patients). BUD 200 and 400 = budesonide 100 μg and 200 μg twice daily; F = formoterol 4.5 μg twice daily. Source: O'Byrne *et al.* (2001).

against clinically significant exacerbations and studies on the impact on airway inflammation would be useful to bolster this observation.

The study by O'Byrne *et al.* aims to extend the observation that the addition of LABA to ICS improves asthma control in patients with moderate–severe asthma, to a group of mild asthmatics. Patients in Group A provide further evidence that ICS improves outcome measures for patients and this should be used in the management of mild asthma. The addition of formoterol provided no further advantage for this group. However, for patients with mild asthma who remain symptomatic despite a low dose of ICS, the addition of LABA does appear to provide further clinical benefit with regard to several important outcome measures.

Leukotriene receptor antagonists

Improvement of aspirin-intolerant asthma by montelukast, a leukotriene receptor antagonist.

Dahlén SE, Malmström K, Nizankowska E, *et al. Am J Respir Crit Care Med* 2002; **165**: 9–14.

B A C K G R O U N D . The aim of this study was to determine if montelukast provided additional benefit to patients with moderate to severe aspirin-intolerant asthma currently requiring moderate to high doses of inhaled corticosteroids.

I N T E R P R E T A T I O N . In patients with aspirin-intolerant asthmatics already requiring moderate to high doses of inhaled corticosteroids, montelukast provides additional improvements in lung function, requirement for rescue medication, improved sleep quality and asthma-specific quality of life score and fewer exacerbations.

Addition of leukotriene antagonists to therapy in chronic persistent asthma: a randomized double-blind placebo-controlled trial.

Robinson DS, Campbell D, Barnes PJ. *Lancet* 2001; **357**: 2007–11.

B A C K G R O U N D . In an attempt to mimic 'real-world' prescribing, Robinson *et al.* explored whether the leukotriene receptor antagonists had further potential as add-on treatment for patients attending chest clinics with difficult to treat chronic asthma.

I N T E R P R E T A T I O N . Compared with placebo the addition of montelukast did not result in any significant change in symptom scores, rescue inhaled β-2 agonist use, twice-daily PEFR or PEFR variability. There was no evidence for response in a subgroup of patients (including aspirin-intolerant asthmatics). The authors concluded that montelukast did not provide additional benefit in patients recruited from their hospital clinic.

Anti-leukotrienes as add-on therapy to inhaled glucocorticoids in patients with asthma: systematic review of current evidence.

Ducharme FM. *Br Med J* 2002; **324**: 1545–8.

BACKGROUND. To evaluate the safety and efficacy of anti-leukotrienes as add-on therapy to inhaled corticosteroids in children and adults with asthma, the author performed a systematic review of randomized controlled trials of children and adults with asthma comparing the addition of anti-leukotrienes or placebo to ICS for a minimum of 28 days.

INTERPRETATION. The addition of antileukotrienes to ICS may modestly improve asthma control but is not as effective as increasing the dose of ICS. A significant reduction in exacerbations was only observed when higher than licensed doses had been used (RR [relative risk] 0.34, 95% CI 0.13–0.88) NNT = 20. The use of anti-leukotrienes was possibly associated with superior asthma control after tapering of glucocorticoids, but it was not possible to quantify the glucocorticoid sparing effect.

Comment

Leukotriene receptor antagonists represent the first new treatment to be developed for asthma for many years. Their development was based on *in vitro* and *in vivo* observations of the role of the cysteinyl leukotrienes in the pathogenesis of asthma. The cysteinyl receptor antagonists, montelukast and zafirlukast (selective $CysLT_1$ antagonists), are the most widely used. These drugs produce a bronchodilator effect additional to that produced by β-2 agonists and in controlled trials have demonstrated benefit in exercise-induced asthma, produced modest improvements in asthma symptoms scores and lung function, and facilitated a reduction of corticosteroid dosage in patients taking oral and high-dose ICSs. They are also known to reduce sputum eosinophilia [31].

From first principles it would seem that they should be particularly effective in patients with aspirin-sensitive asthma. These patients are known to have increased production of cysteinyl-leukotrienes and they are more sensitive to inhalation of leukotrienes than other patients with asthma. Dahlén *et al.* identified 80 aspirin-intolerant asthmatic patients on the basis of history and challenge tests and performed a randomized double-blind trial comparing 4 weeks treatment with montelukast 10 mg/day or placebo and demonstrated that in patients with aspirin-sensitive asthma, the addition of montelukast can provide a small additional benefit to regular ICS. Although no obvious cohort of responders and non-responders emerged, patients and their clinicians should notice benefit within 1 day of commencing therapy. The study was not powered to examine sputum eosinophil counts but a trend toward reduction was observed.

In routine clinical practice clinicians often extrapolate findings from randomized controlled trials with careful inclusion and exclusion criteria to a broader range of patients, many of whom would never have fulfilled the entry criteria for the study. Robinson *et al.* decided to take a pragmatic approach to studying the effects of leukotriene receptor antagonists. However, their broad entry criteria resulted in the recruitment of heterogeneous population including patients with modest reversibility, irreversible airflow obstruction, current smokers (and smokers of more than 10 pack years). Some of these patients might have had chronic obstructive pulmonary disease or hyperventilation syndrome, and no data was provided on compliance with current therapy. Therefore, although their study was disappointing, it may be argued that searching for a bronchodilator response of ≥15% in this patient group was unrealistic.

Ducharme performed a meta-analysis of randomized controlled trials comparing the addition of leukotriene receptor antagonists to placebo or ICS. The concept being that aggregating data from several smaller studies into one larger study may answer questions yet to be addressed by properly powered randomized controlled trials. The quality of trials entered was checked against recognized criteria but the studies were small in number and short in duration, so caution should be exercised with interpretation. We cannot check how the end-points were classified in individual trials and no data is available on airway AHR or inflammatory markers. Again, it will be better to wait for larger, appropriately designed clinical trails that will soon become available.

Monoclonal anti-immunoglobulin E antibody (anti-IgE)

Omalizumab, anti-IgE recombinant humanized antibody, for the treatment of severe allergic asthma.
Busse W, Corren J, Lanier BQ, *et al.* J Allergy Clin Immunol 2001; **108**: 184–90.

BACKGROUND. This was a phase III, double-blind, placebo-controlled clinical trial recruiting 525 patients with severe allergic asthma to evaluate the efficacy and tolerability of omalizumab in the treatment of inhaled corticosteroid-dependent asthma. Following a run-in period of good control on BDP, patients commenced a 16-week study period in which the dose of BDP was kept constant (steroid stable phase). This was followed by a second 12-week period, when the dose of BDP was reduced by approximately 25% of the baseline dose every 2 weeks for 8 weeks until BDP was stopped or worsening of asthma symptoms occurred.

INTERPRETATION. Compared with placebo, omalizumab significantly reduced the number of exacerbations per patient and reduced the percentage of patients experiencing an exacerbation during the steroid stable phase and during the steroid reduction phase. Omalizumab facilitated a greater reduction in BDP and discontinuation of BDP was more likely. Improvements in pulmonary function and symptoms occurred in association with a reduction of rescue β-agonist use. Omalizumab was well tolerated with an adverse events profile similar to placebo.

The anti-IgE antibody omalizumab reduces exacerbations and steroid requirement in allergic asthmatics.
Soler M, Matz J, Townley R, *et al. Eur Respir J* 2001; **18**: 254–61.

BACKGROUND. **This multi-centre, randomized, double-blind, placebo-controlled, parallel-group study administered subcutaneous omalizumab to 546 allergic asthmatic subjects who were symptomatic on entry despite treatment with ICSs in doses equivalent to 500–1200 µg/day of beclomethasone dipropionate. As above, the study was divided into a steroid stable phase (16 weeks) and a steroid reduction phase (12 weeks).**

INTERPRETATION. Patients taking omalizumab experienced fewer exacerbations per patient during both the steroid stable and steroid reduction phase of the study (Table 8.2). The proportion of patients who were able to reduce the BDP dose were significantly greater in the omazilumab group than the placebo group and a ≥50% reduction was achieved in 79% of patients taking omalizumab compared with 55% on placebo (Fig.

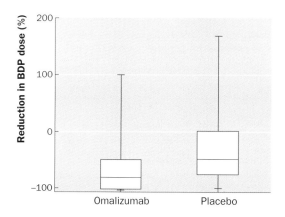

Fig. 8.6 Box and whisker plot showing medians with interquartile range and minimum and maximal values for the per cent reduction in the prescribed dose of inhaled beclomethasone dipropionate (BDP) at the end of the steroid-reduction phase (week 28) compared to the stable-steroid phase. Intent-to-treat population. *P* <0.001.
Source: Soler *et al.* (2001).

Table 8.2 Asthma exacerbations during the stable-steroid and steroid-reduction phases in the intent-to-treat population

	Stable-steroid phase		Steroid-reduction phase	
	Omalizumab	Placebo	Omalizumab	Placebo
Asthma exacerbations per patient	0.28 (0.15−0.41)	0.66 (0.49−0.83)	0.36 (0.24−0.48)	0.75 (0.58−0.92)
Patients with ⩾1 asthma exacerbations	35 (12.8)	83 (30.5)	43 (15.7)	81 (29.8)

Data were analysed by the generalized Cochran–Mantel–Haenszel test (van Elteren test), and presented as mean (95% confidence interval) or n (%) P <0.001.

Source: Soler *et al.* (2001).

8.6). Improvements with respect to placebo were also observed in symptoms scores, use of rescue medication and lung function. Omalizumab was well tolerated and the incidence of adverse events was similar in both groups.

Omalizumab provides long-term control in patients with moderate-to-severe asthma.
Buhl R, Soler M, Matz J, *et al. Eur Respir J* 2002; **20**: 73–8.

B ACKGROUND . This 24-week extension of the above study was designed to investigate the ability of omalizumab to maintain longer-term disease control.

I NTERPRETATION . Omalizumab continued to reduce asthma exacerbations over a longer duration even in the presence of a dose-reduction in ICS. A slightly higher incidence of gastrointestinal adverse events was reported in the omalizumab group, but otherwise the treatment was well tolerated.

Comment

The formation of circulating IgE antibodies to allergens appears to be crucial to the expression of the asthmatic phenotype |**32**|. Indeed, the risk of asthma is not increased in response to house dust mite or cat exposure in the absence of sensitization and the development of IgE antibodies |**33**|. The importance of IgE antibodies is consistent with our current understanding of the immunological model of asthma with activation of Th2 lymphocytes leading to the production of inflammatory cytokines that promote the manufacture of IgE antibodies by B lymphocytes. The recruitment of inflammatory cells such as the mast cells and basophils, which express high affinity receptors for IgE, provides an environment in which allergen exposure leads to activation and release of key inflammatory mediators including histamine, prostaglandins, and leukotrienes. These, and other mediators, orchestrate the early- and late-asthmatic response. Thus, targeting IgE binding should provide an opportunity to intervene in the pathophysiological processes involved in the asthmatic response, regardless of the precipitant.

Omalizumab is a highly specific monoclonal antibody that binds to circulating IgE and prevents receptor binding on effector cells. It is non-analphylactogenic. To date, omalizumab has been shown to reduce dermal wheal and flare reactions, effectively attenuate allergen-induced early and late asthmatic responses, reduce sputum eosinophilia and increase the dose of allergen required to provoke an early response to allergen challenge |34–37|. These studies provide further evidence for the potential of omalizumab to ameliorate IgE mediated reactions regardless of the allergen involved. The treatment appears to be safe, well tolerated and effective at reducing serum total IgE. These studies are also important as they demonstrate that omalizumab can reduce asthma exacerbations. This effect is not lost over an extended period and continues even in the presence of a dose reduction of corticosteroids. Furthermore, other parameters of disease control were improved even with minimal bronchodilator effects indicating that the effects of omalizumab are probably largely anti-inflammatory. Thus, omalizumab is likely to provide a further alternative for asthmatic patients who remain poorly controlled despite appropriate doses of ICSs.

Management plans and education

A qualitative study of action plans for asthma.
Douglass J, Aroni R, Goeman D, Stewart K, Sawyer S, Thien F. *Br Med J* 2002; **324**: 1003–5.

BACKGROUND. The aim of this study was to investigate the patients' perspective on action plans and the implementation of these plans during an asthma attack necessitating an emergency hospital visit.

INTERPRETATION. Over half of the patients did not have an action plan, most commonly because their own doctor had not given them one. However, many patients had developed their own plan, and many of these were medically credible. Most patients who had been given a plan viewed them positively but modified them according to their own experience. Action plans may be improved if doctors take the experience of the patient into account when developing a personal plan.

Evaluation of two different educational interventions for adult patients consulting with acute asthma exacerbation.
Côté J, Bowie DM, Robichaud P, Parent JG, Battisti L, Boulet LP.
Am J Respir Crit Care Med 2001; **163**: 1415–19.

BACKGROUND. The aim of this study was to compare the impact of a comprehensive structured educational (SE) programme on urgent visits for asthma and other clinical parameters, to a more limited programme that included teaching of inhaler technique and prescription of a written self action plan.

INTERPRETATION. The only group to demonstrate a significant improvement in knowledge, willingness to adjust medications, quality of life scores and peak expiratory flows was the SE group. The single prescription of a written self-action plan did not appear to diminish asthma morbidity.

Cost-effectiveness of self-management in asthmatics: a one-year follow-up randomized, controlled trial.
Gallefoss F, Bakke PS. *Eur Respir J* 2001; **17**: 206–13.

BACKGROUND. The aim of this study was to perform a cost-effectiveness analysis of a nurse- and physiotherapist-led patient education in primary care compared to usual care provided by the family physician.

INTERPRETATION. Patient education was associated with improved lung function and quality of life. Direct costs were greater in the educated group but total costs were less, due to lower indirect costs associated with reduced absenteeism from work. In conclusion, education of asthmatic patients is cost-effective and should be part of standard care.

Randomized controlled economic evaluation of asthma self-management in primary health care.
Schermer TR, Thoonen BP, van den Boom G, *et al. Am J Respir Crit Care Med* 2002; **166**: 1062–72.

BACKGROUND. The aim of this study was to perform an economic valuation of a family practice based, comprehensive, physician delivered, self-management programme compared to usual care.

INTERPRETATION. Although the cost-effectiveness of self-management could not be firmly established, it was possible to conclude that guided self-management was safe and efficient compared with asthma treatment usually provided in Dutch primary care.

Comment

The variable nature of the clinical course of asthma suggests that educating patients to enact treatment alterations in response to changes in disease severity should improve clinical outcomes. Thus, guideline statements endorse self-management programmes. Although a number of different programmes have been proposed, the optimum requirements for a self-management plan have not been established.

The study by Douglas *et al.* demonstrates that a significant number of asthmatic patients do not receive a plan from their physician, and some of those that do, do not use them. Those that did receive a plan often modified it according to their own perceptions of asthma. Thus, we need to know more about which type of plans to develop and how best to deliver them to patients. For example, Côté *et al.* suggests that the single prescription of an action plan does not diminish asthma morbidity, probably because patients have not gained enough self-confidence to alter the dose of their medications. They also demonstrated that only one third of patients were willing to monitor their peak flow for more than 1 month, thus plans based on peak flow might be flawed. This is likely to suggest that some form of more intensive educational programme will be necessary to give patients the confidence to alter their own treatment. However, such programmes are likely to be both time-consuming and costly. The latter two studies provide some information on these dilemmas.

Gallefoss *et al.* demonstrated cost-efficiency of a hospital based but nurse- and physiotherapist-led education programme. Schermer employed a more labour intensive, physician-led programme in primary care that was not cost-effective, but demonstrated clinical improvements over usual care. Both studies selected mild asthmatics and hospital admissions were not reported, so recruitment of a more severe population may have allowed the demonstration of clearer benefits. Gallefoss *et al.* demonstrated that a significant few patients account for a substantial proportion of the costs and more intensive regimens may become more cost-effective if they target these patients. Both studies raise the question, as to which part of the programme is most important, and more work needs to concentrate on this. This may also assist in clarifying which members of staff are needed to deliver an effective programme. The costs in Schermer's study could have been reduced had physician-time not been required to deliver the programme. By contrast, the Dutch investigators employed nurses and physiotherapy staff.

References

1. Sporik R, Holgate ST, Platts-Mills TAE, Coswell JJ. Exposure to house-dust mite allergen (*Der p 1*) and the development of asthma in childhood. *N Engl J Med* 1990; **323**: 502–7.

2. Custovic A, Taggart S, Francis H, *et al.* Exposure to house dust mite allergens and the clinical activity of asthma. *J Allergy Clin Immunol* 1996; **98**: 64–72.

3. Tunnicliffe WS, Fletcher TJ, Hammond K, Roberts K, Custovic A, Simpson A, Woodcock A, Ayres JG. Sensitivity and exposure to indoor allergens in adults with differing asthma severity. *Eur Respir J* 1999; **13**: 645–9.

4. Platts-Mills TA, Tovey ER, Mitchell EB, Moszoro H, Nock P, Wilkins SR. Reduction of bronchial hyperreactivity during prolonged allergen avoidance. *Lancet* 1982; **2**: 675–8.

5. Ehnert B, Lau-Schadendorf S, Weber A, Buettner P, Schou C, Wahn U. Reducing domestic exposure to dust mite allergen reduces bronchial hyperreactivity in sensitive children with asthma. *J Allergy Clin Immunol* 1992; **90**: 135–8.

6. Peroni DG, Boner AL, Vallone G, Antolini I, Warner JO. Effective allergen avoidance at high altitude reduces allergen-induced bronchial hyperresponsiveness. *Am J Respir Crit Care* 1994; **149**: 1442–6.

7. Gøtzsche PC, Johansen HK, Burr ML, Hammarquist C. House dust mite control measures for asthma (Cochrane Review). In The Cochrane Library, Issue 4 2002. Oxford: Update software.

8. Henrikson JM, Agertoft L, Pederson S. Protective effect and duration of action of inhaled formoterol and salbutamol in exercise-induced asthma in children. *J Allergy Clin Immunol* 1992; **89**: 1176–82.

9. Dennis S, Sharp SJ, Vickers MR, Frost CD, Crompton GK, Barnes PJ, Lee TH. Regular inhaled salbutamol and asthma control: the TRUST randomized trial. Therapy Working Group of the National Asthma task Force and the MRC General Practice Research Framework. *Lancet* 2000; **3555**: 1675.

10. Inman MD, O'Byrne PM. The effect of regular inhaled albuterol on exercise-induced bronchoconstriction. *Am J Respir Crit Care Med* 1996; **153**: 65–9.

11. Djukanovic R, Wilson JW, Britten KM, Wilson SJ, Walls AF, Roche WR *et al*. Effect of an inhaled corticosteroid on airway inflammation and symptoms in asthma. *Am Rev Respir Dis* 1992; **145**: 669–74.

12. Haahtela T, Jarvinen M, Kava T, Kiviranta K, Koskinen S, Lethonen K, Nikander K, Persson T, Reinikainen K, Selroos O, Sovijärvi, Stenius-Aarniala B, Svahn T, Tammivaara R, Laitinen LA. Comparison of a beta 2-agonist, terbutaline, with an inhaled corticosteroid, budesonide, in newly detected asthma. *N Engl J Med* 1991; **325**: 388–92.

13. Donahue JG *et al.* Inhaled steroids and the risk of hospitalization for asthma. *JAMA* 1997; **277**: 887–91.

14. Eisner MD, Lieu TA, Chi F, Capra AM, Mendoza GR, Selby JV, Blanc PD. Beta agonists, inhaled corticosteroids, and the risk of intensive care unit admission for asthma. *Eur Respir J* 2002; **17**: 233–40.

15. Suissa S, Ernst P, Benayoun S, Baltzan M, Cal B. Low-dose inhaled corticosteroids and the prevention of death from asthma. *N Engl J Med* 2000; **343**: 332–6.

16. Busse WW, Chervinsky P, Condemi J, Lumry WR, Petty TL, Rennard S, Townley RG. Budesonide delivered by turbohaler is effective in a dose-dependent fashion when used in the treatment of adult patients with chronic asthma. *J Allergy Clin Immunol* 1998; **101**: 457–63. (NB: erratum *J Allergy Clin Immunol* 1998; **102**: 511.)

17. Busse WW, Brazinsky S, Jacobson K, Stricker W, Schmitt K, Vanden Burgt J *et al.* Efficacy of inhaled beclomethasone dipropionate in asthma is proportional to dose and

is improved by formulation with a new propellant. *J Allergy Clin Immunol* 1999; **104**: 1215–22.

18. Kelly HW. Establishing a therapeutic index for the inhaled corticosteroids: part 1. Pharmacokinetic/pharmacodynamic comparison of the inhaled corticosteroids. *J Allergy Clin Immunol* 1998; **102**: S36–S51.

19. Szefler SJ, Boushey HA, Pearlman DS, Togias A, Liddle R, Furlong A *et al.* Time to onset of effect of fluticasone propionate in patients with asthma. *J Allergy Clin Immunol* 1999; **103**: 780–8.

20. Kemp J, Wanderer AA, Ramsdell J, Southern DL, Weiss S, Aaronson D *et al.* Rapid onset of control with budesonide Turbohaler in patients with mild-to-moderate asthma. *Ann Allergy Asthma Immunol* 1999; **82**: 463–71.

21. Martin RJ, Szefler SJ, Chinchilli VM, Kraft M, Dolovich M, Boushey HA, Cherniack RM, Craig TJ, Drazen JM, Fagan JK, Fahy JV, Fish JE, Ford JG, Israel E, Kunselman SJ, Lazarus SC, Lemanske RF Jr, Peters SP, Sorkness CA for the National Heart Lung and Blood Institute's Asthma Clinical Research Network. Systemic effect comparisons of six inhaled corticosteroid preparations. *Am J Respir Crit Care Med* 2002; **165**: 1377–83.

22. British guidelines on asthma management. *Thorax* 1997; **52**(Suppl.): S1–S21.

23. Todd G, Dunlop K, McNaboe J, Ryan MF, Carson D, Shields MD. Growth and adrenal suppression in asthmatic children treated with high-dose fluticasone propionate. *Lancet* 1996; **348**: 27–9.

24. Pederson S, O'Byrne PA. A comparison of the efficacy and safety of inhaled cortico-steroids in asthma. *Allergy* 1997; **52**(Suppl. 39): 1–3.

25. Barnes PJ, Pederson S, Busse WW. Efficacy and safety of inhaled corticosteroids. New developments. *Am J Respir Crit Care Med* 1998; **157**(Suppl.): S1–53.

26. van Staa TP, Leufkens HGM, Cooper C. Use of inhaled corticosteroid and risk of fractures. *J Bone Miner Res* 2001; **16**: 581–8.

27. Greening AP, Ind PW, Northfield M, Shaw G, on behalf of Allen & Hanburys Limited UK Study Group. Added salmeterol versus higher-dose corticosteroid in asthma patients with symptoms on existing inhaled corticosteroid. *Lancet* 1994; **344**: 219–24.

28. Pauwels RA, Löfdahl C-G, Postma DS, Tattersfield AE, O'Byrne P, Barnes PJ, Ullman A. Effect of inhaled formoterol and budesonide in exacerbations of asthma. *N Engl J Med* 1997; **337**; 1405–11.

29. Shewsbury S, Pyke S, Britton M. Meta-analysis of increased dose of inhaled steroid or addition of salmeterol in symptomatic asthma (MIASMA). *Br Med J* 2000; **320**: 1368–73.

30. Barnes PJ. Scientific rationale for inhaled combination therapy with long-acting beta-2 agonists and corticosteroids. *Eur Respir J* 2002; **19**: 182–91.

31. Lipworth BJ. Leukotriene receptor antagonists. *Lancet* 1999; **353**: 57–62.

32. Burrows B, Martinez FD, Halonen M, Barbee RA, Cline MG. Association of asthma with serum IgE levels and skin-test reactivity to allergens. *N Engl J Med* 1989; **320**: 271–7.

33. Platts-Mills T, Vaughan J, Squillace S, Woodfolk J, Sporik R. Sensitization, asthma and a modified Th2 response in children exposed to cat allergen: a population-based cross-sectional study. *Lancet* 2001; **357**: 752–6.

34. Togias A, Corren J, Shapiro G, Reimann JD, von Schlegell A, Wighton TG, Alderman DC. Anti-IgE treatment reduces skin test reactivity. *J Allergy Clin Immunol* 1997; **99**: S102.

35. Fahy JV, Fleming HE, Wong HH, Liu JT, Su JO, Reimann J, Fick RB Jr, Boushey HA. The effect of an anti-IgE monoclonal antibody on the early- and late-phase responses to allergen inhalation in asthmatic subjects. *Am J Respir Crit Care Med* 1997; **155**: 1828–34.

36. Boulet LP, Chapman KR, Cote J, Kalra S, Bhagat R, Swystun VA, Laviolette M, Cleland LD, Deschesnes F, Su JQ, DeVault A, Fick RB Jr, Cockcroft DW. Inhibitory effects of anti-IgE antibody on allergen-induced early asthmatic response. *Am J Respir Crit Care Med* 1997; **155**: 1835–40.

37. Milgrom H, Fick RB, Su JQ, Reimann JD, Bush RK, Watrous WJ, for the rhuMAb-E25 study group. Treatment of allergic asthma with monoclonal anti-IgE antibody. *N Engl J Med* 1999; **341**: 1966–73.

Overall section conclusion

The past two years have seen a significant increase in our understanding of asthma but, as always, good research has raised many more questions than answers. The relentless increase in the prevalence of asthma may now be showing some signs of levelling off but clearly further studies surveying other populations will be required over the next few years before a settled optimism will emerge. Nevertheless, the factors that have governed the increase in asthma prevalence already witnessed remain largely elusive. Clues are beginning to emerge from epidemiological studies reporting that apparent protection or susceptibility may be conferred by exposure to various environmental factors. However, our understanding of these remains rudimentary and not at a level where confident advice can be given to individual patients by individual clinicians. Greater insight into the immunological profile of patients who appear to be protected by farming environments or early life exposure to pets or infections will undoubtedly lead to an improved understanding of the immunological mechanisms invoked and also offer the exciting potential to direct research towards effectively manipulating these and abort or ameliorate asthma in susceptible individuals. Such aspirations may be aided by the increasing knowledge that will certainly emerge regarding the interplay of various genes that control the initiation or perpetuation of the disease and contribute to the response to therapy and prognosis.

The assessment of every asthmatic patient should include a search for precipitating or aggravating factors. Traditional culprits include cigarette smoking, exposure to certain pets or occupational exposures, but it is also important to enquire into household conditions, and in particular, the presence of moulds. There is now some tentative evidence that stressful life events may enhance the inflammatory response of the asthmatic airway providing explanation for the observations made by so many patients that their disease becomes more troublesome at such times.

One of the most important goals in the management of asthma is to reduce exacerbations and hospitalizations. The identification of individuals at greatest risk of hospitalization may allow them to be targeted for more intensive management, including provision of patient-centred management plans emphasizing the importance of compliance with inhaled corticosteroids. In addition, we are likely to see the emergence of greater use of tests that reflect the underlying inflammatory state of airways and these may provide a more appropriate target by which to regulate therapy.

Attempts to reduce allergen exposure that have concentrated on house dust mite remain disappointing but larger and longer studies are probably still required before we can advise patients that such manoeuvres are not in their long term interests. Increased confidence with long acting β-2 agonists may see an extension of their role to improving care in even milder asthmatic patients, but more information is needed on this group. β-2 agonists cannot be used as a substitute therapy for inhaled corticosteroids but will facilitate a dose-reduction in corticosteroids without jeopardizing asthma control. This may become more important as more information becomes available on the therapeutic ratio of corticosteroid treatment. More information is needed on the positioning of leukotriene receptor antagonists, in particular identifying patients, such as those with aspirin sensitive asthma, who are likely to benefit from their use. As further studies progress with the new monoclonal antibody to IgE, we may have another new agent to offer patients who remain poorly controlled despite appropriate use of traditional therapy. Finally, we need more information on how best to provide effective and relevant information to patients to enable them to have the confidence to manage the day-to-day changes associated with the variable nature of the condition. Exciting times lie ahead.

Part II

Chronic obstructive pulmonary disease

Chronic obstructive pulmonary disease

Introduction

Chronic obstructive pulmonary disease (COPD) is extremely common, and as mortality from the disease is increasing, COPD is predicted to become the third biggest cause of mortality in the United States by the year 2020 |**1**|. The condition is associated with an enormous economic burden both in terms of direct health care costs and in terms of the consequences of lost productivity |**2**|. As COPD is predominantly caused by smoking, and affects an elderly population, patients often have important comorbidities. For all these reasons, whichever area of health care you are associated with, COPD will impact upon your work in the coming years (and if you are a layperson, or a retired health professional, the wealth and health services of your country are being significantly influenced by COPD as you read this).

A huge amount of research related to COPD was published in 2001–2002. On balance, it seems safe to conclude that, while no single major breakthrough has revolutionized management of COPD over this period, our understanding of multiple facets of this complex, chronic inflammatory disease has been significantly improved. The aim of this section is to give a flavour of the advances achieved across the diversity of problems associated with COPD. Fifty papers that have made significant contributions are summarized. The summaries are designed such that reading the *Background* and *Interpretation* sections should allow the reader to take the 'headline' message from each paper. Thereafter, if more detail is required, a *Comment* section discusses the paper in more depth. Generally the *Comment* sections scrutinize the methods and results more closely, then consider potential limitations of the study (principally with the aim of assessing applicability of the data to 'real life'), and finally an attempt is made to place the study within the framework of existing knowledge.

The section has three chapters. The first considers advances in COPD derived from epidemiological studies of the general population. The second focuses on the patient with stable disease, and is itself divided into sub-sections containing studies evaluating pathogenesis and complications of the disease, studies in which our knowledge of more established treatments has been consolidated, and work relating to new and evolving management strategies. The final chapter deals with advances relating to acute exacerbations of COPD. Wherever possible, if an article in one chapter has particular relevance to an article elsewhere, this will be highlighted in the *Comment* for each paper. A small proportion of the papers considered had commercial sponsorship, and I have identified this in the text whenever it has come to my attention.

The aim of the section is to touch upon important work relating to a wide variety of issues. It is often the case that one or two interesting articles have been selected to highlight an area in which scores of other papers were published in 2001–2002. Three things should therefore be considered. First, there are dozens of excellent articles on COPD that are not covered here and which are left out purely because of limitations on space – the papers selected happened to grab my attention and satisfy the aims of the section. Secondly, the papers discussed should be read as 'stand alone' articles. The *Comment* sections are deliberately not written as mini-reviews (but instead like mini-editorials), and while an attempt is made to place each article in some form of context, the interested reader is invited to consult the literature for more detailed assessment of any of the 30 or more aspects of COPD discussed here. Indeed, in the last couple of years excellent reviews have been written on most of the aspects of COPD dealt with in this section.

Thirdly, the *Comment* sections simply reflect my opinion on 50 papers that I found to be important and stimulating. I have tried to provide some critical evaluation on each in the interests of balance, but emphasize that each of these papers has contributed valuable information to the understanding of COPD.

The compilation of this work has certainly led to changes in my own clinical practice and identified areas that require further research. The hope is that the reader will derive similar benefit. Ultimately, however, the central and overriding theme pervading this section and all of COPD management remains that cigarettes are the predominant cause of the disease and we must all redouble our efforts to prevent (or stop) people smoking.

References

1. Murray CJ, Lopez AD. Alternative projections of mortality and disability by cause 1990–2020: Global Burden of Disease Study. *Lancet* 1997; **349**: 1498–504.

2. Global Initiative for Chronic Obstructive Lung Disease. National Institutes of Health: National Heart, Lung and Blood Institute, USA. Publication Number 2701, 2001.

9

Important observations derived from epidemiological studies

The influence of environmental, biological and genetic factors on COPD can often be teased out using large epidemiological surveys of the general population. Subsets of the population with airflow limitation can be identified, for example, such that associations with a given environmental influence can be compared with the general population. This section considers papers which help us evaluate more clearly the influence on COPD of air pollution, diet and body weight, then goes on to evaluate the risk of β-agonists in patients with co-existing heart disease. Genetic issues such as the risk of COPD in siblings, and the importance of individual α_1-antitrypsin $(\alpha_1 AT)$ genotypes, are also considered. However, we begin with the only paper in the chapter that does *not* specifically deal with COPD, so as to emphasize the most important public health message of all.

Benefits of smoking cessation for longevity.
Taylor DH Jr, Hasselblad V, Henley J, Thun MJ, Sloan FA. *Am. J Pub Health* 2002; **92**: 990–6.

BACKGROUND. **The pioneering work of Doll, Peto and colleagues provided us with unequivocal evidence for a detrimental effect of smoking on mortality, and subsequently allowed us to begin to quantify the beneficial effects of smoking cessation |1,2|. The study under consideration here sought to extend these observations within an enormous American and Puerto Rican population. Specifically the authors aimed to quantify the life-years saved by smoking cessation and to evaluate whether cessation late in life still conferred survival advantage.**

INTERPRETATION. For the specific population studied, the relative risk for all-cause mortality was significantly higher among smokers than those who never smoked. Stopping smoking resulted in a marked reduction in the relative risk of mortality, irrespective of the age at cessation. On average, stopping smoking aged 35 years predicted for at least an extra 6.1 and 6.9 years of life expectancy in men and women respectively, while even stopping at age 65 predicted for an extra 2.7 and 1.4 years respectively.

Comment

The enormous strength of this study centres on the huge population analysed. Data were extracted from the Cancer Prevention Study II, which enrolled 1.2 million adults aged 30 years or over and began in 1982. The current study excluded subjects with incomplete smoking data, those who were ill at the time of enrolment (on the assumption that illness would prompt smoking cessation in many, thus confounding the data), and anyone who had smoked cigars or a pipe. This left 877 243 subjects for analysis. It must be stressed that while enrolment involved all of the United States and Puerto Rico, it was performed by American Cancer Society volunteers and ultimately contained much higher proportions of white, educated, affluent subjects than in the general population. A total of 149 351 subjects died in the 15 years to December 1996, and investigators obtained mortality data in almost 99% of cases, thus allowing mortality according to smoking status at enrolment to be calculated. While inaccuracy of death certificates is a recurring theme in this chapter, this rate of data collection is extremely impressive.

The authors used a Cox proportional hazards model to estimate relative risk of death by age, sex and smoking status. They were further able to calculate approximate projections of life expectancy according to smoking status by extrapolation of risk stratifications from the United States census.

One critical point is that subjects who were smokers at the outset of the study were considered smokers throughout (i.e. they were assumed not to have stopped smoking during the observation period), and those who were ex-smokers at the start of the study were considered ex-smokers throughout (i.e. they were assumed not to have relapsed). As such, the study was designed so that if some subjects considered 'smokers' *had* stopped during the observation period the overall effect would be to underestimate smoking-related mortality; if 'ex-smokers' started smoking again the net effect would be to overestimate mortality among ex-smokers. In this way, any bias was towards an *underestimate* of the benefits of smoking cessation. Limited data available 10 years into the study suggested that over 50% of those who smoked in 1982 had stopped by 1992, while only 3% of former smokers in 1982 had relapsed by 1992 (we are not told whether any 'never smokers' subsequently took up the habit). As such, the crude data in the study would be expected to underplay the benefits of smoking cessation considerably.

Crude mortality figures in the study broadly conformed to previously observed patterns. COPD accounted for approximately 3.4% of all deaths, and it is claimed that 11.2% of deaths attributable to COPD occurred in subjects who never smoked.

Continuing male smokers across the age ranges studied generally had a 2.5 times increased risk of all cause mortality as compared with 'never smokers'. The corresponding risk in women who continued to smoke was approximately 2-fold. Most importantly, stopping smoking resulted in a striking reduction in risk of mortality relative to that in continuing smokers irrespective of the age at which smoking cessation occurred, or the duration of cessation (though to be precise the data is presented for those stopping for at least 3 years). The general trend is for risk to decrease most for those who have stopped longest but even relatively short dura-tions of quitting in patients over 70 years were associated with strikingly significant reductions in mortality risk.

These data were modelled into a predictive equation of life expectancy, based on analogy to US census data. Average life expectancy in never smoking males was predicted at 78.2 years, for continuous smokers the corresponding figure was 69.3 years, for subjects stopping smoking at 35 it was 76.2 years and in those stop-ping smoking at 65 it was 70.7 years. The trend was similar among women. Thus, early smoking cessation almost eliminates the excess mortality risk associated with smoking, but even late quitting has survival advantage.

In taking this hugely important study into our clinical practice, we must acknowledge that this was an affluent American population, while much of the bur-den of disease from smoking unfortunately concentrates on relatively deprived communities. Nevertheless, the trends observed with regard to stopping smoking in this massive study seem likely to apply across populations, and indeed have remarkable parallels with the findings of Peto and colleagues [2]. Therefore, we can now confidently tell young smokers that stopping will increase their life expectancy (and indeed will come very close to normalizing it), and we can tell our elderly patients that there is unequivocal survival advantage in stopping even late in life. The considerable task remaining is to add information on morbidity to these com-pelling data.

Finally, I cannot ignore one fabulous typing error in this paper estimating life expectancy of lifelong non-smoking males at 778 years! I suspect those planning health budgets in the United States had heart attacks when they saw this figure.

Acute effects of particulate air pollution on respiratory admissions. Results from APHEA 2 Project.

Atkinson RW, Anderson HR, Sunyer J, *et al. Am J Respir Crit Care Med* 2001; **164**: 1860–6.

BACKGROUND. The links between particulate air pollution and pulmonary inflammation are gradually being characterized in more detail. In public health terms, it remains important to establish the additional burden on health resources attributable to air pollution, and to determine which particles have the predominant influence on health. Against this background, this study set out to establish the effect of particulate air pollution on hospital admissions for respiratory disease in the Netherlands and in 7 European cities. The authors simultaneously attempted to identify those factors responsible for regional differences in the effects of pollution.

INTERPRETATION. On average, hospital admissions attributable to respiratory disease rose by about 1% per 10 $\mu g/m^3$ increase in the concentration of particles of less than 10 μm diameter (PM_{10}). For analyses incorporating admissions attributable to COPD, there was quite wide geographical variation in the contribution of PM_{10} to the excess hospitalization rate. The average concentration of ozone in any given city seemed to explain some of the geographic variation in admission rates for COPD associated with the levels of PM_{10}.

Comment

This study used pre-determined criteria to quantify admissions for respiratory disease in seven European cities, and in the Netherlands. The hospital admissions studied included asthma in the age range 0–14 years, asthma in the age range 15–64 years, asthma and COPD for ages 65 years and over, and all respiratory disease for ages 65 years and over. Standardized criteria were also used for the measurement of particulate matter. Concentrations of PM_{10}, black smoke, sulphur dioxide, ozone, carbon monoxide, nitrogen dioxide and total suspended particles were measured. Models were created incorporating a variety of meteorological variables, social variables and finally particulate matter data, with the aim of determining the independent contribution of each to admission rates for respiratory disease. In each of the four groups of patients, the contribution of PM_{10} to admissions across the European cities was relatively consistent at approximately 1% increase in the mean number of admissions per 10 $\mu g/m^3$ rise in PM_{10} (for COPD and asthma in those aged 65 years or over the effect was 1% with 95% CI of 0.4–1.5%). Black smoke had a smaller effect (0.2% increase in the mean number of admissions with COPD or asthma among patients aged 65 years or over per 10 $\mu g/m^3$ rise in black smoke concentration). For COPD, the association with PM_{10} appeared to be strongest in Barcelona and weakest in Paris.

The variation in admission rates associated with PM_{10} concentration stimulated creation of a regression model assessing the role of other particles implicated in pollution at each location. In this model, it was determined that ozone had a significant effect on regional variation in the rate of admissions for COPD/asthma associated with PM_{10}. The average concentration of ozone in each city (but not the daily variation in ozone levels) predicted the increased effect of PM_{10} on admission rates.

This study, therefore, adds further weight to the evidence that particulate air pollution contributes to respiratory disease in a dose-dependent manner, at least with respect to PM_{10}. While the overall effect on admissions appears relatively small, the implication is that in more polluted cities the public health costs associated with air pollution may be high. It is likely that in polluted cities many more individuals accrue low-grade inflammation sufficient to produce morbidity but insufficient to warrant hospital admission. A further implication of the study is that individual pollutants may have complex interactions with other airborne particles, and these may contribute to variations in morbidity in different cities. These interactions remain to be elucidated. Continued vigilance in legislation for emissions is clearly required.

As is mentioned elsewhere in this chapter codings for hospital admissions are notoriously inaccurate, and the implications of this study specifically for COPD are unclear, though it seems safe to assume that particulate pollution does contribute to an excess in admissions. The precise locations in cities at which measurements of pollution are made may also influence interpretation but we are told relatively little about this, except that techniques were standardized. However, a significant strength of the study is the use of similar methods in different centres covering an enormous European population (approximately 38 million). Taken together, while it is possible that a degree of error may be built in to the precise effect of air pollution on admissions, the consistent effect across all four groups of patients studied and the consistent methodology employed allow a firm conclusion that PM_{10} have an effect on respiratory health in European cities.

Diet and chronic obstructive pulmonary disease: independent beneficial effects of fruits, whole grains, and alcohol (the MORGEN study).

Tabak C, Smit HA, Heederik D, Ocké MC, Kromhout D. *Clin Exper Allergy* 2001; **31**: 747–55.

B ACKGROUND . **An interaction between diet and COPD has been established for several years. Particular interest has focused on the potential protective action of foods containing antioxidants, but an effect on forced expiratory volume$_1$ (FEV$_1$) has been postulated for a variety of other foods, as well as for alcohol. This study aimed to assess whether fruit (and fruit juices), vegetables, whole grains, fish or alcohol independently affect FEV$_1$ or symptoms of COPD in the general population.**

I NTERPRETATION . After correction for confounding variables and other foods, consumption of fruit and whole grains had a positive effect on FEV$_1$ and was associated with fewer symptoms of COPD in a large cohort of the general population. Low alcohol consumption (but not abstinence) was also associated with fewer COPD symptoms. Curiously, fish consumption had a weak but significant negative association with FEV$_1$. The effects of fruit, whole grain and low alcohol consumption on FEV$_1$ and symptoms were generally additive. Importantly the interaction between these dietary factors and both FEV$_1$ and symptoms was observed in non-smokers and in smokers.

Comment

This cross-sectional Dutch study enrolled subjects aged between 20 and 59 years. Subjects completed questionnaires relating to demographics and to consumption of some 178 food items. Respiratory symptoms were assessed according to the European Community Respiratory Health Survey, and participants underwent physical examination and spirometry. The presence of COPD symptoms was defined as any one from chronic cough, chronic phlegm or breathlessness. The relationship between foods and FEV$_1$ was examined using a multiple linear regression model, the association between foods and symptoms using logistic regression analysis. Complete data, including reproducible spirometry, was obtained for over 13 650 subjects.

After adjusting for confounding variables and for other foods, FEV_1 was higher and COPD symptoms fewer in association with increasing intake of fruits (and fruit juices) and whole grains (which included wholemeal bread, rye bread and unrefined grains). Interestingly low alcohol consumption (1–30 g of alcohol per day) was associated with significantly fewer COPD symptoms than either relative abstinence (less than 1 g of alcohol per day) or moderate to high consumption (defined as greater than 30 g of alcohol per day). Similarly, low alcohol consumption predicted for a higher FEV_1 than did (near) abstinence. No association was found between eating vegetables and either FEV_1 or symptoms.

On the basis of these interesting findings, the authors constructed a model to determine the combined effects of low alcohol consumption (1–30 g of alcohol per day), 'favourable' fruit consumption (more than 180 g/day) and favourable whole grain intake (more than 45 g/day). The arbitrary cut off points for 'favourable' fruit and grain consumption roughly approximate to daily-recommended intakes in Holland. In this model, the effects of favourable fruit, grain and alcohol consumption were effectively cumulative, with respect to the improvement in FEV_1 and with respect to the reduction in COPD symptoms. The magnitude of the protective effect was impressive. For example, among patients with a daily intake of over 45 g of grain *and* over 180 g of fruit *and* 1–30 g of alcohol, the average FEV_1 was approximately 140 ml higher than in subjects with a daily intake of less than 45 g of grain *and* less than 180 g of fruit *and* more than 30 g of alcohol (or indeed less than 1 g of alcohol). Importantly the protective effect was observed in both non-smokers and subjects with a smoking history, implying that some or all of the effects were independent of a confounding effect of tobacco. It will be fascinating in future years to see whether the precise mechanism of dietary protection can be determined, particularly among non-smokers.

One curious result was that fish intake, after correction for confounding variables and other foods, appeared to have a weak negative association with FEV_1. The authors make no further mention of this observation, which may be a statistical quirk, but seems a little at odds with established opinion.

The size of this study, to some extent, should dilute problems associated with inaccuracy in self-reported questionnaires. Of course, it remains impossible to say whether other foods not studied here may have had an influence on FEV_1. One potentially confounding variable that did not appear to be factored in to the study was socio-economic status, when it might be expected that poorer subjects might eat less healthily. However, it should be noted that correction for educational attainment did not alter the study's findings.

Overall, the data in this large and impressive study have important implications for public health. Certainly, this adds substantially to the argument that the general population should be encouraged to eat fruit and wholemeal products as part of a healthy diet. These specific data cannot be extrapolated directly to the elderly individual with advancing COPD until further longitudinal studies are performed in *patients*, but in the absence of any harm associated with these foods, it seems reasonable to recommend adequate to high dietary intakes of fruit and wholemeal bread in patients with COPD. As the authors point out, the significant majority of subjects in the study were already taking quantities of fruit and whole grain above the arbitrary cut off levels associated with protection of FEV_1, and so adequate consumption seems eminently attainable in population terms, at least in the Netherlands.

Prognostic value of weight change in chronic obstructive pulmonary disease: results from the Copenhagen City Heart Study.

Prescott E, Almdal A, Mikkelsen KL, Tofteng CL, Vestbo J, Lange P.
Eur Respir J 2002; **20**: 539–44.

BACKGROUND. All respiratory wards and outpatient departments contain a proportion of patients with COPD who have very low body mass index (BMI), and this group of patients appears to have a poor prognosis. The question of whether nutritional support is worth pursuing aggressively in COPD remains controversial. However, before deciding whether or how best to supplement nutrition in these patients we first need to know the consequences of weight change in COPD. This study, therefore, aimed to determine whether change in BMI independently predicts mortality among patients with COPD.

INTERPRETATION. This large population-based study monitored outcome according to change in weight measured over a 5-year period. Among patients with COPD risk of dying from the disease was independently associated both with marked weight loss over the 5-year period or with being underweight at baseline. All-cause mortality among these patients was also associated with weight loss. The cohort of patients with most severe COPD had the most profound weight loss.

Comment

This study made use of the Copenhagen City Heart Study database, which made independent measurements of BMI on consecutive occasions 5 years apart (the second set of values recorded up to 1983). Information was also available with respect to baseline spirometry, and mortality data for the intervening period were obtained from the national Danish registry. The authors excluded patients with 'self-reported asthma' at either of the two visits. Complete data were available for almost 10 500 subjects of whom 1612 were deemed to have COPD on the basis of an FEV_1/FVC ratio of less than 0.7 at the second visit. It is important to note that this ratio and the patients' denial of asthma were the only criteria required to make a diagnosis of COPD. Certainly, bronchodilator reversibility tests were not performed and it seems likely that some asthma is contained in the COPD group.

The study used the Cox proportional hazards model to evaluate the independent contribution of BMI change to observed mortality, and made strenuous efforts to adjust for age, sex, smoking habit and baseline FEV_1.

At baseline, the patients with COPD had a mean FEV_1 of 67% predicted. When stratified according to FEV_1 at baseline, mean weight loss was observed only in the subgroup with FEV_1 less than 50% predicted. Irrespective of starting FEV_1, weight gain was significantly higher among subjects without COPD.

When all-cause mortality was considered, patients with COPD who lost weight over 5 years had significantly increased relative risk that rose with progressive weight loss. For mortality specifically related to COPD, substantial weight loss (a fall of 3 BMI units or more) increased risk some 114% relative to those with no weight change, whilst low baseline BMI (less than 20 kg/m^2) was also significantly associated with increased risk. Interestingly, being mildly overweight at baseline appeared to protect against risk of death from COPD. It should be noted that the authors performed separate analyses in which the first 2 years of follow-up were excluded, in order to prevent bias from terminal illness, and the results were essentially unchanged.

These data suggest that low weight, and in particular weight loss, have an adverse prognostic effect in COPD. The study data corrects for a number of important potential confounding variables. The main concern with these data, as stated above, is whether the COPD group really had COPD. Interestingly 18% of female 'COPD' patients were never smokers at time of assignment. Furthermore, it is quite possible that undetected COPD was present in the 'non-COPD' group, as over 1% of patients in this group apparently subsequently died of COPD. Indeed the accuracy of death certificates potentially limits interpretation of data on mortality attributable to COPD in this study. A further point is that it may have been useful to include alcohol consumption and socio-economic status in the analysis, and there is no way of knowing how many patients had been deliberately attempting to lose weight between BMI assessments. One final small, nagging doubt also remains about the calculation of changes in BMI in the study. On four separate occasions the authors state that for a height of 1.7 m one unit of BMI change equates to fall in weight of 3.89 kg, but by my calculations this should be 2.89 kg, i.e. 2.89 kg/ (1.7 × 1.7 m) = 1 kg/m^2. One must assume that this was a single arithmetic error made whilst writing the paper and that all data calculations in the study were correct, but the nagging doubt remains.

Overall, the data suggest that low starting BMI and/or weight loss are associated with poor outcome in COPD. The next question is whether weight gain is helpful. Within this study, the data in the COPD group is equivocal—for all-cause mortality there was a non-significant trend for weight gain to be detrimental, for COPD-specific mortality there was a non-significant trend for weight gain to be protective. With regard to baseline weight, for patients with COPD a starting BMI of 25–30 kg/m^2 appeared to be protective. It would seem sensible on the basis of these data to encourage underweight patients with COPD to return to a normal BMI, and to encourage patients with a normal or slightly high BMI to stay in this region. How best to increase BMI in underweight patients with COPD is an altogether more difficult question. Indeed both the best way of adding weight in this context and the benefits of intervention in a prospective trial remain to be proven. It should be noted that the trial by Yeh and colleagues, discussed later in the chapter, deals specifically with the effects of an anabolic steroid on weight gain in patients with COPD and a low BMI.

Association between inhaled β-agonists and the risk of unstable angina and myocardial infarction.

Au DH, Curtis JR, Every NR, McDonnell MB, Fihn SD. *Chest* 2002; **121**: 846–51.

BACKGROUND. **Because cigarette smoking is a risk factor for both ischaemic heart disease and COPD, it follows that these diseases frequently co-exist. As β-blockers reduce the risk of further cardiac events in patients with ischaemic heart disease it seems logical to assume that β-agonists may be detrimental to patients at risk of coronary artery disease. As such, standard β-2 agonist reliever therapy prescribed for COPD may have attendant risks in patients with heart disease. This study aimed to establish the risk of coronary events in patients prescribed metered dose inhalers (MDIs) delivering β-agonists.**

INTERPRETATION. Prescription of inhaled β-agonists in the preceding 3 months predicted for a significantly increased risk of myocardial infarction or unstable angina. This association was independent of potential confounding variables such as age, smoking, diabetes, hypertension and previous history of cardiovascular disease. The increased risk associated with inhaled β-agonists was dose-dependent. The study assumes that most prescriptions of β-agonists were for COPD. The implication appears to be that benefits and risks of β-2 agonists should be weighed particularly carefully in patients with COPD who have pre-existing ischaemic heart disease, or significant risk factors for coronary events. In addition, frequent or increasing use of β-2 agonists should stimulate careful re-assessment of a patient's lung disease along with consideration of whether there is evidence of cardiac ischaemia.

Comment

This study was incorporated within the large Ambulatory Care Quality Improvement Project (ACQUIP) and as such studied patients attending Veterans Affairs (VA) clinics at seven centres in six states in the USA. The present work was a case–control study. Cases were defined as patients discharged from VA hospitals with acute myocardial infarction or unstable angina. Controls were drawn from the ACQUIP database. All patients in the ACQUIP study were sent a health status questionnaire, and the pharmacy records of all patients were obtained over the period of study. For all cases the index date was the first day of admission with acute myocardial infarction or unstable angina; matched controls were given the corresponding index date. The number of β-2 agonist canisters prescribed in the 90 days prior to the index date was established.

In general, potential confounding factors such as age, smoking history, diabetes, hypertension and cardiovascular disease were collated from self-reported questionnaires, but wherever possible the data was corroborated by hospital records or pharmacy data (for example, self-reported diabetes could be confirmed by prescription of insulin). COPD was considered to be present if patients listed the diagnosis, or if they had been prescribed ipratropium more than once. The relative risk of coronary events conferred by β-agonists was calculated by logistic regression analysis, with adjustment for potential confounding variables as above.

The study incorporated 413 cases and 6050 controls. Not surprisingly, diabetes, hypertension, cardiovascular disease and COPD were commoner among cases (COPD was present in 22% of controls and 32% of cases). Curiously, controls had a greater smoking history (25 versus 22 pack years). Average age was approximately 65.

After adjustment for confounding variables use of 3–5 β-2 agonist canisters in the preceding 90 days significantly increased risk of a coronary event (OR 1.57, 95% CI 1.01–2.46), while 6 or more canisters increased risk further still (OR 1.93, 95% CI 1.23-3.03). In contrast, risk associated with 1–2 canisters did not reach statistical significance (OR 1.38, 95% CI 0.86–2.23). In a separate analysis, the authors stratified risk according to whether β-blockers were prescribed. They found that patients taking β-blockers were relatively protected such that only heavy use of β_2-agonist canisters (six or more) was associated with coronary events. Conversely, the relative risk conferred by 3–5, and 6 or more canisters of β-2 agonist in the *absence* of β-blockers was 4.1 and 3.8 respectively.

The authors are quick to point out that a causal relationship between inhaled β-2 agonists and coronary events cannot be inferred from these data. Indeed, they acknowledge that β-2 agonist use could potentially be a non-causal epiphenomenon—patients may have confused the dyspnoea of angina with that of COPD thus increasing β_2-agonist use prior to infarction, or β-2 agonists may have been appropriately used to correct airflow limitation contributing to cardiac hypoxia. However, at least 68.5% of cases had self-reported angina, and it seems unlikely that these effects would be overwhelming among a group of patients 'experienced' in cardiac symptoms.

Two further points remain. Firstly, it is hard to know exactly how many of the patients using β-2 agonists had COPD. While a self-reported diagnosis and regular use of ipratropium were the only diagnostic criteria in this epidemiologic study, the authors argue that the 721 patients using β-2 agonists were drawn from an elderly population, around 80% of whom had a smoking history, and therefore, COPD is most likely to explain β-2 agonist treatment. This seems reasonable, though we shall never know how many patients were inappropriately prescribed β-2 agonists, or how many had genuine asthma. Secondly, VA studies are essentially studies of men, and these results cannot strictly speaking be extended to women at this stage. Results may also be confounded by any participants taking their health care outwith the VA system, but the authors make a good case for this eventuality being unlikely for the vast majority of patients.

Taken together the results of this study are highly relevant to practice and lead to a significant clinical dilemma—how should we modify our prescribing of β-2

agonists in elderly patients with COPD? The first and perhaps most obvious conclusion is that we should encourage patients requiring reliever medication to stop
smoking as a matter of priority. Thereafter, these data suggest that low frequency
use of β-2 agonist carries no statistically significant risk. If a patient is using a lot of
β-2 agonist, or if their use is accelerating, then we are beholden to ask whether this
is worsening COPD, some other respiratory illness, or incipient breathlessness of
cardiac origin, and we should investigate this as appropriate. Finally, in patients
with COPD who have multiple risk factors for ischaemic heart disease, it is necessary to address these risk factors thoroughly, and then to weigh up carefully the
symptomatic benefits of β-2 agonists against the risks inferred from this study.
Further studies on this important subject are awaited with great interest.

Siblings of patients with severe chronic obstructive pulmonary disease have a significant risk of airflow obstruction.
McCloskey SC, Patel BD, Hinchliffe SJ, Reid ED, Wareham NJ, Lomas DA.
Am J Respir Crit Care Med 2001; **164**: 1419–24.

BACKGROUND. Genetic influences other than those made by alpha-1-antitrypsin
(α_1AT) deficiency seem likely to contribute to the pathogenesis of COPD. Rigorous
characterization of the familial risk of developing COPD is a necessary step towards
identifying specific genes influencing evolution of the disease, which in turn is likely to
suggest novel therapeutic approaches. This study therefore aimed to evaluate whether
there is increased risk of airflow obstruction in the siblings of patients with severe
COPD.

INTERPRETATION. The non-smoking siblings of patients with severe COPD had normal
lung function, but among those siblings with a history of smoking 35% had features of
airflow obstruction. The siblings with a smoking history were matched with controls
drawn from the general population and they had a 4.7-fold increased risk of airflow
obstruction.

Comment

Patients were recruited if they had FEV$_1$ below 60% predicted at less than 56 years
of age, below 40% predicted for the age range 56–60 years, and below 20% predicted for the age range 61–65 years. Additionally patients had to have reduced
FEV$_1$/FVC ratio, reduced diffusing capacity for carbon monoxide (Kco) and a
normal serum α_1AT concentration Patients and their siblings filled in a questionnaire and the siblings attended for detailed lung function tests. The control group
in the study was drawn from a large cohort of patients participating in a population-based study of the association between diet, cancer and chronic disease.

The 150 probands studied had a mean FEV$_1$ of 0.9 litres, FEV$_1$/FVC ratio of
approximately 0.36 and an average Kco of 0.47 mmol/min/kPa/l, in keeping with

severe COPD. All were smokers, and all but one Caucasian. One hundred and thirteen probands had identifiable siblings ($n = 221$), and 173 of these completed a questionnaire and lung function testing. Forty-four siblings (25%) had airflow obstruction as defined by FEV_1/FVC ratio less than 0.7 with FEV_1 below 80% predicted. Of these, 39 had reversibility testing to 200 µg salbutamol—32 had unequivocal lack of reversibility. Just over half of the siblings with airflow obstruction had reduced gas transfer. Interestingly, when analysed by smoking status, the siblings who had never smoked ($n = 47$) had a mean FEV_1 of around 98% predicted, while the corresponding figure was 80% among the current or former smokers ($n = 126$).

The siblings with a history of smoking were matched for age, sex and smoking status with the control group (wherever possible 4 controls to each sibling studied). Although no significant difference in FEV_1 was observed between the two groups, 31.5% of the siblings tested had airflow obstruction (defined as FEV_1/VC ratio less than 70% with FEV_1 below 80% predicted) as compared with 9.3% of the control group. When entered into a logistic regression analysis the odds ratio for the risk of airflow obstruction among siblings with a history of smoking was 4.7.

This elegant study provides solid evidence of a familial association for airflow obstruction that is apparent only among those with a smoking history. The implication would appear to be that smoking has a specific interaction with modifier genes, which remain to be fully identified. A significant strength of the study is that a population based, matched control group was used.

Confounding factors seem unlikely to have influenced these findings significantly. We are told that the probands were selected from respiratory clinics, and therefore, selection bias towards probands with a family history of breathlessness could be postulated. However, this seems unlikely. Shared paternity for siblings and probands was not genetically confirmed, but there is no reason to suspect that this should be unusually low. We have no information on how geographically spread the group of siblings was, and we do not know the socio-economic status or rural/urban dwelling status of the two groups, but on balance it seems very likely that the environmental exposures of both were broadly equivalent. Similarly, the racial composition of the control group is unknown, but seems unlikely to have differed significantly from the sibling group. As the authors point out the increased risk of airflow obstruction in the sibling group is highly likely to be explained mostly (and perhaps exclusively) by genetic factors, although shared environmental factors cannot be fully excluded. It is also worth noting that this study included probands with PiMS and PiMZ α_1AT phenotypes, and, therefore, the sibling population would seem likely to contain a slightly higher proportion of patients with α_1AT phenotypes other than PiMM (including the theoretical possibility of rare cases of PiZZ). However, the effect of this small theoretical variation between the groups is likely to be unimportant.

In summary, this study provides firm evidence that COPD is associated with a familial risk of airflow obstruction. The challenge now is to identify which genes mediate susceptibility to cigarette smoke. Genes postulated to influence COPD progression, are also discussed in connection with the paper by Sakao and colleagues.

Changes in lung function and morbidity from chronic obstructive pulmonary disease in α_1-antitrypsin *MZ* heterozygotes: a longitudinal study of the general population.

Dahl M, Tybjærg-Hansen A, Lange P, Vestbo J, Nordestgaard BG. *Ann Intern Med* 2002; **136**: 270–9.

BACKGROUND. A number of different alleles in the α_1AT gene have been described, giving rise to a number of phenotypes other than the normal PiMM phenotype in which adequate serum levels of α_1AT are generated. It is well known that the PiZZ phenotype is associated with severe α_1AT deficiency and a tendency to premature emphysema, especially among smokers. However, the contribution of other non-PiMM phenotypes to the risk of emphysema remains unclear. In particular, the role of the common PiMZ phenotype to COPD requires delineation that is more precise. This study, therefore, aimed to determine whether the *MZ* genotype is associated with accelerated lung function decline and/or COPD in a large Danish population.

INTERPRETATION. Approximately 5% of the general Danish population have the *MZ* genotype. This is associated with plasma α_1AT levels 31% lower than normal, and with an increased average rate of decline in FEV_1 of 4 ml/year. Relative to the population with the *MM* genotype, the *MZ* genotype conferred an increased risk of COPD of around 50%.

Comment

This extremely useful work made use of data from the Copenhagen City Heart Study, which made serial assessments of Danish subjects who were aged 20 years or over at the time of entry. The present study analysed data from participants who had provided blood for genotyping ($n = 9187$), of whom 6248 provided three serial FEV_1 measurements, and 592 representative subjects provided blood for plasma α_1AT estimation. Criteria for airflow obstruction were taken to be FEV_1 less than 80% predicted, and FEV_1/FVC ratio less than 0.7. Data relating to the presence of clinical COPD was from central Danish registries of hospital discharges and causes of death. Genotyping used standard techniques, and tested specifically for the recognized *M, Z, S* and *E* alleles. The study population was almost entirely (99%) of Danish descent.

The *MM* genotype was found in 77% of individuals, but all 10 potential genotypes (the other nine being *MZ, MS, ME, ZZ, ZS, ZE, SS, SE, EE*) were identified in the population studied, albeit that most were rare. *ME* (12%) and *MZ* (4.9%) were the next most common genotypes identified. Mean plasma concentration of α_1AT was 1.59 g/l in the PiMM group, and 1.10 g/l in the PiMZ group. The calculated annual rate of decline in FEV_1 was 21 ml/year in the PiMM group and 25 ml/year in the PiMZ group ($P <0.05$). Interestingly, when the groups were divided into smokers and non-smokers the accelerated rate of decline in the PiMZ group was only maintained among 'non-smokers'. Unfortunately, I found it hard to tell from the paper whether former smokers were included in the non-smoking or smoking group.

The risk of airflow obstruction was higher in patients with PiMZ as compared to PiMM (OR 1.3, 95% CI 1.0–1.7) even when adjusted for age, sex and tobacco exposure. Similarly, the calculated risk of COPD was higher in the PiMZ group (OR 1.5, 95% CI 1.0–2.3) when adjusted for the above variables and FEV_1 at study entry. In passing, it is worth mentioning that the relatively common *ME* genotype was associated with neither accelerated FEV_1 decline nor COPD. In contrast the relatively rare *SZ* genotype (approximately 0.1% of the population) was associated with striking lung function decline in smokers and with a 330% increased risk of COPD (though it must be noted that the number of patients with *SZ* was very small indeed, and as such bias is likely).

Interpretation of the data with regard to COPD may be a little skewed by the accuracy of diagnosis in hospital registries and death certificates, both of which are notoriously inaccurate. Similarly, airflow limitation as defined in the study may well have incorporated asthma (bronchodilator reversibility testing did not feature in the study) and so precise conclusions regarding COPD are hard to draw. Also, the tiny numbers of patients with rarer genotypes leave analysis pertaining to these groups open to huge bias—this does not apply to *MZ* however, as a large number of patients had this genotype. Nevertheless, this study gives one of the best indications to date of the relative importance of *MZ*. It would appear that (certainly in the Danish population), this genotype is common, and while the risk of developing COPD remains relatively small (1.5 times that of the 'normal' *MM* population), in societal terms this genotype may contribute to a significant number of cases of COPD. Indeed the authors estimate that the *MZ* genotype could be responsible for 2.4% of cases of COPD in their population.

What does this mean for clinical practice? At a pragmatic level, these data should not change our treatment of COPD now. In general terms, these data should remind us that α_1AT deficiency is common, and that certain phenotypes other than PiZZ are associated with lung function decline. A better awareness of this situation has implications from the point of view of genetic counselling, as well as our understanding of the genetic factors contributing to clinical COPD. The next step is to work out how patients with PiMZ who have *established* COPD progress—what this study has done is inform us that if one has the *MZ* genotype then the risk of progressing to COPD remains relatively low. Unanswered questions include whether those with PiMZ and established emphysema progress particularly rapidly, and if so, can we prevent progression to established disease by earlier recognition of the (asymptomatic) *MZ* genotype. Finally, it should be noted that the study by Wencker and colleagues, discussed in the next chapter, evaluates the efficacy of α_1AT replacement therapy in patients with severe α_1AT deficiency.

Conclusion

Several important strands of evidence have emerged recently from population-based studies, identifying genetic and environmental influences that may influence the development and/or progression of COPD.

As a result of these studies we are in a stronger position to advise our patients with regard to their weight and their diet. Similarly we are reminded that medications frequently prescribed for COPD may be potentially detrimental if significant (and common) comorbidities exist (for example β-2 agonists in patients with co-existent ischaemic heart disease). Large studies have also provided intriguing insights into genetic factors influencing COPD, allowing us to quantify familial risk more accurately, and clarifying the importance of alternative α_1AT phenotypes in progression of COPD.

Collectively the studies discussed in this chapter are vital to our understanding of the disease. The messages they convey allow us to suggest small interventions that may directly benefit a large proportion of our patients. However, the total beneficial effect for any given patients is likely to be small. This assertion brings us inevitably back to the core issue in COPD, which is that smoking prevention (or cessation) remains by far the most critical intervention of all. All doctors should therefore be assisted by the observations in the first study discussed in this chapter, namely that stopping smoking is beneficial, and remains so regardless of the age at which cessation commences.

References

1. Doll R, Gray R, Haffner B, Peto R. Mortality in relation to smoking: 22 years' observations on female British doctors. *BMJ* 1980; **280**: 967–71.

2. Peto R, Darby S, Deo H, Silcocks P, Whitley E, Doll R. Smoking, smoking cessation, and lung cancer in the UK since 1950: combination of national statistics with two-case control studies. *BMJ* 2000; **321**: 323–9.

10

Advances in 'stable' COPD

Pathogenesis and complications

A more complete picture of the pathogenesis of COPD is beginning to emerge, yet a succession of important questions remains unanswered. While inflammation is central to pathogenesis, debate rages as to which inflammatory cells are most important and which critical interactions between inflammatory cells (and inflammatory mediators) are most important. It is likely that predominant inflammatory influences vary temporally and between different divisions of the airways, and this remains relatively uncharacterized. Clearer understanding of pathogenesis would select rational, novel therapeutic targets and is, therefore, fundamentally important. One of many important studies relating to airway pathology is considered in this section.

Similarly, the central question remains as to why some smokers are susceptible to COPD while most are not. A genetic predisposition to inflammation mediated by smoking is implied, and many groups have investigated the role of candidate genes. The specific role of tumour necrosis factor alpha (TNFα) will be considered because of the central position of this mediator in inflammatory processes.

This section will also consider a paper with no natural home in this chapter, but which is important to clinical practice in challenging our perception of what constitutes bronchodilator 'reversibility' in the clinic. Thereafter the emphasis will move to consider another aspect of the natural history of COPD, namely extrapulmonary complications of the disease. These are increasingly recognized, and clearer evidence is required to optimize their management. Depression, osteoporosis and pulmonary hypertension will be specifically addressed.

Airway inflammation in severe chronic obstructive pulmonary disease. Relationship with lung function and radiologic emphysema.

Turato G, Zuin R, Miniati M, el al. Am J Respir Crit Care Med 2002; **165**: 105–10.

BACKGROUND. The arguments for delineating the inflammatory cells infiltrating airways of patients with COPD, and the interactions between them, have been mentioned above. This study had the specific aim of characterizing and quantifying inflammatory cells in the small airways and pulmonary arteries of smokers with severe

COPD, and comparing these with specimens obtained from smokers who had not developed COPD.

INTERPRETATION. Patients with severe COPD had significantly higher numbers of CD4+ and CD8+ T lymphocytes in small airway walls, and higher numbers of intra-epithelial macrophages than did patients without COPD who were closely matched for age and smoking history. In contrast pulmonary arteries showed similar profiles of inflammatory cells in each group.

Comment

This study examined surgically resected specimens from two distinct groups of patients. The first comprised smokers attending for lung-volume reduction surgery (LVRS), with entry into the study being conditional upon forced expiratory volume$_1$ (FEV$_1$) less than 50% predicted. The second group contained smokers with mild (or no) airflow limitation (FEV$_1$ 70% of predicted or greater) having lung tissue resected for 'localized pulmonary lesions'. The patients ($n = 9$ in each group) had detailed lung function tests and a chest X-ray performed prior to surgery. Resected tissue was scrutinized for the presence of intact airways with an internal perimeter of under 6 mm (diameter less than approximately 2 mm) and muscular pulmonary arteries of internal perimeter under 2 mm (diameter less than approximately 0.5 mm). At least four such airways and 15 such arteries were studied in each patient using immunohistochemical staining of inflammatory cells.

Importantly, while there were only 9 patients in each of the groups, these were very well matched for smoking history (approximately 45 pack years) and age (approximately 62). In contrast, as expected, lung function abnormalities and radiological severity of emphysema were significantly more advanced in the group with severe disease (FEV$_1$ 29% predicted versus 86% predicted, transfer factor for carbon monoxide 30% predicted versus 82% predicted). The authors go to significant lengths to demonstrate that both the airways and arteries examined in each group were of comparable size and morphology.

The patients with severe COPD had more than twice as many leukocytes in the walls of small airways (corrected for airway size) as did controls. The difference was largely explained by there being approximately twice as many CD4+ cells and CD8+ cells in the walls of patients with severe disease. Similarly, approximately three times as many inflammatory cells were found in the airway epithelium of patients with severe COPD, which contained four times as many macrophages as were seen in control epithelium. Interestingly no changes in inflammatory cell numbers were observed in pulmonary arteries from the two groups. The authors describe significant correlations between severity of lung function abnormalities and the number of leukocytes in small airways when these two very different sets of patients are grouped together, but unfortunately the data for each separate group is not presented.

This is the most authoritative analysis of inflammatory cell types in the small airways and pulmonary arteries of patients with COPD to date. The data adds further to the body of evidence implicating tissue macrophages and CD8+ cells in at least the progression of COPD. As with the study by Hattotuwa and colleagues described later in the chapter, the very nature of the samples obtained has implications for detailed interpretation. We are told very little about the surgical procedures performed, but it is highly likely that the upper lobes were removed from all patients in the severe group and that other lobes were removed in half or more of the control group. Therefore, it seems reasonable to assume that the region of lung most susceptible to emphysema was not examined in most of the controls. Risk of significant bias would be less if resected tumours confined to the upper lobes had been a prerequisite for the control group. Furthermore, we are told remarkably little about the control group—one must assume that all 9 had an operable tumour but this is not explicitly stated. Similarly we are not told how long each patient was anaesthetized for—anaesthetics can themselves induce inflammation, though on balance this would be unlikely to explain the differences observed. Furthermore no information is provided about recent infection rates or occupation, each of which could potentially influence the degree of airway inflammation. Finally the number of leukocytes in airway walls, which are central to the paper, appear to be underestimated technically as in both groups the sum of the individual inflammatory cells exceeds the total 'number of leukocytes' quite considerably.

However, despite these considerations the inflammatory changes in the patients with severe COPD are very striking, and consistent with the emerging picture in the literature. The strength of the study lies in its originality and the matched smoking history of the two groups. On balance then, this study fits snugly into the jigsaw indicating that macrophages and CD8+ cells are important in progression of COPD. The task ahead is to determine the sub-sets of patients in which individual cells such as the neutrophil, the CD8+ lymphocyte and the macrophage are important. Perhaps more crucially still we need to establish how the different cell types interact, such that rational targets for therapy can be developed.

Association of tumor necrosis factor-α gene promoter polymorphism with low attenuation areas on high-resolution CT in patients with COPD.

Sakao S, Tatsumi K, Igari H, *et al. Chest* 2002; **122**: 416–20.

BACKGROUND. Unanswered questions such as why only a minority of smokers develop emphysema, why emphysema progresses much more rapidly in some patients as compared with others, and why there are racial differences in the frequency of emphysema remain pivotal to our future understanding of COPD. It seems rational to postulate that genetic factors may have a part to play in answering these questions. As inflammation is central to the progression of COPD, polymorphisms in genes encoding inflammatory mediators (or their inhibitors) are worthwhile candidates for further study. Against this background Sakao and colleagues recently identified an association between a polymorphism in the promoter region of the TNFα gene and development of COPD in a Japanese population |1|. TNFα is a potent inflammatory mediator, and the polymorphism in question results from a single base change at the −308 position of the promoter region, adenine (TNFα −308*2) substituting for the commoner guanine residue (TNFα −308*1). The mutation is said to result in higher concentrations of TNFα *in vitro* |2|. In the present study Sakao and colleagues aimed to identify whether this polymorphism was specifically associated with emphysema as evidenced by high resolution CT scanning.

INTERPRETATION. The TNFα −308*2 polymorphism was twice as common among patients with emphysema deemed to be severe on high resolution computerized tomography (HRCT) as it was among patients with less marked emphysema. However, the difference did not reach statistical significance. Larger studies are required to determine whether this trend is likely to have biological significance.

Comment

The study recruited 84 outpatients with COPD according to American Thoracic Society (ATS) criteria |3|. The patients were cigarette smokers with an FEV_1 of less than 80% predicted. Patients with a history compatible with chronic bronchitis were excluded. All patients gave a blood sample and proceeded to an HRCT scan of thorax.

DNA was prepared from peripheral blood lymphocytes using standard techniques, and a segment of the promoter region for the TNFα gene (−331 to +14) was amplified by polymerase chain reaction. The amplified segment was digested using the restriction enzyme *Nco1* and run out on a gel such that two bands were observed for the TNFα −308*1 allele (325 and 20 base pairs respectively) but only one for the TNFα −308*2 allele, (345 base pairs). Three pre-determined regions of HRCT scans were scored for emphysema whereby no radiological emphysema scored 0, 1–25% emphysema scored 1, 26–50% scored 2, 51–75% scored 3 and 76–100% scored 4. Scoring was performed for each lung at each level and, therefore, the possible range of scores was 0–24. Each scan was independently scored by 3 chest physicians blinded to the other results of the study, and the average score used. Two groups of patients were identified, those with a score greater than 10 (severe emphysema) and those scored at 10 or under.

The severe and non-severe groups were well matched for age (approximately 64 years) and smoking history but FEV_1 was significantly lower in the severe group (40 and 54% of predicted values respectively). Taking all patients together, emphysema score correlated significantly with the FEV_1/FVC ratio. The total frequency of the TNFα −308*1 allele was 85.1% as opposed to 14.9% for the TNFα -308*2 allele. Breaking this down by emphysema score, the TNFα -308*2 allele frequency was 19.3% in the severe group and 10% in the non-severe group, but this trend did not reach statistical significance ($P = 0.09$).

There are a few points to make in relation to these findings. Although the *allele* frequency for TNFα −308*2 was 19.3% in the severe group, there were still only three homozygotes for TNFα −308*2 in the severe group (and none in the non-severe group). Two separate conclusions arise from this. The first is that this study would have been more interesting if TNFα levels in bronchoalveolar lavage fluid (BALF) had been measured (i.e. is TNFα really increased in TNFα -308*2 homozygotes and perhaps, more importantly, is it increased in heterozygotes?). Either way, but particularly if heterozygotes do not generate an excess of TNFα in the lungs, the second conclusion must be that a much larger study would be required to establish whether this polymorphism has an effect on emphysema, and even then it would need to be demonstrably independent of confounding influences such as smoking. A further point is that extrapolation of these data to Western populations would be unwise, especially as the polymorphism was not associated with severity of disease in a Caucasian population |4|. In fact, the genetic background of the population studied here is not explicitly stated, but is assumed to be approximately 100% Japanese.

In summary this study had good scientific rationale and used sound methodology, yet we are again left in the frustrating situation where still bigger studies are required to establish the importance of biologically plausible genetic factors. In the broader context it should be noted that this is only one of an increasing number of studies assessing the impact of polymorphisms in genes encoding a whole variety of potent inflammatory mediators implicated in the pathogenesis of COPD. No clear pattern has yet emerged.

Evaluation of bronchodilator responses in patients with 'irreversible' emphysema.

O'Donnell DE, Forkert L, Webb KA. *Eur Respir J* 2001: **18**: 914–20.

BACKGROUND. O'Donnell *et al.* question the reliability with which FEV_1 gives a global and accurate reflection of expiratory airflow limitation. In particular, they argue that gas trapping is a significant consequence of airflow limitation and therefore lung volumes may provide a sensitive index of expiratory airflow that may be more sensitive to change than FEV_1. If this were the case, then lung volumes may detect responses to treatment that would be missed by reliance upon reversibility in FEV_1. With this in mind, the aim of this study was to evaluate the reduction in lung volume induced by salbutamol in patients deemed to have 'irreversible' airflow limitation according to change in FEV_1.

INTERPRETATION. Among patients with moderate to severe 'irreversible' COPD, residual volume (RV) and functional residual capacity (FRC) showed strikingly significant acute reductions in response to 200 μg salbutamol. Intriguingly, the effects were most marked in patients with most severe gas trapping. While these data suggest that gas trapping can be ameliorated pharmacologically, they are currently insufficient to say whether these effects are sustainable, reproducible, or clinically important with respect to symptoms or outcome.

Comment

This intriguing study recruited 84 patients who had FEV_1 of 50% predicted or less, FEV_1/FVC ratio of less than 70% predicted, diffusing capacity for carbon monoxide 50% predicted or less, a smoking history of at least 20 pack-years, and a rise in post-bronchodilator FEV_1 of less than 10% predicted. The patients went on to have spirometry for measurement of FEV_1, FVC and inspiratory capacity, and constant-volume body plethysmography for measurement of RV and FRC. In each case, measurements were obtained before and between 15–30 min after administration of 200 μg salbutamol. In all cases, patients were asked not to take short acting β-2 agonists within 4 h of reversibility testing. A fall in RV or FRC of greater than 10% predicted was deemed clinically important.

At baseline, patients had fairly advanced emphysema, with average FEV_1 0.77 litres (32% predicted), diffusing capacity for carbon monoxide 37% predicted, and RV 5.2 litres (253% predicted). Mean age was 66 years. In response to salbutamol the mean effect was for RV to fall by 18% of the percentage predicted RV, and for the FRC to fall by 10% of the percentage predicted FRC. In contrast (and as expected) the FEV_1 rose by only 3.4% of the percentage predicted FEV_1. The majority of patients showed an improvement in RV in response to salbutamol, and this effect was more pronounced among patients with severe COPD (i.e. those with FEV_1 less than 30% predicted). Interestingly, a similar trend was observed for the inspiratory capacity—considering all 84 patients the average increase was 190 ml (from mean baseline 1410 ml), but the effect was greater (270 ml) in patients with severe COPD.

These data suggest that subtle pharmacological effects are missed when we rely on the standard bronchodilator reversibility test. The next question to be answered is how important are changes like those detected in RV? As the authors point out the study was not placebo controlled, nor do we know that the effects are reproducible. Furthermore, it would be useful to know whether these changes are sustained and whether they can be improved incrementally with other treatments. One point to consider is that for arithmetic reasons, a small absolute change in a massively increased RV results in an apparently impressive change in the percentage predicted. That is, the patients in this study had predicted RV of around 2.1 litres, an observed RV of 5.2 litres, and an improvement with salbutamol of some 0.37 litres; thus while the per cent predicted change is 0.37/2.1 (a massive 18%), the real change is from 5.2 to 4.83 litres, which is still over twice predicted. In other words, are these apparently impressive changes clinically important? With regard to symptoms the implied answer appears to be no, otherwise most of our patients with severe COPD would feel much better with salbutamol. However, only trials assessing improvements in RV, FRC or inspiratory capacity against symptoms and outcome can properly answer this question. The final point to make is that measurements such as RV remain technically more difficult than FEV_1, and for routine clinical practice easier, alternative tests for subtle reversibility would be required (interestingly the results here suggest that inspiratory capacity could be suitable in this regard).

In summary, this study neatly draws attention to the limitations of conventional reversibility testing, and reminds us that subtle effects of bronchodilators are worth exploring. The challenge now is to demonstrate whether these changes are clinically meaningful.

The emphasis of this section now swings towards the prevalence of complications of COPD, with particular reference to depression, osteoporosis and pulmonary hypertension.

Risk of depression in patients with chronic obstructive pulmonary disease and its determinants.

van Manen JG, Bindels PJE, Dekker FW, Ijzermans CJ, van der Zee JS, Schadé E. *Thorax* 2002; **57**: 412–16.

BACKGROUND. Depression is associated with several chronic diseases. However, previous studies designed to determine whether COPD is specifically associated with depression have been equivocal. The study by van Manen *et al.* aimed to establish whether depression is more common among patients with COPD than controls, and to determine those aspects of COPD (if any) specifically related to depression.

INTERPRETATION. Despite some potential methodological problems it appears that when data is adjusted for comorbidity and demographic factors, depressive symptoms are significantly more common in patients with severe COPD than in controls. Severe physical impairment, minimal bronchodilator reversibility and living alone appeared to be significant determinants of depressive symptoms among patients with COPD.

Comment

This study was performed in a primary care setting in the Netherlands and enrolled large numbers of patients and controls. Patients aged 40 years or over with suspected obstructive airways disease on clinical grounds completed a Center for Epidemiologic Studies Depression (CES-D) questionnaire and had detailed spirometry with reversibility testing to salbutamol. One hundred and sixty-two patients fulfilled the entry criteria which included adequate completion of the CES-D questionnaire, along with FEV_1 less than 80% predicted, reversibility to salbutamol of less than or equal to 12% of predicted FEV_1, a smoking history, and FEV_1/FVC ratio more than 1 standard deviation below predicted before and after salbutamol. Three-hundred and fifty-nine controls were derived from a group of subjects aged 40 years or over in whom there was no clinical evidence of asthma or COPD. All patients and subjects provided demographic data and completed a standard Dutch questionnaire for the detection of comorbidities. Patients with COPD completed the symptoms and activity components of the St George's Respiratory Questionnaire (SGRQ).

Participants were considered by the authors to be depressed if the CES-D score was greater than 15. In determining the prevalence of depression among patients and controls, logistic regression analyses were performed to adjust for demographic factors and comorbidity. A similar strategy was employed specifically among patients with COPD to determine those variables most closely associated with depression.

CES-D greater than 15 was found in 22% of patients with COPD and 17.5% of controls. Among patients with more advanced COPD (FEV_1 less than 50% predicted) the equivalent rate was 25%. When adjusted for comorbidity and demographic factors, depression was found to be significantly higher among patients with severe COPD (2.5 times more common than in controls). Interestingly, no significant difference was found when comparing the overall population with COPD and controls.

Among the cohort of patients with COPD those factors associated with depression after adjustment for all variables studied were living alone (adjusted odds ratio [OR] 2.8), reversibility to salbutamol of less than or equal to 1.1% of predicted FEV_1 (adjusted OR 3.7) and severe physical impairment as judged by a score on the SGRQ activities dimension of over 68.7 (adjusted OR 5.6). Severe symptoms on the SGRQ also showed a trend towards a significant association with depression.

This study is important principally because it included a control group derived from a similar population, and a sufficient number of participants to allow meaningful conclusions. The study provides persuasive evidence for a specific association between COPD (in particular more advanced disease) and depression. The data also strongly suggest that increasing disability and social isolation predict for depression in COPD. On the assumption that depression is under-recognized in clinical practice, the implication must be that we need to identify depression and its determinants more readily in our patients with COPD. The best form of intervention for these patients remains to be determined, but the clear links with isolation and physical impairment imply an important potential role for pulmonary rehabilitation.

While this study has several strengths, a few methodological points should be noted in making an overall interpretation. First, controls were recruited from only 13 of the 28 practices from which patients were derived, and were recruited during spring and summer months (patients were recruited all year round and over a much longer period). It seems plausible that the rate of depression may vary with geographical location, time of year and calendar year, though the expected differences should be small. Secondly, lung function was not performed on the controls and unrecognized COPD may exist in that group (indeed 24 subjects were excluded on the basis of 'self-reported' COPD/asthma). Thirdly, as the authors concede, CES-D measures depressive *symptoms*, not clinical depression (while clinical depression is very common with CES-D scores greater than 15, this is not universal, and therefore, 'depression' is overestimated in the study). Furthermore, many CES-D forms were incomplete, and two of the CES-D questions (impaired appetite and sleep disturbance) are common features of COPD, thus potentially overestimating the number of patients with COPD labelled as depressed. The authors readily acknowledge and discuss most of these points. On balance it seems likely that the association between severe COPD and depressive symptoms would be preserved with correction of these issues, but that the increased risk would be a little less than the 2.5 times described above.

In summary, this study adds some weight to the link between COPD and depressive symptoms, and it seems prudent to advise that we encourage a high index of suspicion for depression in patients with severe COPD, especially those who are disabled and socially isolated.

Bone loss in patients with untreated chronic obstructive pulmonary disease is mediated by an increase in bone resorption associated with hypercapnia.

Dimai HP, Domej W, Leb G, Lau K-HW. *J Bone Miner Res* 2001; **16**: 2132–41.

BACKGROUND. Osteoporosis is associated with COPD, but the mechanisms underlying the association have not been established. Opportunities to address this question are complicated by factors such as relative immobility, cigarette smoking and corticosteroid use, each of which is independently associated with osteoporosis. This study aimed to establish whether chronic hypercapnia and/or acidosis contribute to loss of bone mineral density (BMD) in COPD, and if so whether the principal effect was related to inhibition of bone formation or promotion of bone resorption.

INTERPRETATION. In this study patients with relatively advanced COPD were compared with age- and weight-matched controls. For reasons that were unclear, patients with COPD were not receiving treatment for the condition. BMD was significantly lower in patients with COPD. Furthermore those patients with hypercapnic COPD had significantly lower BMD than those with normal $PaCO_2$. In contrast BMD was equivalent among acidotic and non-acidotic patients with COPD. In general, BMD loss in COPD correlated with markers of bone resorption. The data confirm the association of COPD and osteoporosis and suggest an independent contribution from hypercapnia.

Comment

This study recruited male patients with COPD (according to WHO criteria) who had received no treatment in the preceding 3 months, and who had never been treated with corticosteroids. Patients with primary or tertiary hyperparathyroidism, high creatinine or diabetes mellitus were excluded. Patients had partial quantitative computed tomography (CT) scanning of the distal, non-dominant forearm for calculation of BMD. A history was taken, spirometry was performed, and both arterial and venous blood were drawn for a variety of measurements including calcium, magnesium, parathyroid hormone, calcitonin, ICTP (a marker of bone resorption) and osteocalcin (a marker of bone formation).

Seventy-one patients and 40 'apparently healthy' male controls were recruited. We are told that the controls were matched for age, weight and BMI but we are not told how—given that there are more patients than controls it could be that controls were recruited after patients, which could potentially introduce bias. It is also a little unusual that the 'healthy' controls were drawn 'from the same clinic' (i.e. a respiratory unit) as the patients, but we are told little more about their respiratory health. The COPD group had significantly lower FEV_1/FVC ratio (0.56 versus 0.85), PaO_2 (65 versus 91 mmHg) and pH (7.38 versus 7.40), and higher $PaCO_2$ (47 versus 40 mmHg) as compared with controls. The BMD was dramatically reduced in the COPD group as compared with controls (24% reduction in total BMD, 33% reduction in trabecular BMD, $P < 0.001$ in each case). Among the COPD group BMD was significantly correlated with pH ($r = +0.58$), $PaCO_2$ ($r = -0.44$) and ICTP ($r = -0.44$), but not with osteocalcin. On the basis of these findings patients with COPD were subdivided into those with high ($n = 35$) or normal ($n = 36$) $PaCO_2$ (cut off 45 mmHg). In the hypercapnic group BMD was reduced significantly (Fig. 10.1) and ICTP significantly increased, with no difference in osteocalcin. When subgroup analysis was performed in hypercapnic patients with ($n = 15$) and without ($n = 20$) acidosis (cut-off pH 7.35) no statistically significant difference was found in any parameter, including BMD, ICTP or osteo-calcin.

The conclusion seems to be that a deficit in BMD is common in COPD and more so among hypercapnic patients. Bone resorption would appear to contribute, but inhibition of bone formation has not been rigorously excluded.

The great strength of this paper is the inclusion of patients whose BMD is not influenced by steroid (or other forms of) therapy, allowing study of patients with advanced COPD. However this feature is almost the most controversial aspect of the work, in that it seems remarkable that patients with this severity of disease were

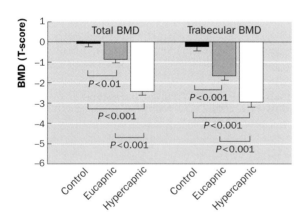

Fig. 10.1 Comparison of total (left panel) and trabecular (right panel) BMD among the subgroup of patients with untreated COPD with eucapnia (middle bars), the subgroup of patients with untreated COPD with hypercapnia (right bars), and age- and weight-matched control subjects (left bars). Source: Dimai et al. (2001).

not on treatment for their COPD. Similarly, the authors use a physical activity index that averages exercise over 15 years in order to demonstrate similar physical activity in patients and controls (because exercise is likely to influence BMD over many years). We are not told the *recent* exercise capacity of these patients and again it would seem very surprising if the COPD patients had not been significantly more immobile for several months or even years, which would potentially favour loss of BMD. Theoretically smoking may also have influenced the results, the COPD patients having over three times higher tobacco exposure, though this is less likely to have influenced the difference between hypercapnic and eucapnic patients with COPD, as the tobacco exposure was higher in the latter. It is not clear whether these collective concerns could explain the study's findings, but on balance, it seems unlikely that they could account for all of the dramatic differences in BMD noted.

Against this background, the effect of hypercapnia on BMD requires confirmation in larger studies. Even then we are left with several questions for clinical practice. First, does low BMD actually translate to meaningful end-points (i.e. increased fracture risk) in COPD, and if so, how can we best restore BMD in COPD? In part this demands clearer delineation of whether enhanced resorption or diminished formation is at the heart of the changes in BMD. Intervention through exercise (for example, pulmonary rehabilitation) and/or pharmacological means would appear worthy of further study also.

'Natural history' of pulmonary hypertension in a series of 131 patients with chronic obstructive lung disease.

Kessler R, Faller M, Weitzenblum E, *et al. Am J Respir Crit Care Med* 2001; **164**: 219–24.

BACKGROUND. It is well established that in patients with very advanced COPD, severe hypoxaemia is associated with the progressive development of pulmonary hypertension. However, less data exists for us to predict whether pulmonary hypertension will ensue in patients with moderate COPD. The current study set out to determine the rate of progression to pulmonary hypertension among a cohort of patients with COPD in which pulmonary artery pressure (PAP) at baseline was normal. An associated aim was to determine those factors at baseline that predict for subsequent pulmonary hypertension.

INTERPRETATION. In patients with moderate COPD resting PAP generally increases very slowly. Indeed only 25% of patients developed pulmonary hypertension over a mean follow up of 6.8 years and in the majority of these PAP was only just above normal. Relative hypoxaemia was retrospectively observed in those patients progressing to pulmonary hypertension, and in this group a more rapid temporal decline in PaO_2 was observed. Resting and exercise PAPs were independently associated with future pulmonary hypertension, but the predictive value of these parameters was disappointingly low.

Comment

This study prospectively evaluated the change in PAP among patients with COPD in whom baseline-resting PAP was known to be normal (less than 20 mmHg). The diagnosis of COPD appears to have been well founded, and patients were only enrolled if their disease was relatively stable, with no recent exacerbations. Patients with obesity, sleep apnoea, left sided heart disease, or co-existent lung disease were excluded, as were patients taking vasoactive drugs or long-term oxygen. Resting and exercise PAPs were performed at the time of the initial right heart catheterization, along with collection of demographic and spirometric data. Patients were invited to have a second right heart catheterization and exercise test after an interval of at least three years.

At baseline, mean age was 55 years, FEV_1 was 1.46 litres and mean PaO_2 was 67 mmHg. Abnormally high exercise PAP was defined at a level of over 30 mmHg; 58% of patients exceeded this pressure at baseline but the mean exercising PAP for the whole group was only 32.4 mmHg. Thus exercise PAP is commonly (but minimally) elevated among patients with normal resting PAP.

The mean interval to the second evaluation of PAP was 6.8 years. Only 60% of patients completed an exercise test the second time round. The changes in PAP with time were statistically significant but clinically very small, the mean resting PAP rising from 15.2 to 17.8 mmHg and the mean exercise PAP rising from 30.7–33.3 mmHg. Overall 25% of patients had developed pulmonary hypertension by the second visit, and this was clinically borderline in most cases. The development of resting pulmonary hypertension was more common among patients with high exercise PAP at the first visit.

Similarly patients who went on to develop pulmonary hypertension were found to have a lower baseline PaO_2. Furthermore, there was a small but significant temporal fall in PaO_2 among these patients, whereas those who remained free of pulmonary hypertension maintained a steady PaO_2 throughout the observation period. The authors went on to perform logistic regression analysis and found that the only independent predictors of subsequent pulmonary hypertension were the resting and exercise PAP at baseline. Unfortunately, the model generated by logistic regression analysis was unhelpful in identifying individual patients progressing to pulmonary hypertension.

The importance of this study for clinical practice is largely derived from the reassuring observation that PAP increases very slowly in patients with moderately severe COPD. The data also informs us that patients with advancing arterial hypoxaemia appear to be at increased risk of pulmonary hypertension, as would be expected clinically. However, one important caveat should be considered in attempting to interpret these data, namely that it is not clear from the paper how many patients undergoing initial study did *not* have follow up, either because they refused, could not be contacted or died. One would anticipate that the number is high. Certainly, it seems likely that the 131 patients described are a self-selecting group, and as such may not be representative of patients with moderately severe COPD in practice.

Inevitably, a paper of this nature generates questions for further study. In particular it would be most interesting to know whether clinical outcome in terms of FEV_1, symptoms and mortality is any different among those patients with and without mild pulmonary hypertension in association with moderate COPD. Such a study would require large numbers and considerable planning but would answer the important question of how much clinical significance to attach to low grade abnormalities in resting and exercise PAP. Similarly, it will be important to determine the effects of pulmonary rehabilitation on outcome, among patients with demonstrable, but mild exercise hypertension such as those described in this study.

Re-evaluation of established treatments for COPD

In general smoking cessation, anticholinergic therapy and short-acting β-2 agonists are central components in the management of stable COPD. Although there is considerable experience with each of these, the optimal way to provide them has not yet been established. This section will consider the introduction of bupropion for smoking cessation in COPD and will discuss studies on tiotropium, a novel anticholinergic agent that will become widely available in the UK very soon.

Certain other treatments are widely accepted under particular circumstances. They include inhaled and oral corticosteroids, long-acting β-2 agonists, methylxanthines, oxygen therapy and pulmonary rehabilitation. Generally speaking our knowledge of exactly who these treatments should be given to (and how) is even less clear, and several studies have addressed such issues in the last two years. A number of these will be considered in this section. Finally, two specific and important areas will be discussed briefly at the end of the section, namely self-management programmes for COPD and palliative care for patients with the disease.

Given the crucial importance of cigarette smoking to the pathogenesis of COPD, it seems appropriate to begin with one of the most important smoking cessation studies published to date.

Smoking cessation in patients with chronic obstructive pulmonary disease: a double-blind, placebo-controlled, randomized trial.
Tashkin DP, Kanner R, Bailey W, et al. Lancet 2001; **357**. 1571–5.

BACKGROUND. Smoking cessation and the administration of long-term oxygen to hypoxaemic patients are the two interventions associated with a reduction in mortality among patients with COPD. The best way in which to effect smoking cessation remains unclear. Bupropion has been shown to increase smoking cessation rates significantly among 'healthy' smokers |5|. This study aimed to establish the efficacy of bupropion in patients with COPD.

INTERPRETATION. Bupropion significantly enhanced complete abstinence measured over weeks 4–8 of a 12-week treatment period. Continued smoking cessation remained significantly higher in the bupropion group after stopping treatment, with 16% of bupropion-treated patients abstinent at 6 months as compared with 9% of patients who received placebo. Bupropion was generally well tolerated, with insomnia the most common attributable adverse event.

Comment

This elegant and important trial recruited by advertisement. Those screened were aged 35 years or over, had smoked at least 15 cigarettes per day in the previous year, and had smoked for at least 9 months of that year. All patients had clinically defined COPD as per ATS criteria. Exclusion criteria included 'major depression' (which is not defined) or other significant comorbidity. Patients in the trial were not permitted theophyllines or corticosteroids.

This was a multicentre (11 USA centres), randomized, double-blind, placebo-controlled trial. During a 1-week screening period, patients targeted a date for smoking cessation, which automatically became day 7 of the treatment period. Patients were advised not to attempt to stop before this date, and therefore, by definition were smoking for the first week of the actual trial. Patients were randomized to slow release bupropion (150 mg daily for 3 days and then 150 mg twice daily for the remainder of the 12-week treatment period), or to placebo. Patients received counselling from a trained smoking cessation counsellor three days after target date and at each subsequent trial visit. Participants kept diary cards describing daily smoking habits, and attended trial visits for assessment of variables such as adverse events and exhaled carbon monoxide (CO). The primary end-point was continuous abstinence from the start of week four to the end of week seven as defined by diary card records of smoking and exhaled CO of less than 10 parts per billion. However, follow up proceeded to 6 months. Data were analysed on an intention to treat basis, which assumed particular importance given that 31% of participants did not complete 6 months of the trial. The authors acknowledge the involvement of the manufacturer of bupropion in the trial.

Four hundred and four patients were included. Patients were well matched at baseline. Smoking histories amounted to around 52 pack years in each group, with recent smoking of around 28 cigarettes per day, and average age was around 54 years. Mean FEV_1 was approximately 70% predicted. However, it should be noted that 95% of patients were white (as opposed to around 80% of the general population) and that a 'history of depression' appeared more common in the placebo group (23 versus 18%). Continuous smoking cessation for the 4–8 week period was 28% in the bupropion group and 16% in the placebo group ($P = 0.003$). Importantly the significant difference was maintained to 6 months, though cessation rates were generally low in each group (Fig. 10.2). Subgroup analysis suggested that heavier smokers were more recalcitrant to cessation but that older patients were more receptive to stopping. There is also a suggestion (though not statistically significant) that advancing severity of COPD predicted for less success in stopping.

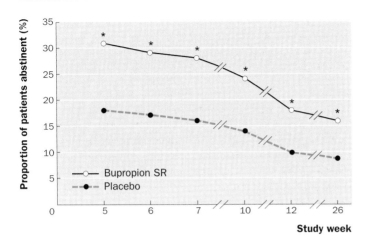

Fig. 10.2 Rates of continuous abstinence for weeks 4–12 and 4–26. *$P < 0.05$. Source: Tashkin *et al.* (2001).

Adverse events were of comparable frequency with only insomnia and marked anxiety being obviously more common in bupropion-treated patients. This resulted in 9 of the 14 withdrawals of bupropion because of adverse advents; there were 13 withdrawals due to adverse events in the placebo group and thus, there were 27 adverse-event withdrawals in total and not 7 as quoted in the paper's abstract. Importantly, no bupropion-treated patients had seizures, which is one theoretical concern.

In general the findings of this trial seem applicable to patients with mild to moderate COPD. However, the fact that a disproportionate number of white patients were enrolled could hint that the trial selected subjects from a generally more affluent background, and the very use of advertisements may select out more motivated patients. A further caveat is the potential to pick out false positives for smoking cessation—especially at 6 months patients (who may feel guilty at having smoked again) would only need to record no smoking in their diaries and abstain for long enough prior to the study visit to record less than 10 parts per billion of exhaled CO. While this effect should be similar in each group, it does hint that even the low cessation rates at 3–6 months could be overestimates. Finally, it may be relevant that there was a higher 'history of depression' in the placebo group. Bupropion has antidepressant properties, and it is conceivable that bupropion improved low-level depression in the treated arm of the study, improving motivation to stop, while the higher rate of low-level depression (itself associated with smoking) may have contributed to continuation of smoking in the placebo group. Such a bias favouring an effect of bupropion may be small, but then so were cessation rates at the end of the study, and it would have been interesting to see validated depression scores before and after treatment for both groups.

Despite these potential concerns, it must be firmly concluded that this landmark trial gives us evidence on which to base our use of bupropion in smokers with mild to moderate COPD. Bupropion effects increased abstinence up to 6 months at least but at this point cessation rates are depressingly low, and only 7% above those with placebo (i.e. 32 versus 18 patients were continuously abstinent at 6 months). In this setting, the remaining question is whether these rates justify use of the drug. In my opinion, at the present time they do, as the effects of continued smoking are so important. All patients should be offered a concerted trial of available smoking cessation strategies to include nicotine replacement therapy, counselling, smoking cessation clinics and bupropion (obviously, these are not mutually exclusive). A direct comparison of bupropion against nicotine replacement therapy (and against the combination of these and/or other anti-smoking treatments) is required in patients with COPD, as are long-term cost–benefit analyses.

Inhaled corticosteroids and the risk of mortality and readmission in elderly patients with chronic obstructive pulmonary disease.

Sin DD, Tu JV. *Am J Respir Crit Care Med* 2001; **164**: 580–4.

BACKGROUND. A recurring theme in this chapter is the controversy surrounding the use of inhaled corticosteroids in COPD. The large multi-centre trials on which most of our evidence is based suggest that inhaled steroids do little if anything to influence the rate of decline of FEV_1, but that they may (especially in patients with more severe disease) influence other disease-specific variables such as the rate of exacerbations and quality of life |6–9|. Little convincing evidence previously existed to support a beneficial effect of inhaled steroids on mortality. This study, therefore, aimed to establish the association between use of inhaled steroids and both mortality and hospital re-admission in a group of elderly patients with severe COPD.

INTERPRETATION. In this large, observational study following the progress of patients discharged from hospital after an exacerbation of COPD, inhaled steroids were associated with a 24% reduction in the risk of hospital re-admission for COPD and a 29% reduction in risk from all-cause mortality. The apparent protective effect was maintained after correction for potentially important confounding variables. Therefore, allowing for the significant restraints of observational studies, inhaled steroids appeared to confer benefit in elderly patients discharged from hospital after an exacerbation of COPD. However, this association requires to be confirmed within the framework of a prospective, randomized, placebo-controlled trial.

Comment

This retrospective, longitudinal cohort study identified patients aged 65 years or over, who were admitted to hospital with a principal reason for admission consistent with COPD (derived from hospital discharge, database systems). The study recruited over a 5-year period, each patient being followed for up to a year post-discharge, the primary end-points being death (as recorded by the regional registry) or re-admission to hospital during that year. Patients were excluded if they died within 30 days of discharge. The 'inhaled steroid group' comprised patients receiving a prescription for inhaled steroids within 90 days of discharge from the index admission (prescription monitoring was evaluated from a regional therapeutic database, which also provided information on other medicines prescribed for COPD).

A remarkable number of 22 620 patients were studied, and categorized into two groups depending on whether inhaled steroids were prescribed. The inhaled steroid group (51% of all patients) were receiving significantly more COPD treatments (including β-2 agonists, anticholinergics, oral steroids, antibiotics and theophyllines), had visited the emergency room more often in the year prior to the index admission, but were slightly younger (74.7 versus 75.5 years) and had slightly less comorbidity as assessed by the Charlson Index.

Crude analysis revealed a 10% reduction in repeat admission for COPD or death (95% CI 6–15%) in the group receiving inhaled corticosteroids. When adjusted for a number of covariates the adjusted relative risk was 0.74 (95% CI 0.71–0.78) (Fig. 10.3). When studied separately the reduction in risk for all cause mortality was 29%, whilst that for readmission for COPD was 24%. The analysis was repeated

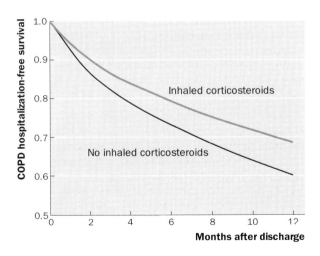

Fig. 10.3 Adjusted probability of hospitalization-free survival in patients with COPD who did and did not receive inhaled corticosteroids post-discharge (within 90 days of discharge). Source: Sin and Tu (2001).

with stratification for age and number of comorbidities, and the protective effect was maintained even in patients above 84 years or with advanced comorbidity. Importantly, when other COPD medications were studied in the same model β-2 agonists and anticholinergics had no influence on outcome. Antibiotics and theophyllines were associated with a significant increase in re-admission (but not mortality), while oral corticosteroids were associated with a striking and significant increase in both parameters (see the discussion of the paper by Schols *et al.* later in this section).

This intriguing study set out to study elderly, ill patients specifically because an effect on mortality was more likely to be observed in this group. Indeed the authors contend that previous large studies may not have observed a protective effect of inhaled steroids precisely because they included patients with milder disease. The results here are strikingly and significantly in favour of inhaled steroids. In patients with more severe COPD, inhaled steroids do appear to reduce exacerbations |12|, and it may be that this explains the changes observed by Sin and Tu. This begs the question of whether we should use inhaled steroids in such patients. Before trying to give a view on this, a few limitations of the study (which the authors readily attest to) are worth mentioning.

First, hospital databases, pharmacy registries, death registries, and insurance databases are notoriously inaccurate, and the reliability of diagnosis in particular must be called into question. The observational nature of the study does not allow confirmation of the diagnosis of COPD (or indeed objective confirmation of severity, though we obviously know that these patients had at least one admission and a high rate of attendance at outpatients/emergency rooms). This raises the possibility that the protection is conferred by treating 'hidden' asthma that is over-represented in the group receiving inhaled steroids. Certainly, 'anti-asthma' treatment is much higher in the inhaled steroid group, and the prevalence of inhaled steroids themselves seems suspiciously high for the treatment of COPD, given that the study occurred prior to the publication of major trials investigating efficacy of these drugs in COPD. If a lot of late onset asthma were inadvertently labelled as 'bronchitis' in hospital coding, a confounding effect would explain at least some of the protection observed. Similarly, we have no information on socio-economic status, and it could be postulated that health care access and provision could have been poorer in the 'non-inhaled steroid group'. Extending this theme, we have no information on smoking status or heart disease—it could be plausible that more patients in the control group smoked and/or had more clinically apparent heart disease/left ventricular failure such that inhaled steroids for 'chronic breathlessness' were (appropriately) not prescribed. Indeed this epitomises the problem of observational studies, in that such speculation could go on and on.

As mentioned above the authors are the first to acknowledge these restraints, and make good cases against some of these potential confounding variables. They also make the powerful argument that this fascinating data demands a prospective, randomized, controlled trial of inhaled steroids in elderly patients, and this appears to be exactly what is required. In the meantime, it should be cautiously concluded that this study adds to the body of evidence supporting use of inhaled steroids in elderly patients with severe COPD.

Effects of withdrawal of inhaled steroids in men with severe irreversible airflow obstruction.

O'Brien A, Russo-Magno P, Karki A, *et al. Am J Respir Crit Care Med* 2001;
164: 365–71.

BACKGROUND. Although the evidence to support the use of inhaled corticosteroids in COPD is equivocal, a high proportion of patients with the disease end up on this therapy. In a significant proportion of these patients a persuasive argument can be made for discontinuation of inhaled steroids on the grounds of cost and potential side-effects in the face of limited proven efficacy. Very little is known about the effects of withdrawing medication in this setting. This study aimed firstly to identify the prevalence of 'unnecessary' prescriptions for inhaled steroids, and secondly to establish the effect of withdrawing inhaled corticosteroids in male patients with COPD.

INTERPRETATION. No clear indication for maintenance inhaled steroids could be found in 35% of patients in the authors' institution. In a prospective, randomized, placebo-controlled, crossover study, withdrawal of inhaled steroids was associated with a small but significant reduction in pre-bronchodilator FEV_1 and with an increase in exertional dyspnoea. However, the design and small size of this study makes interpretation of these findings more difficult.

Comment

In the first part of this study, a random sample of patients receiving repeat prescriptions for inhaled steroids was identified. Medical records were scrutinized for predetermined indications for inhaled steroids that were taken to include one or more from asthma, bronchodilator reversibility, bronchial hyper-reactivity and documented responsiveness to steroids, prescription of oral steroids, blood eosinophilia and elevated total IgE. None of these criteria was satisfied in 35% of patients. Even allowing for difficulties inherent in retrospective case record analysis, this figure is impressive.

In the second part of the study all patients receiving inhaled steroids at the authors' hospital were identified, and their medical records used to describe those with irreversible airways disease. We are told nothing about the ensuing screening process, nor the numbers involved, but 24 patients consented to further study. Patients discontinued their inhaled steroid and they were then randomized into two groups. The first group received placebo metered dose inhaler (MDI) four times daily for six weeks and then crossed over to beclomethasone dipropionate (BDP) MDI 84µg four times daily for a further six weeks. In the second group the order of BDP and placebo was reversed. Compliance was evaluated by weighing of

MDI canisters. Assessment occurred at baseline and then at three-week intervals, and incorporated spirometry, six-minute walk with assessment of dyspnoea, and assessment of quality of life using the Chronic Respiratory Diseases Questionnaire (CRDQ). Importantly, analysis included data only from patients completing the trial, and was not, therefore, on an intention to treat basis.

The starting cohort of 24 patients comprised men with at least 20 pack-year smoking histories. The mean age was 67 years, mean FEV_1 was 1.6 litres. Nine patients withdrew (6 failed to return after one visit, 3 had exacerbations) leaving 15 for analysis. Mean pre-bronchodilator FEV_1 fell 100 ml from baseline after placebo (1.7–1.6 litres) and rose 40 ml from baseline (1.63–1.67 litres) after treatment with BDP ($P <0.05$). Only 7 patients completed a six-minute walk. Among these there was a fall in the Borg dyspnoea scale while on BDP and a rise while on placebo ($P <0.05$), though it should be noted that the baseline Borg scale before BDP was 20% lower than that before starting placebo. No differences were observed with respect to quality of life or walking distance. Finally, all 3 patients withdrawn from the study with exacerbations were receiving placebo at the time, but it is impossible to draw any conclusion from this, not least because the study was not analysed on an intention to treat basis.

This study addresses an important clinical issue. Thousands of doctors will contemplate stopping inhaled steroids for COPD every year. On balance it seems reasonable to conclude that we should monitor our patients in the period following discontinuation of inhaled steroids, but these data should not prevent the withdrawal of unnecessary treatment. Further interpretation seems extremely difficult mainly because of the very low numbers. As mentioned above it is hard to understand why numbers were so low—from the data in the paper it would appear that well over 100 patients ought to have been eligible. In addition, patients with concurrent co-morbidity such as heart disease and sleep apnoea were not excluded (indeed exclusion criteria do not appear to be explicitly stated). Quite aside from these methodological considerations, the question is whether a fall in FEV_1 of 100 ml (in the absence of any change in symptoms as assessed by CRDQ) or a rise in exercise Borg dyspnoea score of 0.85 clinically significant?

In summary, this study looked at a prevalent and important clinical issue, and much larger studies incorporating a longer observation period should be designed. We should continually question whether inhaled steroids are necessary in individual patients with COPD, as it seems a high proportion of patients continue to receive these unnecessarily. We should stop inappropriate inhaled steroids with the reassurance that this leads to only a very small average clinical detriment, but we should monitor our patients over this period.

The effects of inhaled fluticasone on airway inflammation in chronic obstructive pulmonary disease: a double-blind, placebo-controlled biopsy study.

Hattotuwa KL, Gizycki MJ, Ansari TW, Jeffery PK, Barnes NC. *Am J Respir Crit Care Med* 2002; **165**: 1592–6.

BACKGROUND. The drive to characterize the predominant inflammatory cell types infiltrating the airway during stable COPD (and exacerbations of the disease) is stimulated by the desire to identify new, logical therapeutic targets. As discussed already evidence to date suggests a relatively prominent involvement of CD8+ T lymphocytes and tissue macrophages in COPD. This study aimed to determine whether inhaled corticosteroids beneficially alter the inflammatory profile in the airways of patients with COPD, and to evaluate whether there were corresponding changes in symptoms.

INTERPRETATION. Using a randomized, double-blind, placebo-controlled design, this study demonstrated that the ratio of CD8+:CD4+ T lymphocytes in the bronchial epithelium, and the number of mast cells in the sub-epithelium were significantly reduced as a consequence of fluticasone administered for 3 months, though it should be noted that significance was lost after correction for multiple comparisons. The frequency of exacerbations, cough and reliever bronchodilator use was also reduced in the steroid-treated group.

Comment

This study addressed a pivotal question for understanding the pathology of COPD. Patients were recruited from respiratory clinics and by advertisement and were eligible if aged 40–75 years, with a smoking history, FEV_1 of 25–80% predicted with no reversibility to 200 µg salbutamol (i.e. less than 15%/200 ml rise in FEV_1 from baseline), and no recent exacerbations. Patients stopped any prescribed inhaled steroids and then had an 8-week run-in after which they had bronchoscopy with biopsy of second order carinae from all lobes. Within 2 weeks of this, patients were randomized to receive twice daily placebo or 500 µg of fluticasone propionate via Accuhaler for three months, after which bronchoscopy with biopsies was repeated. Patients then had a one-month wash out period prior to a trial of oral prednisolone for 2 weeks. The authors acknowledge that the manufacturer of fluticasone funded the study in part.

Biopsies were stained using labelled monoclonal antibodies directed at inflammatory cell markers, and samples were analysed for epithelial integrity and the number of inflammatory cells within epithelium and sub-epithelium (to a predetermined depth). Patients kept diary cards and were invited for regular spirometry. Thirty-seven patients were enrolled. Five withdrew/were withdrawn (3 of whom required systemic steroids for exacerbation), 1 died, and 1 had incomplete biopsies, leaving 30 patients in the final analysis (i.e. data analysis was not on an intention to treat basis). It should be noted that a further 7 patients in the placebo group and 3 in the steroid group had exacerbations and these patients received antibiotics and more intensive bronchodilators but remained in the study.

The primary end-point of the study was determination of macrophage and CD8+ T lymphocyte numbers. Neither of these cell types were significantly altered by fluticasone, nor were neutrophils, CD4+ T lymphocytes or eosinophils. Indeed the only significant changes observed were in epithelial mast cells and sub-epithelial CD8:CD4 ratio (both reduced in the steroid group). However, when Bonferroni's correction for multiple comparisons was applied, even these differences were non-significant. Little information is given about epithelial integrity, but it appears to have been largely preserved in each group. The number of exacerbations was significantly lower in the fluticasone group (but appears to have been analysed on an intention to treat basis), as was cough, use of reliever medication and sputum score.

Studies of this nature are notoriously difficult to design, perform and interpret and there is little doubt that this study made strenuous efforts to minimize such problems. The data presented readily illustrates the inter-individual variation in inflammatory cell numbers in biopsies, and (judging by the placebo group) the within individual/between biopsy variation, which may in part explain an apparently significant increase in CD4+ cells in the epithelium and sub-epithelium of the placebo group. Other factors beyond the authors' control may well have influenced the study, including the increased use of antibiotics in the placebo group, the slightly higher prevalence of current smoking in the placebo group, and the fact that 11 patients (7 placebo, 4 steroid-treated) had bronchodilator reversibility at the end of the study. If this had been manifest at the start, these patients would have been excluded. Unfortunately the unavoidable conclusion is that greater patient numbers will be required (in exactly this sort of study) to see differences in inflammatory cell numbers. The wide variation in COPD severity at entry strengthens this point. The other potentially relevant question is whether one is looking at a level of airway epithelium that is important in any given individual's disease. As the authors point out, the pathology of COPD intrinsically affects small airways and alveolar tissue, and (other than in patients with features of chronic bronchitis) the importance of inflammatory changes in tissue as proximal as that studied here is difficult to assess.

The overall conclusion on the basis of this evidence is that the symptomatic improvement effected within 3 months by fluticasone does not correlate with major changes in those cells implicated in the inflammatory process. However, there is a tantalising suggestion that this interpretation would change in larger studies conducted with the same design strategy. Inflammatory changes in the airways were also considered when discussing the paper by Turato *et al.* in the previous section.

Dose-dependent increased mortality risk in COPD patients treated with oral glucocorticoids.

Schols AMWJ, Wesseling G, Kester ADM, *et al. Eur Respir J* 2001; **17**: 337–42.

BACKGROUND. **While the use of oral corticosteroids in exacerbations of COPD is both widespread and established, the place of maintenance oral corticosteroids for patients with severe disease is far more contentious. Interestingly there is little hard evidence to support or discourage the use of maintenance oral corticosteroids in this context. Against this background, this retrospective study aimed to evaluate the association between maintenance oral corticosteroids and mortality in moderate to severe COPD, whilst specifically adjusting for confounding variables associated with poor outcome in the disease.**

INTERPRETATION. This study demonstrated that oral corticosteroids are independently associated with a significantly increased risk of all-cause mortality in patients with moderate to severe COPD. The risk appears to be dose-dependent, and manifest from a dose of 10 mg prednisolone per day (or equivalent). Intriguingly, concomitant use of inhaled corticosteroids is associated with a reduction in the relative risk of mortality attributable to oral corticosteroids.

Comment

This important study retrospectively analysed outcome among patients with COPD who had been admitted to a single Dutch institute for a period of pulmonary rehabilitation between 1987 and 1991. The patients were deemed clinically stable at the time, and were eligible for the present study if they satisfied ATS criteria for COPD with FEV_1 less than 70% predicted and less than 15% increase in predicted FEV_1 in response to salbutamol. Furthermore, patients were excluded if they had significant comorbidities known to affect mortality (including cancer, cardiovascular disease and insulin-dependent diabetes).

Five hundred and fifty-six patients were analysed. It is assumed (though not explicitly stated) that these were the only patients fulfilling study criteria. Data pertaining to smoking habit, spirometry, resting arterial blood gases, and BMI were obtained. All-cause mortality was determined for the group, but we are not told how.

The group had an average age of 65 years, pre-bronchodilator FEV_1 of 36% predicted, PaO_2 of 8.9 kPa and $PaCO_2$ 5.4 kPa. Interestingly, after adjustment for FEV_1, BMI, arterial blood gases, age and smoking habit in a multivariate model, maintenance oral corticosteroids at 10 mg prednisolone per day (or equivalent) had a relative risk for all-cause mortality of 2.3 (95% CI 1.2–4.4, $P < 0.01$) as compared with taking no steroids. This rose to 4.0 for 15 mg prednisolone per day (95% CI 2.0–8.1, $P < 0.001$) but was not significant for 5 mg prednisolone per day (relative risk 2.3, 95% CI 0.9–5.8, $P = 0.08$). The corresponding survival curves are

shown in Fig. 10.4. Intriguingly the co-existent administration of inhaled corticosteroids led to a relative reduction in the risk associated with 10 mg prednisolone
(to 1.6, not significant) and 15 mg prednisolone (to 1.6, not significant). When
patients taking inhaled corticosteroids alone were analysed, mortality was not

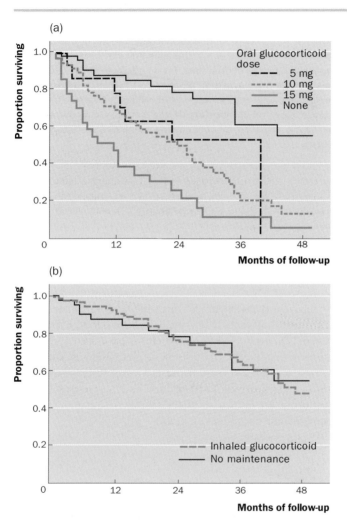

Fig. 10.4 Kaplan–Meier plot: (a) oral glucocorticoid use categorized by dose (5 mg,
10 mg and 15 mg) compared to no maintenance glucocorticoid treatment; (b) inhaled
glucocorticoid use compared to no maintenance glucocorticoid treatment. Oral GC 0 mg:
$n = 43$, log rank test; 5 mg: $n = 16$, Chi-squared $= 3.65$, $P = 0.056$; 10 mg: $n = 59$,
Chi-squared $= 14.75$, $P = 0.0001$; 15 mg: $n = 32$, Chi-squared $= 24.88$, $P = 0.000$.
Inhaled GC: $n = 156$, Chi-squared $= 0.05$, non-significant. Source: Schols *et al.* (2001).

significantly different when compared with individuals not taking steroids of any description.

The authors readily acknowledge that there are limitations in the study, particularly with regard to retrospective design and the fact that there is no information pertaining to the duration or initial indication for steroids. This may be important, as it remains possible that those patients prescribed maintenance oral steroids were precisely those who had multiple exacerbations and were, therefore, at highest risk of death in the first place. Indeed, in an ideal world it would have been interesting to see the influence of exacerbation frequency, duration of corticosteroid therapy and the influence of other prescribed medications (for example, theophyllines) on the model described in this study. Furthermore, it would have been interesting to know more about cause of death, even within the limitations of information derived from death certificates. In particular, it would have been interesting to know how many patients died as a direct consequence of COPD.

Overall, however, this study is timely and welcomed, providing us with valuable clinical information. It strengthens considerably the argument against giving maintenance prednisolone in COPD (certainly at or above 10 mg prednisolone and probably at 5 mg prednisolone) unless under exceptional clinical circumstances. The study makes a relatively neutral contribution to the debate on using inhaled corticosteroids in moderate to severe COPD. The authors go on to provide interesting speculation regarding the mechanism by which oral steroids might increase risk of mortality. They argue that myopathy (and perhaps impaired immunity) may contribute, but of course have no data to support these hypotheses. The remaining question is why inhaled corticosteroids appear to protect against the increased mortality associated with maintenance oral corticosteroids? Whilst a specific effect of inhaled steroids might be invoked, it should be noted that patients receiving oral steroids alone took a higher average dose (equivalent to 10.2 mg) than those concomitantly taking inhaled steroids (oral dose equivalent to 8.9 mg prednisolone). This apparent protective effect of inhaled steroids, therefore, requires to be confirmed in other large studies.

A long-term evaluation of once-daily inhaled tiotropium in chronic obstructive pulmonary disease.

Casaburi R, Mahler DA, Jones PW, *et al. Eur Respir J* 2002; **19**: 217–24.

BACKGROUND. The theoretical advantages of tiotropium for the management of COPD have been known for some time. In particular, by prolonged engagement of M3 muscarinic receptors tiotropium should exert a more prolonged bronchodilator effect than conventional anticholinergic drugs. This study aimed to demonstrate the efficacy and safety of tiotropium given for one year to patients with COPD.

INTERPRETATION. This was a multi-centre, double-blind, placebo-controlled trial comparing 18 µg of tiotropium once daily with placebo. Tiotropium resulted in a rapid and significant rise in pre-bronchodilator FEV_1 of around 110 ml and this was maintained over the 1-year follow-up period. Patients taking tiotropium were significantly less breathless, appeared to have fewer exacerbations, and had a statistically significant improvement in quality of life. The predominant adverse effect associated with tiotropium was dry mouth, experienced by 16% of patients as opposed to 2% among those taking placebo.

Comment

This study recruited outpatients aged 40 years or over who satisfied ATS criteria for COPD, had at least a 10 pack-year history of smoking, an FEV_1 65% of predicted or lower, and in whom disease had been deemed stable. Exclusion criteria included any suggestion of allergy, significant heart disease, a requirement for domiciliary oxygen, or maintenance oral corticosteroids equivalent to 10 mg prednisolone per day or more. Fifty centres were involved in the study, though unusually the paper does not list these. We are not told how many patients were screened. The authors acknowledge that the manufacturers of tiotropium were the sole funding body for the trial.

Patients had a 2-week baseline period during which one must assume (though it is not explicitly stated) that the 55% or more of patients taking anticholinergics had these stopped, and that long acting β-2 agonists were discontinued also (it is not clear how many patients were receiving these prior to the trial). Those patients already on theophyllines, inhaled corticosteroids (ICS) or oral corticosteroids (if less than the equivalent of 10 mg prednisolone per day) were allowed to continue these, and were allowed albuterol as required for symptom relief. Patients were randomized to receive one year of tiotropium 18 μg, or placebo, each delivered once a morning via a dry powder inhaler. Patients kept diary cards that included peak expiratory flow (PEF), symptom scores and bronchodilator use. In addition regular visits incorporated measurements such as spirometry, assessment of dyspnoea (using the Transition Dyspnoea Index), and assessment of generic and disease-specific health status using the Short Form 36 (SF-36) and SGRQ respectively. Exacerbations and adverse events were reported during assessment visits.

The two groups were well matched at baseline. Mean FEV_1 for all participants was 1.02 litres (just below 40% predicted) and the average age was 65. The study randomized on a 3:2 ratio such that more patients were in the tiotropium arm ($n = 550$) than in the placebo group ($n = 371$), on the basis that this would be more informative with respect to adverse events. Importantly, throughout the study tiotropium was associated with a pre-treatment FEV_1 approximately 110 ml higher than that at baseline or that recorded in the placebo group (Fig. 10.5). It should be noted that theophyllines, β-2 agonists and inhaled corticosteroids were stopped for several hours before spirometry, and the bronchodilator effect, therefore, can be attributed to tiotropium. In general, PEF measurements also conformed to a pattern of rapid and sustained bronchodilatation in the tiotropium group. Dyspnoea index was significantly better in the tiotropium group throughout and patients reported less wheeze (but not cough). Tiotropium significantly improved each aspect of the SGRQ relative to placebo, but the mean effect fell just short of a 4-point difference (which is considered clinically significant). Exacerbations and self-reported albuterol use were significantly reduced in the tiotropium group. Adverse events were common in both groups—dry mouth explained all of the excess adverse events in the tiotropium group but less than 1% of patients had to withdraw because of this.

This large trial provides compelling evidence for efficacy of tiotropium in moderately severe COPD. These data, coupled with the convenience of once daily dosing make it likely that tiotropium will make a big impact on clinical practice, if costs can be kept affordable. However, while this trial is overall, very convincing, certain aspects (and some frustrating omissions as mentioned above) require attention. First, we are told that 'bronchodilator responsiveness was not an entry criterion' but we are not told how many patients did have bronchodilator reversibility, nor the frequency and magnitude of this. While the authors exclude asthma from the study, the PEF for the placebo group is notably lower in the mornings than the evenings, and there is some 10 litres/minute variation in the morning values. The suspicion, in the absence of further information, is that some patients with an

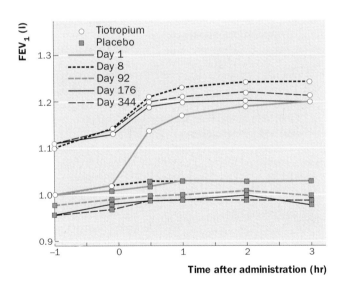

Fig. 10.5 Mean response to tiotropium or placebo on days 1, 8, 92, 176 and 344 of the 1-year trial. Note that the elevation over baseline prior to drug administration on days subsequent to the first treatment day in the tiotropium group is evidence of tiotropium's 24-h duration of action. The SEM for the mean differences between groups ranged 0.01–0.02 L. FEV_1: forced expiratory volume in 1 second.
Source: Casaburi *et al.* (2002).

'asthmatic phenotype' have crept in to the study, making a demonstrable broncho-dilator effect for tiotropium more likely. Second, we are told that 24% of patients discontinued the trial at 9 months because of drug expiry, which seems amazing! Third, it seems possible that exacerbations will have been under-reported as the rate was dependent on patients' memory at interview and the rate of exacerbation seems a little lower than in other studies. Fourth, it is a pity that compliance was not measured, given the advantages of once daily dosing, and that we are told nothing about 16 adverse events attributed to tiotropium that were not due to dry mouth. Finally, we are told that this study is the amalgamation of two identical trials, one of which was designed to assess efficacy, the other safety—the purists might contend that it is hard to justify adding data specifically designed to look at efficacy to a trial assessing safety (and vice versa) without definitive evidence that the two trials were identical in all respects.

Despite these issues, tiotropium appears to be a welcome addition to the thera-peutic arsenal for COPD.

A 6-month, placebo-controlled study comparing lung function and health status changes in COPD patients treated with tiotropium or salmeterol.

Donohue JF, van Noord JA, Bateman ED, et al. Chest 2002; **122**: 47–55.

BACKGROUND. The optimal means by which to effect sustained, symptomatically beneficial bronchodilatation in COPD remains undetermined. The emergence of efficacious long acting β-2 agonists and anticholinergics demands a comparison of these in the management of COPD. This study, therefore, aimed to compare the safety and efficacy of tiotropium bromide and salmeterol over a 6-month period.

INTERPRETATION. Tiotropium produced significantly higher pre-bronchodilator FEV_1 than both salmeterol and placebo at 24 weeks. At this time-point tiotropium also improved symptomatic dyspnoea and health-related quality of life (as measured by standard, validated questionnaires) as compared with salmeterol and placebo. Dry mouth affected 10% of patients taking tiotropium but did not lead to any patients discontinuing the study.

Comment

It should be noted from the outset that this study was funded by (and all authors were/had been affiliated to) the manufacturer of tiotropium. The study was con-ducted in 39 centres from 12 countries, though the relative contribution from indi-vidual countries/centres is not apparent. This was a randomized, placebo-controlled, double-blind, double-dummy, parallel-group study, and the doses of tiotropium and salmeterol used are likely to be their optimal clinical doses. Entry criteria includ-ed FEV_1 of 60% predicted or less, FEV_1/FVC ratio of 0.7 or less, age 40 or over, and a smoking history of over 10 pack-years. Bronchodilator reversibility did not feature in entry criteria. Patients were excluded if they had experienced recent infection, if they had evidence of allergy, or if they had significant comorbidity.

During a 2-week run-in patients discontinued any prescribed long-acting β-2 agonists and any anticholinergics. Other maintenance treatments were continued. Patients were then randomized to tiotropium dry powder device (DPD) 18 μg daily (plus placebo MDI twice daily, $n = 209$), salmeterol MDI 50 μg twice daily (plus placebo DPD once daily, $n = 213$), or placebo (placebo DPD once daily plus placebo MDI twice daily, $n = 201$) for a further 24 weeks. Assessments included spirometry as well as a standardized questionnaire assessing breathlessness (the baseline and transtion dyspnoea indices, BDI and TDI) and the SGRQ (as an index of health-related quality of life). In addition patients kept diary cards for PEF and rescue (short acting) β-2 agonist use. It appears that the study was not analysed on an intention to treat basis (though this is not stated).

The three groups were very well matched at baseline, with average age 65 years, pre-bronchodilator FEV_1 1.08 litres (40% predicted), and broadly similar use of medication. Both salmeterol and tiotropium effected rapid and sustained broncho-dilatation, but at 24 weeks, both pre- and post-bronchodilator FEV_1 was significantly higher in the tiotropium group (Fig. 10.6). A few points are worth noting here. First, the effectiveness of salmeterol appears greater at week 2 than at week 24 (Fig. 10.6), implying tachyphylaxis for salmeterol but not tiotropium. Second, that FEV_1 falls back to pre-bronchodilator values by 12 hours in the salmeterol group and not the tiotropium group is unsurprising because tiotropium has a longer duration of action. Third, the magnitude of increase in the tiotropium group is hard to assess—while the figure suggests pre-bronchodilator FEV_1 is about 100 ml greater at 24 weeks than at baseline (Fig. 10.6), another table in the paper puts the baseline pre-bronchodilator FEV_1 in this group at 1.11 litres, which would make the absolute change at 24 weeks rather less impressive. Fourth, the authors measured pre-bronchodilator FEV_1 60 and 10 minutes before treatment—for some reason the value increased over this 50 minute period in all groups, suggesting inherent variability in baseline or some additional placebo/'training' effect of up to 40 ml. Evening (but not morning) PEF was significantly higher in the tiotropium group than in the salmeterol group.

The transition dyspnoea index (TDI) improved significantly in the tiotropium group as compared with both other groups. While the magnitude of the difference when compared with salmeterol was statistically significant, the mean difference was less than 1 (the level of change considered clinically significant). Similarly the total change in SGRQ was significantly improved in the tiotropium group by 5 points (a change of 4 is deemed clinically significant) but the mean difference as compared with salmeterol or placebo was only 3 points. We are told nothing about the symptom or activity domains of the SGRQ. Both salmeterol and tiotropium reduced reliever β-2 agonist use to a similar extent. Remarkably little is written about adverse events, except that discontinued participation because of these was significantly less in the tiotropium group. Indeed the only drug related adverse event we are told about is dry mouth, present in 10% of the tiotropium group, but not necessitating withdrawal in any patient.

This is a large and well-designed study. There are a few points to discuss however. First, each of the longitudinal analyses in the paper uses slightly different numbers of patients (for each group, this tends to be somewhere between the number at enrolment and the number finishing the trial). We are told that some missing spirometric values 'were estimated using other values recorded for the patient on that test day'. However, on the assumption that the data were not

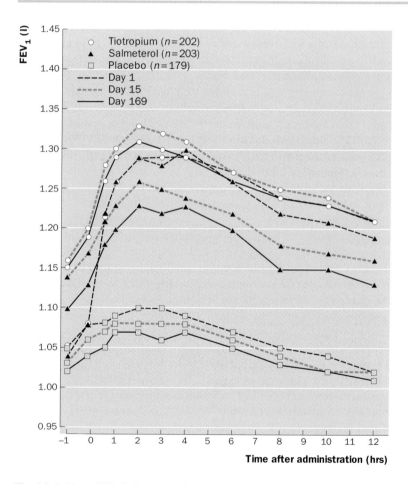

Fig. 10.6 Mean FEV_1 before and after administration of tiotropium, salmeterol and placebo on days 1, 15 and 169 of treatment. $P < 0.001$ for tiotropium vs placebo on all test days post-treatment; $P < 0.05$ for tiotropium vs salmeterol on all test days except day 1 and −1 h on day 15. Source: Donohue *et al.* (2002).

analysed on an intention to treat basis, it is difficult for the reader to work out exactly how the numbers in each analysis were derived. While this is unlikely to affect interpretation of the overall data very much, it is a little confusing. Second, for the practicing chest physician it is frustrating (though ultimately understandable) that a fourth arm combining tiotropium with salmeterol was not included. Third, it should be noted that over 50% of patients in the study had maintenance anticholinergics stopped in the run-in period whilst β-2 agonists (in the form of salbutamol) were continued. It is theoretically conceivable that up-regulated anticholinergic responsiveness early in the study would have favoured a response to tiotropium (though this would not explain findings later in the study). Finally, the costs of each treatment were not evaluated.

Overall, however, this study makes a persuasive argument for tiotropium being more effective than salmeterol in the maintenance treatment of COPD. It remains to be seen whether additional benefit is conferred by using both treatments together.

The addition of salmeterol 50 μg bid to anticholinergic treatment in patients with COPD: a randomized, placebo controlled trial.

Chapman KR, Arvidsson P, Chuchalin AG, *et al. Can Respir J* 2002;
9: 178–85.

B A C K G R O U N D . **In recent years increasing evidence has emerged to support a role for long acting β-2 agonists in the treatment of COPD. The potential for these drugs to make a significant additional contribution to concurrent therapies for COPD is less well established. Therefore, the aim of this study was to evaluate the efficacy and tolerability of salmeterol added to the treatment of patients already established on anticholinergic therapy.**

I N T E R P R E T A T I O N . This relatively large and well-designed study demonstrated a rapid and statistically significant rise in both morning (pre-treatment) FEV$_1$ and PEF with the introduction of salmeterol 50 μg twice daily, this effect being maintained throughout 24 weeks of study. FEV$_1$ and PEF were significantly higher in salmeterol-treated patients than in placebo-treated patients to 16 weeks, but the effect was lost at 24 weeks. Quality of life was significantly improved within the salmeterol group, but this was not significantly different when compared directly with placebo. Salmeterol appeared to be well tolerated.

Comment

Good studies to determine the efficacy of new therapies in COPD should involve multiple centres with sufficient recruitment. This study went to significant lengths to satisfy these criteria, incorporating 52 centres from six developed countries in North America and Europe, screening some 506 patients. The authors acknowledge that the manufacturer of salmeterol supplied sole funding for the trial.

This was a randomized, double-blind, placebo-controlled, parallel-group trial. Inclusion criteria were rigorous and ensured that the trial contained patients aged 40 years or over already established on anticholinergic therapy in whom there was evidence of smoking history, airflow obstruction, reversibility to salbutamol of 5–15% of predicted FEV_1, and ongoing symptoms compatible with COPD. Recent infection, concurrent respiratory disease, or inadequate inhaler use were grounds for exclusion. A 4-week run-in period was used to convert all standalone β-2 agonists (short and long acting) to salbutamol as rescue medication. Curiously, however, preparations containing β-2 agonists in combination with anticholinergics were allowed to continue. All other medications for COPD were continued. After the run-in period 408 patients were randomized to receive salmeterol 50 μg twice daily ($n = 201$) or placebo twice daily. Assessment was performed at baseline, then at 4, 8, 16 and 24 weeks. Thereafter there was a follow-up period of 2 weeks (no further mention appears to be made of the follow up period in the manuscript).

Patients completed diary cards (PEF, use of rescue medication, day and night symptom scores), and visits incorporated interview, spirometry, and (in 42 centres) SGRQ data relating to quality of life. Data were analysed on an intention to treat basis.

The two groups were well matched at baseline though mean FEV_1 in the salmeterol group (1.19 litres) was 90 ml lower than in the placebo group. Similarly, in the salmeterol group use of inhaled corticosteroids (68%) and methylxanthines (24%) were higher than in the placebo group (55% and 17% respectively).

Importantly, salmeterol effected a significant and rapid but small (80 ml) increase in mean morning (pre-treatment) FEV_1 (Fig. 10.7). This effect was maintained throughout 24 weeks of study, and therefore, salmeterol tachyphylaxis can be excluded effectively in this study (compare with the previous study by Donohue

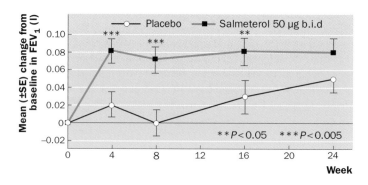

Fig. 10.7 Adjusted mean change from baseline in FEV_1 in a study investigating the role of salmeterol in patients with moderately severe COPD already receiving anticholinergic therapy. Source: Chapman *et al.* (2002).

et al.). The change in FEV_1 from baseline was significantly higher in the salmeterol group than in the placebo group at all assessment visits except at 24 weeks. Two points are worth making here. First, the absolute FEV_1 after treatment is not shown in this paper, but given that baseline FEV_1 started 90 ml higher in the placebo group, the implication is that salmeterol allowed FEV_1 to 'catch up' but not overtake the absolute FEV_1 in the placebo group. Second, the absence of a significant difference between salmeterol and placebo at 24 weeks appears to be due to a spontaneous rise in FEV_1 in the placebo group, which is not mirrored in the salmeterol group. The cause for this is unclear; the authors suggest that participation in a trial may have improved compliance with all medications in the placebo group, but other COPD treatments (and in particular inhaled corticosteroids) were already more prevalent in the salmeterol group, in whom the same argument would apply. Interestingly the trend for FEV_1 was mirrored very closely by morning (but not night-time) PEF.

The other statistically significant finding in this study was an improvement in quality of life as judged by SGRQ. The total score and symptom component were significantly improved after 24 weeks within the salmeterol group, but not within the placebo group. However no significant difference was noted when directly comparing values in the salmeterol and placebo groups (again apparently because of a small, non-significant improvement in quality of life associated with placebo).

In addition to the above findings, salmeterol treatment was associated with non-significant trends towards reduced rescue bronchodilator use and fewer exacerbations, but no changes were noted in uptake of health care during the study.

The unfortunate problem in interpreting this trial clinically appears to relate to the unexpected spontaneous improvement in FEV_1 and spirometry in the placebo group late in the study period. This remains unexplained, and emphasizes the frustration of clinical trials, even those as rigorously and carefully executed as this one. Therefore, the jury would unfortunately appear to remain out with regard to the benefits of adding salmeterol to anticholinergics in this context. On the one hand, it is hard to recommend additional treatment which effects a small rise in FEV_1 and which is no more effective than placebo at 24 weeks with regard to FEV_1, PEF or quality of life. On the other hand, there are clear trends throughout this paper towards an effect of salmeterol. Ultimately, the frustratingly predictable conclusions would appear to be that a further trial is required to answer this question, and that such a trial should ideally be still larger, partly to remove any confounding effects of other medications such as inhaled corticosteroids.

Formoterol in patients with chronic obstructive pulmonary disease: a randomized, controlled, 3-month trial.

Aalbers R, Ayres J, Backer V, *et al. Eur Respir J* 2002; **19**: 936–43.

BACKGROUND. In many ways this study extends the observations of Chapman and colleagues with the exception that a different preparation of β-2 agonist was used for a shorter period, and that pre-existing anticholinergics were discontinued. Specifically, the authors aimed to evaluate the efficacy of formoterol in COPD.

INTERPRETATION. Formoterol, especially at a dose of 18 μg twice daily, appeared to result in small but significant improvements over placebo in terms of FEV_1, symptom scores, symptom-free days and use of reliever medication. In general formoterol was well tolerated. Unfortunately, however, interpretation of the data is hampered by inclusion of a significant proportion of patients who did not meet initial inclusion criteria.

Comment

This was a randomized, parallel-group, double-blind, dose-ranging, placebo-controlled trial assessing the efficacy and safety of formoterol. Patients aged 50–80 years were recruited if they had a smoking history of 10 or more pack-years, a clinical diagnosis of COPD, and active symptoms during the run-in period. They were also required to have FEV_1 greater than 700 ml and between 40 and 70% predicted, along with FEV_1/FVC ratio below 88% and 89% predicted for males and females respectively. Exclusion criteria included significant comorbidity, recent exacerbation, and allergy. Eighty-six centres in nine countries participated. The authors acknowledge that the manufacturers of formoterol funded the study.

During a 2-week run-in period suitable patients' medications were adjusted such that the only allowed treatments were terbutaline as reliever β-2 agonist, and any pre-existing inhaled or oral corticosteroid. Patients were randomized to 12 weeks of either inhaled (via a turbohaler device) placebo ($n = 173$) or formoterol at a dose of 4.5 μg twice daily ($n = 171$), 9 μg twice daily ($n = 166$), or 18 μg twice daily ($n = 177$). Patients used diary cards to record a variety of symptoms and use of reliever bronchodilator. Other assessments included spirometry, assessment of adverse events, and shuttle walk test.

The patients were well matched at baseline, with average FEV_1 1.48 litres (54% predicted) and age 62 years. The primary outcome measurement is not clear but appears to have been symptom score. The lowest dose of formoterol had no significant effect on any of the symptoms (sleep disturbance, dyspnoea, cough, chest tightness, total symptoms), but 18 μg twice daily reduced total symptoms by 13%, chest tightness by 8% and breathlessness by 9% relative to placebo. Similarly, this dose improved symptom free days by 5.7%. In other words, by the end of the trial patients taking placebo had symptoms on 93.4% of days while those on formoterol still had symptoms on 87.7% of days. It would be interesting to know if patients regarded this as clinically significant, but no health-related quality of life assessment was performed. Bronchodilator use was also statistically significantly reduced by formoterol and the implication is that the decrement was less than one puff per day on average. At all doses of formoterol a significant rise in FEV_1 over placebo was observed, the magnitude being around 5% (approximately 75 ml). No significant effect was observed for walking distance.

Formoterol was generally well tolerated. Tremor, tachycardia and hyperglycaemia were each noted in 2% of patients taking 18 µg twice daily, but in no patients taking placebo. Interestingly, at this dose the rate of adverse events described as 'deterioration of COPD' was equal to that in the placebo group.

While this study suggests a small but significant effect for formoterol, there are three problems worthy of note. First, given that the clinical effects were small (but statistically significant), health-related quality of life indices would have been helpful in informing us whether these differences are meaningful to patients (which in turn may drive compliance). Secondly, the range of bronchodilator reversibility in the study is huge (−35 to +92% for all subjects), and while no specification relating to reversibility is made in the entry criteria, this raises the possibility that a proportion of patients had asthma. Furthermore, there is a hint that more patients in the formoterol 18 µg twice-daily group had greater reversibility, as compared to the placebo group. Thirdly, and most importantly, an unspecified number of patients in the study do not appear to satisfy entry criteria. The authors themselves concede that 'miscalculations' led to several patients with FEV_1/FVC greater than 90% predicted entering the study, but in addition to this, there are clearly patients with FEV_1 under 40% predicted, or aged under 50 years. The authors say that excluding the miscalculations for FEV_1/FVC and those patients with reversibility of over 10% predicted FEV_1 does not influence results. However, given the small differences in end-points, it is impossible to say whether these effects would persist (and how *clinically* significant they would be) if *all* inclusion criteria had been adhered to. Therefore, the real effect of formoterol in this trial is hard to interpret.

Effect of theophylline on induced sputum inflammatory indices and neutrophil chemotaxis in chronic obstructive pulmonary disease.

Culpitt SV, de Matos C, Russell RE, Donnelly LE, Rogers DF, Barnes PJ. *Am J Respir Crit Care Med* 2002; **165**: 1371–6.

BACKGROUND. Theophyllines are widely used in COPD. However, debate continues as to which of theophylline's pharmacological actions are important in COPD, and exactly how theophyllines exert their effects. Furthermore relatively little is known about whether theophylline can significantly influence inflammatory processes at the core of COPD pathogenesis. This study therefore aimed to assess the effect of theophylline on neutrophil chemotaxis.

INTERPRETATION. This study demonstrated that theophylline reduces neutrophil numbers in induced sputum. Furthermore, theophylline significantly reduced the responsiveness of neutrophils to important chemotactic stimuli and decreased the chemotactic activity of sputum from patients with COPD.

Comment

This was a randomized, double-blind, placebo-controlled, crossover study. The authors acknowledge support from the manufacturer of theophylline. Patients satisfied ATS criteria for COPD and had to have less than 15% increase in predicted FEV_1 in response to two weeks of 30 mg of prednisolone, as well as a greater than 20 pack-year smoking history. Use of oral or inhaled corticosteroids or an exacerbation in the previous 6 weeks obviated entry to the trial. After a 2-week run-in period, patients were randomized to 4 weeks of either oral theophylline (150–300 mg twice daily) or placebo. A 2-week washout period was followed by crossover so that the patients who had received theophylline received placebo for 4 weeks, and vice versa. Induced sputum was collected before and after each 4-week period, along with venous blood (for isolation of peripheral blood neutrophils).

Twenty-five patients (11 smokers, 14 ex-smokers) were recruited and all completed the study. Compliance appears to have been excellent, based on theophylline serum levels. Mean age was 62, and mean FEV_1 1.36 litres.

Theophylline significantly reduced the number of neutrophils in sputum (it should be noted that the neutrophil was the predominant cell in sputum in virtually all patients), without affecting macrophage numbers. Furthermore the sputum concentration of interleukin (IL)-8 (a neutrophil chemo-attractant), myeloperoxidase (from azurophil granules in neutrophils) and lactoferrin (from specific granules in neutrophils) were all significantly reduced by theophylline.

The authors also isolated peripheral blood neutrophils from 10 patients and demonstrated that theophylline reduced neutrophil responsiveness to maximally chemotactic concentrations of IL-8 and the bacterial chemo-attractant fMLP. A less pronounced effect on leukotriene B_4-mediated chemotaxis was observed. In an extension of these experiments sputum from patients receiving theophylline was significantly less chemotactic for neutrophils (extracted from healthy volunteers) than was sputum from patients receiving placebo. Unfortunately, no experiments were performed to determine which chemotactic agents in sputum were influenced by theophylline.

This extremely elegant and well-designed trial suggests a potentially important effect of theophylline on neutrophil recruitment and adds important information on the function of methylxanthines. The question ultimately is whether this effect is prolonged, and if so, can it alter the natural history of the disease? In this short study theophylline exerted a small (but statistically significant) rise in FEV_1 and PEF. These questions demand a longer and much larger trial. Other unanswered questions include whether theophylline has equal efficacy among patients who are not sputum producers, and exactly how theophylline exerts its effects on IL-8 expression and on neutrophil responsiveness?

Interestingly, we are told very little about adverse effects, other than that theophylline induced self-limiting nausea in 5 patients and sleep disturbance in one. Given that theophylline inhibited responsiveness of peripheral blood neutrophils, it would be extremely interesting to know specifically whether extra-pulmonary infection is commoner among patients receiving theophylline. It is also interesting that among theophylline treated patients the median total number of inflammatory cells in sputum was 1.8×10^6/ml, while the corresponding numbers for neutrophils and macrophages were 1.1×10^6/ml and 0.4×10^6/ml respectively. This may be an arithmetic quirk, but it appears that many more 'other' inflammatory cells (perhaps lymphocytes and/or eosinophils) were present after theophylline therapy, and it would be interesting to know if there were any consequent adverse effects.

Overall, however, this study provides strong evidence for an effect of theophylline on neutrophil recruitment in COPD. Once again, we are left asking which cells are most important in COPD when the neutrophil is the predominant cell isolated from sputum but there is increasing evidence to implicate lymphocytes and macrophages in tissue specimens from airways (see the discussions relating to papers by Turato and colleagues and Hattotuwa and colleagues).

Ambulatory oxygen improves quality of life of COPD patients: a randomized controlled study.

Eaton T, Garrett JE, Young P, *et al. Eur Respir J* 2002; **20**: 306–12.

B ACKGROUND . While there is good evidence to support the use of long-term oxygen supplementation in chronically hypoxaemic patients |10,11|, there is less consensus on whether ambulatory oxygen significantly benefits those patients with exertional dyspnoea and desaturation. Immediate benefit after using oxygen does not necessarily indicate continued responsiveness over weeks or months. With this in mind, this study aimed to assess the effect of ambulatory oxygen on health-related quality of life in patients with COPD who did not qualify for long-term domiciliary oxygen therapy.

I NTERPRETATION . When compared with ambulatory air-filled cylinders, ambulatory oxygen was associated with small but significant improvements in health-related quality of life, along with a reduction in anxiety. Interestingly 41% of patients considered to have responded to ambulatory oxygen chose not to continue with the treatment upon completion of the trial.

Comment

This was a well-designed randomized, double-blind, controlled, crossover trial comparing ambulatory oxygen with ambulatory air. Patients were eligible if they had COPD according to ATS criteria, with a PaO_2 of 7.3 kPa or greater at rest breathing room air (i.e. precluding domiciliary oxygen), but with exertional dyspnoea limiting activities of daily living and a corresponding desaturation to SaO_2 88% or less on exercise whilst breathing room air. In addition, patients had to be ex-smokers who had been clinically stable for over 2 months and had participated in a 6-week pulmonary rehabilitation programme. Patients with significant comorbidity limiting exercise were excluded.

Those recruited had a 2-month run-in period followed by randomization to 6 weeks of either oxygen or air (administered via a portable 2-kg aluminium cylinder delivering 4 litres/minute intranasally, for use in any activity with which the patient anticipated breathlessness). The two treatments were crossed over for the next 6 weeks. Primary outcome measures to assess short-term efficacy included the CRDQ (as a disease-specific health-related quality of life measurement), the SF-36 (as a generic health-related quality of life measurement), and the Hospital Anxiety and Depression Scale, measured at 0, 6 and 12 weeks. As an adjunct to the trial, the 6-minute walk test was used to measure *immediate* efficacy, comparing the distance walked using air or oxygen. Patients continued with their usual COPD treatments during the trial.

Fifty patients entered the trial with 9 withdrawals (6 for 'personal reasons', 3 because of comorbidities presenting during the trial) leaving complete data for 41 patients with a mean age of 67 and FEV_1 26% predicted. The *immediate* response to ambulatory oxygen revealed a statistically significant improvement in 6 minute walking distance (40 m) and Borg dyspnoea index (0.7 units), but in each case the mean gain over that seen for ambulatory air was less than the difference considered clinically significant for any individual (54 m and 1 unit respectively). Turning to the primary end-points of the trial, a similar effect was observed, with all 4 components of the CRDQ significantly improved, but the differences as compared with ambulatory air being less than those considered clinically significant in any individual. There was also a small significant improvement in anxiety and in elements of the SF-36. Using pre-determined criteria, 34 of 41 patients were considered to have responded to immediate and/or short-term ambulatory oxygen. Interestingly, however, only 20 of the responders wished to continue with ambulatory oxygen after completion of the trial. Finally, the authors used logistic regression analysis to try and determine predictors of short-term responsiveness to ambulatory oxygen, but none could be identified.

This is a well-designed and extremely useful study, in which there were few potential biases, aside from a small carry-over effect, which the authors acknowledge. We are not told how many patients had used oxygen and recognized benefit from it during previous exacerbations/rehabilitation, and this could have influenced results in favour of ambulatory oxygen. It is a little curious that exacerbations were not responsible for withdrawals from the trial over a 3-month period in a group of patients with moderate to severe COPD. It is frustrating that one figure in the paper suggests only 39 patients completed the trial when the text states 41, but aside from this, the study has a most valuable message. That is, ambulatory oxygen does indeed improve quality of life in the majority of patients with exertional dyspnoea/desaturation, though a proportion of such patients will find the treatment unacceptable (perhaps due to clumsiness or weight of the cylinder). Overall these data suggest that a trial of ambulatory oxygen is worthwhile in patients with exertional dyspnoea/desaturation, with continued treatment offered to those who derive clear benefit. The challenges ahead are to determine whether these effects are beneficial in the longer term with regard to physiology, symptoms and quality of life, while identifying more confidently those who may benefit most.

Patients at high risk of death after lung-volume-reduction surgery.

National Emphysema Treatment Trial Research Group. *N Engl J Med* 2001; **345**: 1075–83.

BACKGROUND. Lung-volume reduction surgery (LVRS) is an effective therapy for a proportion of patients with emphysema. However, LVRS carries high attendant risks of morbidity and mortality. We would be able to inform our patients more thoroughly if we had good evidence with which to identify those patients likely to benefit, and those likely to do badly after surgery. This study is derived from the larger National Emphysema Treatment Trial (NETT) which randomized patients to receive LVRS or best medical care with the intention of comparing exercise capacity and mortality at 2 years, but also with the aim of identifying optimal selection criteria for LVRS. Critically, from the outset independent monitors for NETT scanned data to identify subgroups of patients with unacceptable rates of surgical mortality (pre-determined as 30-day mortality of over 8%). On this basis patients with FEV_1 of 20% predicted or less and either homogeneous emphysema on high HRCT or a diffusing capacity for CO of 20% predicted or less were identified to have unacceptable surgical risk. Enrolment of these patients ceased in May 2001 (41 months into the trial). The present study for discussion analyses data on the 140 patients satisfying the above criteria who had already enrolled in the trial.

INTERPRETATION. In patients with FEV_1 of 20% predicted or less and either homogenous emphysema on HRCT or diffusing capacity for CO of 20% predicted or less, LVRS was associated with 16% 30-day mortality (95% CI 8.2–26.7), while all patients receiving medical treatment were alive at 30 days. Overall mortality was also higher among the surgical group than in the medical group (relative risk of overall mortality 3.9). Among those patients who survived to 6 months, those in the LVRS group had statistically significant improvements in walking distance and FEV_1, but the clinical significance of these small changes seems negligible. On the basis of these data, patients with the poor prognostic factors listed should only be offered LVRS under exceptional circumstances.

Comment

This study is hugely significant in providing us with clear data with which to advise sick patients with advanced emphysema. In so doing, it removes some significant doubts about where we should "draw the line in the sand" for LVRS referral.

It is worth going over the basic entry criteria for NETT to make best use of the data. The trial recruited patients with an FEV_1 between 15 and 45% predicted who had convincing evidence of hyperinflation (e.g. residual volume [RV] 150% predicted or more) with baseline PaO_2 45 mmHg or more and $PaCO_2$ 60 mmHg or less.

The other technical point to make relates to the definition of 'homogeneous emphysema'. HRCT slices were obtained at three pre-determined anatomical points and a radiologist scored emphysema at each given level using a system whereby no emphysema scored 0, 1–25% emphysema scored 1, 26–50% scored 2, 51–75% scored 3 and 76–100% scored 4. A variation in score of 2 or more in either lung when comparing the three slices was regarded as heterogeneous emphysema, with lesser variation in emphysema being regarded as homogeneous.

In this particular study, there were 140 patients with FEV_1 of 20% predicted or less and either homogenous emphysema on HRCT or diffusing capacity for carbon monoxide of 20% predicted or less. Seventy had been randomized to the LVRS group and 70 to medical therapy. The groups were well matched at baseline. At 30 days, 11 patients undergoing surgery had died, and all medical patients were still alive. Overall mortality (to an average of approximately 3 years of follow up) was 33/70 in the LVRS group and 10/70 in the medical group (Fig. 10.8). The Kaplan–Meier curve for overall mortality shows a steep rise to 3 months in the surgical

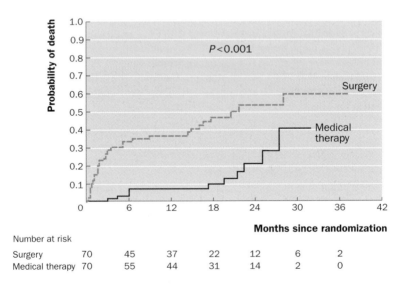

Number at risk							
Surgery	70	45	37	22	12	6	2
Medical therapy	70	55	44	31	14	2	0

Fig. 10.8 Kaplan–Meier estimates of the probability of death among high-risk patients, according to whether they were randomly assigned to undergo lung-volume-reduction surgery or receive medical therapy. This intention-to-treat analysis shows the overall results for the high-risk group. The difference between groups was significant ($P < 0.001$) by the log-rank test. Source: National Emphysema Treatment Trial Research Group (2001).

group, suggesting that prolonged post-operative complications contributed. Death was due to respiratory failure in 90% of patients who died in each group. There is a trend for the survival curves to come together after 2 years, but the difference in overall mortality remains unequivocally significant. Interestingly the combination of FEV_1 of 20% predicted or less and homogeneous emphysema was associated with particularly high risk of mortality and persistent deviation of survival curves. FEV_1 of 20% predicted or less and diffusing capacity of 20% predicted or less had a relative risk for death 3 times higher than medical patients with survival curves tending to converge after 2 years. This may be of some importance pragmatically, as greater specialist knowledge is required to interpret an HRCT result as compared to a diffusing capacity result.

A further important issue in this subgroup analysis relates to functional outcome measures at 6 months in each group. On an intention to treat basis, no significant difference was seen in exercise capacity, change in FEV_1, 6-minute walking distance or quality of well-being score. For each measurement, more patients undergoing LVRS showed some improvement, but the numbers were small. When only those patients completing 6 months of the trial were analysed (i.e. excluding those who died or those with incomplete data) there was a clearer trend for advantage in the LVRS patients, with significant differences in the change in 6-minute walk distance and FEV_1. However, the actual mean differences between the groups were 36.5 metres and 6% of predicted FEV_1 respectively. The overall summary must be not only that mortality is unacceptably high in these patients, but that the potential benefits are disappointingly low.

The authors acknowledge that any subgroup analysis is open to claims of bias. However, as they also point out, this subgroup was identified using the pre-determined concept that 30-day surgical mortality of 8% or more was unaccept-able. The setting of this arbitrary level can be argued either way, but it would have been interesting to determine whether other susceptible groups would have been detected if 8% had been 7% or 6%, etc. My only minor quibble with the paper probably relates to a typographical error—the methods section describes NETT recruiting patients 70 years or over and I presumed this should read 70 years or *under*. This remains uncertain as while the mean age of patients at baseline was about 64 years the standard deviation hints at patients over 70 years of age being included. This may seem pedantic but would assume importance if the risk of mortality with LVRS is markedly stratified by age, i.e. what does one say to a 50–55 year old patient who has failed medical therapy, has an FEV_1 of exactly 20% predicted and apparently homogeneous emphysema on HRCT, especially when organs for transplant are rare? As the authors discuss in another context, LVRS is not absolutely contraindicated in such patients—instead the risks have to be discussed properly.

In summary, this paper gives us clear grounds to say that patients with FEV_1 of 20% predicted or less and either homogeneous emphysema on HRCT or diffusing capacity for carbon monoxide of 20% predicted or less have high mortality after LVRS.

Cost–benefit and cost-effectiveness analysis of self-management in patients with COPD—a 1-year follow-up randomized, controlled trial.

Gallefoss F, Bakke PS. *Respir Med* 2002; **96**: 424–31.

BACKGROUND. As the prevalence of COPD rises in coming years, so it is inevitable that the costs attendant upon managing the disease will increase substantially. This is likely to impact profoundly on health care systems, and strategies to reduce costs without compromising the effectiveness of treatment are badly needed. Gallefoss and Bakke have published widely on the effect of patient education and self-management on outcome measurements in COPD, and the aim of this particular study was to determine the effects of the same interventions on health related costs over a one-year period of follow up.

INTERPRETATION. Those patients randomized to intensive education and self-management were 5 times less likely to visit their GP during the year of follow up, and were significantly more satisfied with their medical care. Furthermore, the total cost of care was 47% lower in the educated group, though this was not statistically significant. The implication is that carefully designed education and self-management plans seem cost-effective in moderately severe COPD.

Comment

This study randomized patients to receive standard care alone, or patient education and a customized self-management plan followed by standard care. The first of two 2-hour education sessions was conducted by a doctor and a pharmacist, the second by a nurse and physiotherapist. Educated patients also received a detailed education booklet. Patients were recruited from a respiratory outpatient clinic and were eligible if aged below 70 years, with FEV_1 between 40 and 80% predicted, and no significant comorbidity. Sixty-two patients were enrolled. Both groups were followed up for one year and measured outcomes included the use of reliever medication as well as the (self-reported) number of GP visits, days of absenteeism or days in hospital attributable to COPD. Direct and indirect costs were calculated and incorporated estimations of the cost of education (from the price of the patient's travel and clinic visit right down to the cost of the education pamphlet), loss of productivity, hospital costs, medication costs and GP visits. Nine patients did not complete the study (5 in the treatment group) for a variety of reasons. Data appear to have been analysed according to trial completion rather than on an intention to treat basis.

The groups were well matched at baseline. FEV_1 for the whole study group was 57% predicted, and the mean age was 60 years. Outcome appeared to be significantly improved by education and self-management with 73% of the control group visiting their GP in the ensuing year, as compared with 15% of the intervention group. Patient satisfaction was higher in the intervention group, and rescue medication less (though the 11% of patients who did not take up prescriptions at all were not factored into the statistical analysis for some reason). The calculated cost per patient in the control group was almost 20 000 Norwegian krone, whereas it was just over 10 500 krone in the intervention group (recruitment was from 1994–1995), though this difference was not statistically significant in light of the wide inter-individual variation in costs, and the small study size. The costs of hospital admissions and lost productivity explained the vast majority of the difference in costs. We are not told how many hospital days or lost working days were incurred, but the data strongly suggests that a very small proportion of control patients are responsible for most of the extra cost, as would be expected.

The authors went on to calculate a cost–benefit analysis and on the basis of these findings concluded that for every krone spent on the education process, there was a saving of 4.8 krone.

The biggest difficulties in analysing these findings relate to the small sample size and to the unavoidable fact that the study is not blinded. Therefore, it is possible that patients in the intervention group were biased towards not seeking a GP's help. A further issue is that as many as 20 patients in the study appear to have greater than 20% reversibility in FEV_1 in response to bronchodilators, suggesting that some patients had asthma. It might also be argued that the outcome measure of 'number of GP visits' could have been replaced by symptom scores or quality of life data.

The small sample size also exaggerates the effects of the small number of control patients who contributed most to excessive costs. Furthermore, any service setting up an education system of this type will incur costs inherent in training health professionals to deliver the education and this does not appear to figure in the cost analysis, thus potentially favouring a difference between the groups.

In summary this trial emphasizes that education and self-management plans are worthy of greater scrutiny and attention in COPD. The trial suggests that this form of intervention could make huge savings in the cost of COPD while improving at least some markers of outcome. Overall, however, the unavoidable conclusion is that much larger studies are required to confirm this effect (possibly using a wider range of outcome measurements).

The effectiveness of outpatient pulmonary rehabilitation in chronic lung disease: a randomized controlled trial.

Finnerty JP, Keeping I, Bullough I, Jones J. *Chest* 2001: **119**: 1705–10.

BACKGROUND. Pulmonary rehabilitation programmes have been shown to benefit patients with COPD |12|. Their widespread introduction in the last few years has been a significant part of modernization of care for COPD. However, these schemes tend to be time consuming for the staff involved and expensive for health care providers. The challenge is to develop rehabilitation programmes which are less demanding on resources but which retain full effectiveness. Short outpatient programmes may be appropriate in this context. This study, therefore, aimed to assess the efficacy of a 6-week outpatient pulmonary rehabilitation programme.

INTERPRETATION. This randomized study compared a 6-week outpatient pulmonary rehabilitation programme to standard outpatient care comprising 3-monthly clinic visits. Patients receiving pulmonary rehabilitation had a significant improvement in health-related quality of life and walking distance at 3 months, with the improvement in quality of life being maintained at 6 months.

Comment

This study recruited patients with a diagnosis consistent with COPD attending a respiratory outpatient department. No formal cut-off appears to have been made with regard to disease severity, but patients generally appear to have had moderate to severe disease. Exclusion criteria included dementia, depression and significant comorbidity. All patients had stopped smoking or had made a commitment to try stopping. After explanation of the trial, patients were randomized to 6 weeks of outpatient pulmonary rehabilitation, or to ongoing standard outpatient care. The rehabilitation programme was based on twice-weekly sessions, one of which comprised 2 hours of education, and the other a 1-hour exercise visit. The principal contact was with a trained physiotherapist (every week) but the patients also had contact with a doctor, occupational therapist, specialist nurse, dietician and liaison nurse counsellor, such that dietary issues, coping strategies, sleep problems, etc. were all addressed. Patients were assessed at baseline, 3 months and 6 months, and the primary outcome variable was health-related quality of life as measured by the SGRQ. The 6-minute walk test was a secondary outcome variable.

One hundred and eight patients were screened of whom 100 were randomized ($n = 50$ in each group). Twenty-seven of these did not attend the baseline visit, a further 8 patients were withdrawn on account of diagnostic misclassification, and 10 patients failed to complete the study, leaving 55 patients for analysis of SGRQ at 3 months (32 in the rehabilitation group).

The groups were well matched at baseline with average age around 69 and FEV_1 approximately 1.03 litres (41% predicted). The total SGRQ in the control group began at 59.3 and was 58.5 at 3 months. In contrast, the corresponding figures in the rehabilitation group were 59.9 and 47.4 respectively ($P < 0.01$ as compared with the control group). A change of 4 points is considered clinically significant. The total SGRQ remained significantly lower in the rehabilitation group at 6 months (50.6 vs 57.1), but it should be noted that only 24 rehabilitation patients were included at 6 months, while an additional two patients (i.e. $n = 25$) had appeared in the control group! It should be noted that all three components of the SGRQ (activity, symptoms and impact) were considerably improved in the rehabilitation group but not the control group. Similarly, at 3 months, walking distance had improved around 20% in the rehabilitation group but remained essentially unchanged in the control group ($P < 0.05$), but at 6 months (when again a number of rehabilitation patients were unavailable) the difference, while apparently sustained, no longer achieved statistical significance.

Interpretation of this study is slightly difficult because so little is said about the care received by the control group, but one must assume they turned up for medical assessment alone at 3-monthly intervals and, therefore, had two routine visits during the observation period. We are not told how many visits were missed. Similarly, we are not told what clinic arrangements the rehabilitation patients returned to after the 6 weeks of study. Furthermore, given that by its very nature this study was not blinded, it is conceivable that staff (and patient) enthusiasm for a new treatment regimen may have impacted positively on a subjective measurement like the SGRQ while, conversely, those randomized to receive standard care may have been relatively disgruntled. Finally, we are not told how many individuals in the rehabilitation group improved (though one assumes nearly all did so). This study is admirable in seeking to show the general applicability of rehabilitation in non-specialized centres. In this regard, knowing how many participants improved would have been helpful—in particular, analysis was not on an intention to treat basis, and if we assume that those who dropped out had no benefit then we would have been able to assess how many of the original 50 in the rehabilitation group actually benefited from intervention.

These considerations aside, however, the improvement in SGRQ is very striking both at 3 and at 6 months. The implication is that short, outpatient pulmonary rehabilitation programmes are effective, though cost–benefit and cost-effectiveness analyses remains to be performed. As the authors point out, the challenge now is to optimise the evidence base for individual components of such programmes, and to evaluate longer-term efficacy.

A comparison of the palliative care needs of patients dying from chronic respiratory diseases and lung cancer.
Edmonds P, Karlsen S, Khan S, Addington-Hall J. *Palliative Med* 2001; **15**: 287–95.

BACKGROUND. Palliative care services, certainly in the UK, have traditionally evolved around patients with cancer. Furthermore, cancer services are allocated a higher proportion of funding budgets than are services dedicated to chronic disabling conditions such as COPD. For these reasons, it might be expected that patients dying with cancer receive more health care resources than patients dying with chronic respiratory disease do. A disproportionate weighting of palliative services for patients with cancer would only be justifiable if the palliative requirements of those patients were disproportionately high also. This study aimed to compare the symptoms and psychosocial issues affecting patients dying with chronic lung disease and patients dying with lung cancer.

INTERPRETATION. Patients dying with chronic respiratory disease (the majority of whom had COPD) have a high prevalence of symptoms, principal among which are breathlessness, pain, insomnia, anorexia and low mood. The prevalence of symptoms is broadly comparable to those in patients with lung cancer, though breathlessness is significantly more common in chronic respiratory disease, while anorexia and constipation are more common in lung cancer. In general, patients with chronic respiratory disease had symptoms for longer, and had a greater requirement for assistance with self care. As compared with patients with lung cancer a significantly lower proportion of patients with chronic respiratory disease knew they were dying, significantly fewer died at home, and the principal carer was significantly less likely to be present at the time of death. It should be concluded that terminally ill patients with chronic respiratory disease have very considerable palliative care needs.

Comment

This study gathered information from randomly selected death certificates issued in 20 health districts in England. Sampling was deliberately biased towards the detection of death associated with cancer. The authors contacted individuals known to, and closely involved with, the care of each deceased patient, and invited them to complete an interview relating to the patient's final illness. Information was obtained for 449 patients with lung cancer and 87 patients with chronic lung disease, of whom 82 were said to have died from COPD according to the death certificate. The two groups were closely matched with regard to demographic variables with the exception that patients with chronic lung disease were older and less likely to have a surviving spouse.

For patients with chronic lung disease, respondents reported a wide range of symptoms experienced in the last year of life. Those symptoms with a reported prevalence of over 60% included breathlessness (94%), pain (77%), low mood (71%), anorexia (67%) and insomnia (65%). A broadly similar pattern was observed for lung cancer, though breathlessness was significantly more common among patients with chronic lung disease, while anorexia and constipation were significantly commoner in patients with lung cancer. Almost 50% of patients with chronic lung disease or lung cancer saw a GP 10 or more times in their final year, though interestingly patients with lung cancer were more likely to receive district nurse care. Extending this theme, no patients with chronic lung disease saw a Macmillan or hospice nurse. Despite these observations, patients with chronic lung disease were reported to have a significantly higher requirement for help with self-care.

An important trend emerged suggesting poorer preparation for death among patients with chronic lung disease. For example, only 62% of patients with chronic lung disease appeared to know they were dying (significantly less than for lung cancer), and of those who had acknowledged that they were dying, the realization first occurred within one month of death in 62% (as compared with 42% for lung cancer). When compared with patients with lung cancer significantly more patients with chronic lung disease died in hospital (72% versus 51%), significantly fewer at home (12% versus 27%) and none in a hospice (14% of patients with lung cancer died in a hospice). The respondent was significantly less likely to be present at the time of death for patients with chronic lung disease (43%) than for patients with lung cancer (70%). The most likely explanation for the apparent lack of preparation for death in chronic lung disease is that death resulted from a rapid deterioration as part of an exacerbation, but it remains possible (and indeed likely) that the culture of dying at home was promoted more actively among patients with lung cancer.

There is no doubt that technical problems are inherent in a retrospective study of this nature. For example, the study is reliant upon information recorded in death certificates, which are notoriously inaccurate, and the data is dependent upon the memory and perceptions of respondents, introducing further potential inaccuracy. In addition, there is little opportunity in a retrospective study to assess how rigorous the diagnosis of COPD was. Further problems in interpreting the data are that many of the patients with lung cancer probably had co-existent COPD. If anything exclusion of these patients would probably have exaggerated the high palliative requirements of patients with chronic lung disease relative to those of patients with lung cancer, and patients with chronic lung disease were significantly older. Adjustment for age would obviously be likely to reduce symptoms in the chronic lung disease group relative to lung cancer patients. However, these limitations were largely unavoidable. One final point to note before considering the clinical applicability of these findings is that the study data refers to patients who died in 1990.

On balance, these technical considerations do little to detract from the powerful message of this study, which is that patients with COPD have far-reaching and important palliative requirements. It seems highly likely that these requirements are both under-recognized and relatively unmet. The study should heighten our awareness of the common symptoms of terminal COPD, many of which are readily treatable. The study should encourage us to consolidate mechanisms of support for patients with terminal disease, and reinforce the need to explain patients' diagnosis and prognosis in a clear way that allows them to plan for, and come to terms with, the last days of their lives.

New and evolving treatments for COPD

In many ways, this section gives a glimpse of the future management of COPD. Alpha$_1$-antitrypsin therapy for α_1AT deficiency is incorporated in this section because its benefit has not been unequivocally proven and its use is generally limited to a few countries worldwide—as such, it was not considered 'established' therapy in COPD. The other treatments to be considered are derived from four distinct rationales. The first is particularly fascinating in attempting to reverse the hitherto irreversible lung damage characteristic of emphysema by stimulating regeneration of alveolar tissue. The second concentrates on identifying and neutralizing mediators central to pulmonary inflammation. The third concentrates on clearance of bronchial mucus. The fourth relates specifically to the stimulation of muscle strength and bulk with the expectation that this will improve weight and exercise tolerance.

We begin with α_1AT because experience with this treatment in the context of COPD is considerably greater than that with the other therapies discussed.

Longitudinal follow-up of patients with α_1-protease inhibitor deficiency before and during therapy with intravenous α_1-protease inhibitor.

Wencker M, Fuhrmann B, Banik N, Konietzko N. *Chest* 2001; **119**: 737–44.

BACKGROUND. Alpha$_1$-antitrypsin (α_1AT) is the predominant antiprotease in human airways (α_1AT is synonymous with α_1-protease inhibitor; while α_1-protease inhibitor is the better descriptive term, α_1AT is still more commonly used and, therefore, will be applied in the remainder of this discussion). The original observation that premature emphysema develops in patients deficient in α_1AT |13| led to the protease-antiprotease theory of emphysema, which contends that a relative excess of proteases (in particular human neutrophil elastase) is central to the pathogenesis of the disease. Intravenous replacement therapy with α_1AT is both logical and feasible, yet definitive evidence that the treatment significantly alters the course of the disease is still awaited. The first randomized, placebo-controlled trial of α_1AT replacement showed a non-significant trend towards benefit |14|. As the authors of the present study point out, larger, randomized, placebo-controlled trials are extremely difficult to organize because of the disease being rare and sensitive outcome measurements for emphysema lacking. Therefore, they set out to analyse lung function decline in patients observed both before and after institution of α_1AT replacement therapy.

INTERPRETATION. Among 96 patients with α_1AT deficiency the rate of decline in FEV$_1$ fell significantly from 49 ml/year to 34 ml/year after introduction of α_1AT replacement therapy. When the group was stratified by lung function at the start of the observation period, a single subgroup was identified in which α_1AT therapy made a significant difference. This subgroup comprised patients with well-preserved lung function at the beginning of observation in whom there was precipitous decline in (pre-treatment) FEV$_1$. As such early detection of α_1AT deficiency is important, and those patients with rapid decline in lung function would appear to benefit from early introduction of replacement therapy.

Comment

This study had access to databases recording spirometry and demographic data on patients with severe α_1AT deficiency both before and after initiation of α_1AT replacement therapy. The present study included patients who had at least two sets of spirometry (at least a year apart) both before and after the start of α_1AT therapy. By definition these patients could only enter the present study if they had fulfilled entry criteria for treatment with α_1AT, which were a serum level of α_1AT below 35% of normal, absence of smoking in the 3 months prior to treatment, and a FEV$_1$

of less than 65% predicted or a fall in FEV_1 of over 120 ml/year. Exclusion criteria for treatment included hypersensitivity to blood products and smoking. The authors acknowledge financial support from the supplier of $\alpha_1 AT$.

For the present study 96 patients (from a registry of 442 patients compiled by 26 centres) had sufficient lung function data. The mean durations of observation before and after treatment were 47 and 50 months respectively, incorporating an average of 4.9 and 7.7 measurements of FEV_1 respectively. The mean first available FEV_1 was 1.4 litres (41% predicted), 89% of patients had the PiZZ phenotype, and 13% of patients had never smoked. It should be noted that all patients were treated with a weekly intravenous dose of $\alpha_1 AT$ at 60 mg/kg.

When studying the whole group of 96 patients, treatment was associated with a significant reduction in the rate of decline in FEV_1 (Table 10.1). Interestingly, when the patients were stratified by FEV_1 at the time that observation first began, only the subgroup with FEV_1 greater than 65% predicted showed significant improvement with treatment. Within this subgroup, a further small set of patients was identified in whom FEV_1 had fallen rapidly prior to treatment, and in this group, treatment slowed the decline in FEV_1 dramatically.

The very nature of this study introduces potential biases. For example, 14 of the patients smoked during the pre-treatment observation, presumably influencing rate of decline of FEV_1. Furthermore, it seems possible that those patients who attended for at least two sets of spirometry after treatment were regular attendees who had benefited from $\alpha_1 AT$; conversely those ineligible because they had less than two sets of lung function may have been non-attendees because they were ill (or dead!), or because they were unhappy with their treatment. It is also possible that a decline in the rate of lung function reflects the natural history of the disease, in which case an effect of treatment would best be demonstrated by stopping $\alpha_1 AT$ and observing accelerated decline in these patients (which, of course, would be

Table 10.1 Decline in FEV_1 for non-treatment and treatment periods*

Variables	ΔFEV_1 before therapy with α_1-Pi, ml/yr	ΔFEV_1 during therapy with α_1-Pi, ml/yr	Difference between treatment and non-treatment	P value
Total (n = 96)	−49.2 ± 60.8	−34.3 ± 29.7	14.9 ± 61.4	0.019
First available FEV_1				
<30% (n = 25)	−15.3 ± 38.5	−19.0 ± 18.0	−3.7 ± 48.6	NS
30 to 65% (n = 60)	−49.3 ± 43.4	−37.8 ± 25.0	11.6 ± 48.8	0.066
>65% (n = 11)	−122.5 ± 108.4	−48.9 ± 54.9	73.6 ± 107.0	0.045
Rapid decliners (n = 7)	−255.7 ± 70.4	−52.7 ± 61.3	203.0 ± 99.2	0.001
Slow decliners (n = 4)	15.9 ± 128.8	−10.6 ± 66.0	−26.4 ± 89.5	NS

Δ = change; α_1-Pi = alpha$_1$-protease inhibitor. * Data are presented as mean ± SD.
Source: Wencker et al. (2001).

extremely hard to justify ethically). Each of these potential confounding factors would be extremely difficult to control for in this type of study.

Overall, this is an immensely important study in the context of α_1AT deficiency. As always in studies like this, several questions present themselves. For example, we do not know whether the fall in lung function observed with treatment is associated with improvement in exercise tolerance, symptoms or mortality, i.e. what do isolated observations of lung function mean in this context? This may be an important question when α_1AT is such an expensive, life-long therapy. The huge strength of this study lies in its identification of a subgroup of patients for which an indication for treatment seems incontrovertible. The main conclusions are therefore two-fold. First, we must try to identify patients with severe α_1AT deficiency early. Second, it seems logical to monitor patients closely (and especially those with preserved lung function at time of diagnosis), and initiate treatment in those with early evidence of precipitous decline in lung function, with careful ongoing monitoring of lung function thereafter.

A pilot study of all-*trans*-retinoic acid for the treatment of human emphysema.

Mao JT, Goldin JG, Dermand J, *et al. Am J Respir Crit Care Med* 2002; **165**: 718–23.

BACKGROUND. The seminal work of Massaro and Massaro |15| demonstrating regeneration of alveolar tissue in emphysematous rats after administration of retinoic acid provided the first convincing indication that human emphysema may be potentially reversible. The enormous implications of that work stimulated the study of all-*trans*-retinoic acid (ATRA) in patients with COPD. The present study aimed to assess the safety and pharmacokinetics of ATRA in patients with emphysema, whilst also evaluating potential changes in lung function, pathology and symptoms.

INTERPRETATION. Side-effects associated with ATRA were common but generally mild. The optimal dosing schedule for ATRA remains to be established. ATRA was not associated with any demonstrable beneficial change in lung function, CT appearances or symptoms in this pilot study. Formal trials to study the efficacy of ATRA in COPD are awaited with huge interest.

Comment

The authors performed a double-blind, placebo-controlled, crossover study in which patients received oral ATRA (25 mg/m² dose twice daily) or placebo (twice daily) for 3 months, with subsequent crossover to the other preparation. Assessments incorporated lung function tests, HRCT scans, and quality of life assessment using the SGRQ. Patients were eligible if they had emphysema on HRCT scan along with any two from the following list—FEV_1 less than 60% predicted, total lung capacity greater than 110% predicted, or diffusing capacity for carbon monoxide less than 60% predicted. Patients were also required to have been abstinent from tobacco for 6 months to allay potential fears regarding the risk of lung cancer with concomitant retinoids and cigarette smoking. A range of stringent exclusion criteria were in place, largely to exclude significant comorbidity and to avoid patients with very advanced emphysema (for example, those with resting hypoxaemia). Twenty patients were enrolled and all completed the study.

The mean baseline FEV_1 was 1.24 litres and PaO_2 approximately 75 mmHg. With placebo treatment none of the lung function variables altered. Unexpectedly residual volume and total lung capacity *increased* by a small but significant amount in the patients treated with ATRA in the first 3 months. No changes were seen for ATRA or placebo with respect to serial quantitative CT analysis or quality of life as judged by SGRQ.

As ATRA is known to promote its own metabolism, the authors measured serum levels of ATRA 3 hours after the doses given at baseline, 3 weeks and 8 weeks of each half of the trial. In general, the serum concentration fell with time, though the response in individual patients was unpredictable. Indeed levels of ATRA in some individuals were so low that it would have been useful to know the pre-dosing concentrations. Poor bioavailability with this dosing schedule may partly explain the observed lack of efficacy of ATRA. It might also have been useful to know the concentration of ATRA in BALF, which one must assume was generally low at any given point.

Adverse effects were strikingly more common during ATRA treatment. Although the incidence of adverse effects in the placebo group was lower than in most trials, this does not detract from the high frequency in the ATRA group. More than half of patients receiving ATRA had skin changes, headache or hyperlipidaemia, and a quarter or more developed itch, musculoskeletal pain, fatigue or transaminitis. All of these effects were generally mild and tolerable, but it does seem likely that achieving long-term compliance in future trials may be challenging because of side effects. Of course, this problem simply compounds the difficulties in achieving satisfactory serum (and BALF) levels of ATRA in future trials.

It is impossible not to feel disappointed that no beneficial effects of ATRA were seen in this study, and slightly worrying that lung volumes went up during treatment (though the latter effect may well be a statistical quirk). However, as the authors stress, this was by definition a pilot study and efficacy was not the most important parameter being scrutinized this time around. In fact, any significant efficacy changes would have been quite remarkable given the time-course, the dosing problems and the (presumed) relative insensitivity of measurements like CT scores to change over this period. In summary, this well-designed study lays important ground for the development of larger trials studying efficacy. It is hard to escape the conclusion that long-term trials of retinoids in this context will require an agent which has fewer side-effects and which gives more predictable concentrations in the blood (and BALF).

Erythromycin and common cold in COPD.
Suzuki T, Yanai M, Yamaya M, *et al. Chest* 2001; **120**: 730–3.

BACKGROUND. The observation among Japanese patients that erythromycin significantly attenuates pulmonary inflammation in diffuse panbronchiolitis, stimulated huge interest in whether macrolides may have anti-inflammatory properties quite distinct from their antimicrobial activity. Exacerbations of COPD commonly occur secondary to the inflammatory reaction invoked by upper respiratory tract viral infection such as is seen in the common cold. In the absence of a cure for the common cold, the present study aimed to determine whether erythromycin could decrease the frequency of both the common cold and exacerbations among patients with COPD.

INTERPRETATION. This randomized, controlled trial compared the ability of erythromycin and riboflavin (as control) to impact upon the frequency of exacerbations of COPD, and frequency of symptoms associated with the common cold, over a one-year period. Self-reported symptoms consistent with the common cold were approximately four times less common in the erythromycin-treated group. Exacerbations of COPD were reduced to a similar level.

Comment

This quite remarkable study recruited patients with COPD according to ATS criteria. Patients were allowed to participate if they were taking anticholinergic treatment or sustained-release theophyllines (indeed it appears that all patients were taking these), but not corticosteroids. Patients with bronchiectasis or diffuse pan-bronchiolitis were excluded. The details of treatment are a little vague but it appears that patients were randomized to receive either erythromycin (200–400 mg/day, $n = 55$) or riboflavin (10 mg/day, $n = 54$) which they appeared to take for 13 months, with the study period constituting the last 12 months. Patients kept daily diary cards in which they recorded (on a scale 0–3) symptoms of nasal congestion, malaise, sneezing, nasal discharge, headache, chills, fevers, sore throat, hoarse voice and cough. Investigators defined a common cold as a symptom score of over 5. Patients visited hospital every 2 weeks and an exacerbation of COPD was defined as 'acute and sustained worsening of COPD symptoms requiring changes to regular treatment'. An exacerbation was considered severe if hospital admission was required.

The two groups were well matched at baseline, with average age around 70 and FEV_1 of approximately 1.39 litres—unfortunately, we are told nothing about smoking history, bronchodilator reversibility or predicted values for FEV_1. The average weight in this Japanese study was much lower than in most Western studies, at around 54 kg.

The erythromycin group had significantly fewer common colds or exacerbations of COPD (Table 10.2). This study and its dramatic results require further scrutiny. First, it must be noted that this was not a blinded study, nor strictly speaking was it placebo-controlled. Second, the outcome measures are all subjective, and in par-

Table 10.2 Number of common colds and exacerbations and the severity of exacerbations in each treatment group

Measures	Control group (n = 54)	Erythromycin group (n = 55)	P value
Total common colds, No.	245	67	0.0002
Total patients with two or more common colds, No.	41	7	<0.0001
Total number of exacerbations, No	64	14	<0.0001
Mild/moderate	53	14	0.0087
Severe	11	0	0.0007
Total patients with one or more exacerbations, No.	30	67*	<0.0001
Mild/moderate	20	6	0.0004
Severe	10	0	0.0004

*It is assumed that there is a misprint in the original paper and that this value should read 6.

Source: Suzuki et al. (2001).

ticular, there is no objective evidence to support a diagnosis of viral infection in any of the participants. Third, all patients were taking theophyllines which are known to interact with oral erythromycin, increasing theophylline levels and potentially reducing erythromycin plasma levels. Under these circumstances, it would have been interesting to know more about adverse effects (we are told only that one patient was excluded from the erythromycin group on grounds of diarrhoea and anorexia) and the plasma levels of erythromycin. Fourth, we are shown no evidence to confirm compliance with erythromycin. Fifth, it would have been fascinating to know whether lung function and exercise tolerance were significantly maintained in the erythromycin group, i.e. does erythromycin alter the natural history of the disease by preventing exacerbation?

These considerations aside, this remains a remarkable result. How should we interpret it, and is it applicable to our clinical practice? The most influential clinical studies on anti-inflammatory effects of macrolides have also been performed in Japanese populations, and it does seem necessary to reproduce these findings in other populations in case genetic effects favour a response in Japanese patients. Furthermore, as the authors point out, it is counter-intuitive to most teaching on antimicrobial drugs to give these long-term, because of fears relating to emerging resistance. It is a pity that the present study did not study microbial resistance, or the economic benefits entailed by erythromycin treatment. It should be noted that no patients died in the study, so no proven benefit exists for mortality.

If it is assumed that long-term macrolides would not be prescribed unless overwhelming evidence excluded resistance while demonstrating reduced morbidity and cost, then the next question is whether erythromycin is superior to placebo in *treating* (rather than preventing) the common cold. Additional questions are whether erythromycin or penicillins (or a combination) are superior in treating existing exacerbations of COPD, and (crucially) whether erythromycin can alter the natural history of the disease. Meanwhile the mechanism of action of erythromycin in the context of preventing upper respiratory tract infection (and inflammation generally) requires to be fully elucidated.

In summary, this fascinating study suggests a potent anti-inflammatory effect for erythromycin, but clinical application is likely to require more subtle strategies than continuous prescription because of the inherent risk of microbial resistance.

Cilomilast, a selective phosphodiesterase-4 inhibitor for treatment of patients with chronic obstructive pulmonary disease: a randomized, dose-ranging study.

Compton CH, Gubb J, Nieman R, *et al. Lancet* 2001; **358**: 265–70.

BACKGROUND. Most of the commonly used pharmacological agents for the maintenance treatment of COPD have been shown to improve symptoms and lung function, but the effects are generally modest at best. Development of novel therapeutic agents for COPD is, therefore, required and is a fertile area for research. Phosphodiesterase-4 is thought to be the principal enzyme in the degradation of cyclic AMP. As cyclic AMP mediates bronchodilator and anti-inflammatory effects in the airway, inhibition of phosphodiesterase-4 is a logical target in COPD. Cilomilast is a specific inhibitor of phosphodiesterase-4. Therefore, this randomized, double blind, placebo-controlled, parallel group study aimed to evaluate the efficacy, tolerability and dose-response of cilomilast in patients with COPD.

INTERPRETATION. In this large and very well-designed study, cilomilast at a dose of 15 mg twice daily was associated with an improvement in FEV_1 from the first administration. At this dose the FEV_1, FVC and PEF tended to rise steadily over the 6-week study period and each variable was significantly elevated at the end of the study, though the improvements were relatively modest. Cilomilast was clinically ineffective at lower doses. There was a non-significant trend towards improved quality of life parameters with cilomilast at 15 mg twice daily. In general, cilomilast was well tolerated, though there were trends towards dose dependent nausea, diarrhoea and abdominal discomfort.

Comment

This meticulous study screened 604 patients from 60 centres in five North European countries. The authors acknowledge that the manufacturer of cilomilast was the study's sole sponsor.

The study employed robust methods. Entry criteria incorporated strict conditions compatible with the diagnosis of COPD, including ongoing symptoms, FEV_1 after bronchodilator therapy of between 30 and 70% predicted, and fixed airflow obstruction defined as a rise in FEV_1 of less than 15% predicted or less than 200 ml after 200 µg of salbutamol. Exclusion criteria included asthma, recent poor control of COPD and significant comorbidities. The study also incorporated a 2-week run-in period during which patients were asked to stop all treatments for COPD with the exception of short acting β-2 agonists and anticholinergics. During the run-in period patients also received placebo in a single-blind fashion as a means of establishing compliance (by tablet counting), and those with poor compliance were excluded. In total 180 patients were excluded from the study.

After the 2-week run-in period patients were randomized to receive oral cilomilast at 5 mg ($n = 109$), 10 mg ($n = 102$) or 15 mg ($n = 107$), or placebo ($n = 106$), with each taken twice daily. Regular assessment over the 6-week study period incorporated spirometry, PEF, interview, physical examination, recordings of bronchodilator use, and quality of life assessment using the SGRQ. The primary end-point for efficacy was the pre-treatment FEV_1, with secondary outcome parameters including pre-treatment PEF and vital capacity (VC) as well as measurements of airflow after the first treatment dose. Data were analysed on an intention to treat basis.

Patients were ideally matched at baseline (overall average FEV_1 was approximately 1.4 litres or 47% predicted). Cilomilast at 15 mg twice daily had a rapid effect, causing an 80 ml increase in FEV_1 at 4 hours. In general this dose resulted in a time-dependent increase in FEV_1 (Fig. 10.9), FVC and PEF. At lower doses cilomilast appeared to induce a small early improvement in airflow relative to placebo, but this invariably returned to baseline by week 6. In view of these data it would be

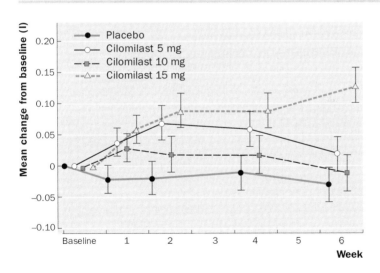

Fig. 10.9 Mean (SE) change from baseline in trough pre-bronchodilator FEV_1. Improvement with 15 mg twice daily was significantly greater than placebo at week 1 ($P = 0.011$), week 2 ($P = 0.002$), week 4 ($P = 0.016$), and week 6 ($P < 0.0001$). Source: Compton et al. (2001).

interesting to know whether efficacy of the 15 mg dose rises further beyond 6 weeks or whether it loses effect with time as the lower doses appeared to do (i.e. is there tachyphylaxis?). Interestingly, at 15 mg of cilomilast twice daily, the improvements in FEV_1, FVC and PEF all appeared to be just below 10% of the pre-treatment value. It is also interesting that all parameters fell over time in the placebo group— this raises the outside possibility of delayed washout of the medicines withdrawn prior to the study period. There was a trend towards improved health related quality of life and rescue bronchodilator use in the cilomilast 15 mg twice-daily group, but this did not attain statistical significance.

The overall rate of total and serious adverse effects was similar in all four groups. Nevertheless, there appeared to be a dose-dependent increase in abdominal pain, diarrhoea and mild nausea in the cilomilast group (8, 9 and 11% for each symptom respectively at 15 mg twice daily, as compared to 3, 1 and 1% respectively in the placebo group). It remains to be seen whether these side-effects limit long-term tolerability.

In summary cilomilast was ineffective below 15 mg twice daily. At this dose, it was generally well tolerated. Cilomilast works rapidly and at 15 mg twice daily, produces a sustained (and apparently increasing) effect over 6 weeks, though the effect is relatively small. Further work is required to determine the long-term efficacy and the clinical interaction with other COPD treatments. The results of ongoing clinical trials are, therefore, awaited with interest.

A randomized, placebo-controlled trial of a leukotriene synthesis inhibitor in patients with COPD.
Gompertz S, Stockley RA. *Chest* 2002; **122**: 289–94.

BACKGROUND. Our understanding of inflammation in COPD is becoming more complex every year, yet the neutrophil still appears to have a prominent place in the pathogenesis of the disease. Neutralization of inflammatory mediators involved in neutrophil recruitment to the lung is, therefore, a logical therapeutic target. Leukotriene B_4 (LTB_4) is a potent neutrophil chemo-attractant derived from the metabolism of arachidonic acid. Five lipoxygenase activating protein (FLAP) plays a central part in generating leukotrienes from arachidonic acid and this study therefore aimed to assess the efficacy of a specific inhibitor of FLAP on the generation of LTB_4, total neutrophil chemo-attractant activity and myeloperoxidase (MPO, secreted from azurophil granules of neutrophils during activation) in stable COPD.

INTERPRETATION. In this small randomized, double-blind, placebo-controlled trial, LTB_4 concentrations in sputum showed a small but significant reduction in those patients treated with a FLAP inhibitor. However, the LTB_4 sputum concentration at the end of the trial period was not significantly different from that in the control group. No differences were observed either within or between groups with regard to MPO or chemo-attractant activity. Larger trials are required to determine the importance of these findings.

Comment

This was a phase II study of the FLAP antagonist BAYx1005. The authors acknowledge support from the manufacturer of BAYx1005. Recruited patients were aged between 40 and 75 years, and had a history of chronic bronchitis with an FEV_1 less than 65% predicted. Patients were excluded if they had symptoms compatible with an exacerbation in the previous 4 weeks, if they had used corticosteroids (inhaled or oral) or other anti-inflammatory drugs in the previous 4 weeks, if their FEV_1 rose by more than 15% predicted in response to bronchodilators, or if they had a history of significant comorbidity (which included atopy, bronchiectasis or $\alpha_1 AT$ deficiency. With the exception of anti-inflammatory drugs and other drugs known to affect leukotriene synthesis, patients remained on their maintenance therapy.

After a run-in period of 1 week, patients were randomized to receive BAYx1005 (500 mg twice daily; $n = 8$) or placebo ($n = 9$) for 2 weeks. At the start of the run-in, and at the beginning and end of the study period, sputum was collected for isolation of the sol phase. LTB_4 concentration, MPO activity and sputum chemotactic activity were determined using standard techniques. The groups were similar at baseline and had reduced diffusing capacity for carbon monoxide, indicating a degree of emphysema. However, it should be noted that 6 of 8 patients in the BAYx1005 group were current smokers as opposed to only 4 of 9 in the placebo group, while 2 patients (1 in each group) appear never to have smoked. In addition, pre-bronchodilator FEV_1 was 30% predicted in the treatment group and 40% in the placebo group.

The authors went to some length to assess the variability inherent in LTB_4 and MPO measurements over time, assessing an additional 6 patients with chronic bronchitis who provided periodic sputum samples. It is not clear whether these subjects satisfied entry criteria for the study. This subgroup analysis confirmed marked inter-individual variation for these parameters, but it is hard to tell the degree of variation with time within individuals from the available data.

In the main study sputum LTB_4 was 8 nM before BAYx1005 and 4.2 nM after treatment ($P < 0.05$), with corresponding values of 5.4 and 8.3 nM respectively in the placebo group. However, it should be noted that there was no significant difference *between* the two groups either before or after treatment, that intra-individual variation in both groups was large, and that the variation in mean group LTB_4 in the separate variability study was 1.5 nM. No significant differences were observed between the groups with respect to MPO or total chemotactic activity, though MPO did fall in 6 of 8 patients in the BAYx1005 group.

A few small points are worth making. First, the study only used one dose of BAYx1005, which may not be the optimal dose. Second, by measuring an inherently variable mediator like sputum LTB_4 only once after treatment started, the study potentially made significant differences even harder to demonstrate in such a small study. Third, chemotactic activity was measured using neutrophils from healthy volunteers while neutrophils from patients with COPD often behave quite differently. As always when a novel anti-inflammatory agent emerges, the final question is whether inhibition of a single mediator (or handful of mediators) can make a significant impact upon a process as complex as the inflammation found in COPD. The answer would appear likely to be no, but that should not prevent important trials like these, particularly if they were to be combined with other targets (for example, other important neutrophil chemo-attractants such as IL-8).

Even with these considerations in mind, the small but significant fall in sputum LTB_4 in the BAYx1005 group is impressive given the small group size and the other points noted above, and functional activity *in vivo*. Ultimately, as the authors acknowledge, a much larger and longer study is required to determine whether FLAP antagonists have a role in COPD.

Use of a mucus clearance device enhances the bronchodilator response in patients with stable COPD.

Wolkove N, Kamel H, Rotaple M, Baltzan MA Jr. *Chest* 2002; **121**: 702–7.

BACKGROUND. Oscillatory devices, or 'flutter valves', are widely used to aid sputum expectoration in patients with bronchiectasis. The principle behind these is that when patients breathe out, the valve generates fluctuations in pressure and flow. Potential benefits include generation of positive end-expiratory pressure (PEEP) as well as agitation and dispersal of mucus, which in turn is easier to expectorate. Wolkove and colleagues hypothesized that this technique may improve access to inhaled bronchodilators in patients with COPD. The aim of this study was, therefore, to determine whether a particular oscillatory mucus clearance device (MCD) could improve spirometry, exercise tolerance and dyspnoea after administration of bronchodilators in COPD.

INTERPRETATION. In this small study a hand-held MCD, when compared to a sham device, resulted in a significant improvement in FEV_1 2 hours after administration of bronchodilator. The MCD was also associated with small but significant improvements in 6-minute walk distance and breathlessness.

Comment

This was a randomized, crossover, sham-controlled study. Recruited patients were in hospital as part of a pulmonary rehabilitation programme or after a recent exacerbation of COPD and had FEV_1 less than 50% predicted and FEV_1/FVC ratio less than 0.65. All were deemed clinically stable (including those with recent exacerbations). Patients were studied on three separate mornings. The first was used for training in the use of the MCD. On the second visit, patients were randomized to receive either the MCD or a sham device (in which the ball-bearing producing 'flutter' was removed). Spirometry was performed before and after 10 minutes with the relevant device, bronchodilator (400 μg salbutamol base, 80 μg ipratropium via MDI) was administered, and spirometry measured again at 30, 60 and 120 minutes.

Between 30 and 60 minutes a 6-minute walk test was performed, with assessment of dyspnoea using a modified Borg scale. The third visit was a duplicate of the second except that patients previously receiving the MCD got the sham device and vice versa.

Twenty-three patients participated. The mean FEV_1 was 0.74 litres (34.5% predicted), and average age was 72 years. Sixteen of the patients reported cough on most days of the year, and all but one of these said the cough was productive.

Interestingly, immediately after using the MCD (i.e. before bronchodilator) there was a 50 ml rise in FEV_1, as compared with less than 10 ml after the sham device. However, this difference did not reach statistical significance. The general trend was for FEV_1 to rise with time after both devices, but for the rise to be greater after the MCD, the difference becoming statistically significant at 2 hours (improvement in FEV_1 over pre-treatment levels 186 ml for the MCD and 130 ml for the sham device). Similarly the walking distance in 6 minutes was improved after MCD (174 vs 162 m, $P <0.01$), as was the oxygen saturation after exercise (92.3 vs 91.4%, $P <0.05$) and the Borg dyspnoea index both before (1.6 vs 1.9, $P <0.05$) and after (4.0 vs 4.4, $P <0.01$) exercise.

These interesting results clearly suggest a beneficial role for the MCD. It should be pointed out, however, that while the results are statistically significant the clinical improvements are small. It is a pity that the timescale was not extended further to 6 hours to determine whether the effect was sustained over the duration of action of ipratropium. It would also be interesting to know whether the benefits are sustained (and perhaps even increased) if the MCD is used over several weeks or months. Furthermore, we are told that the observed differences (as might be expected) were greater among patients producing sputum, and in this regard, it seems strange that patients without cough were included at all. Similarly, bronchodilator reversibility appears not to have been tested, and one might anticipate best results in those with demonstrable reversibility. Finally, it would be impossible to blind patients to the device being used as there is obviously no physical sensation of 'flutter' with the sham device, and this could have biased patient performance in favour of the MCD.

Nevertheless, these results are of considerable interest and deserve further study in the longer term. It will be most interesting to determine whether the MCD benefits patients principally through sputum disaggregation, through alveolar recruitment consequent upon additional PEEP, or both, as this may influence the sub-groups of patients most likely to benefit in future trials. From a clinical perspective, it is likely that any proven benefit of MCDs would translate to an inexpensive addition to bronchodilator therapy.

Neltenexine tablets in smoking and non-smoking patients with COPD. A double-blind, randomized, controlled study versus placebo.

Cattaneo C. *Minerva Med* 2001; **92**: 277–84.

BACKGROUND. Chronic bronchitis is characterized by mucus hypersecretion and by expectoration of sputum. The question of whether pharmacological agents capable of reducing mucous secretion or sputum viscosity have any useful place in the management of COPD has been a source of considerable controversy over the years. Neltenexine is said to reduce mucous hypersecretion, and to aid expectoration of sputum. This study was performed to evaluate the efficacy and safety of neltenexine in patients with COPD.

INTERPRETATION. The study appears to demonstrate a significant effect of neltenexine on symptoms such as breathlessness and cough, as well as on sputum volume, FEV_1 and PaO_2. In general, the improvements noted were more pronounced among non-smokers taking neltenexine. However, interpretation of the data is hampered by a paucity of clinical information.

Comment

This was a randomized, double-blind, placebo-controlled, single-centre (and apparently single-observer) trial. Inclusion criteria included age 40 years or over, COPD diagnosed at least 3 years previously (and free from exacerbation at enrolment), FEV_1 between 70% and 80% predicted and FEV_1/VC ratio less than 0.9. Exclusion criteria included co-existent respiratory diseases such as asthma or pneumonia, and the use of glucocorticoids, β-2 agonists, anticholinergics, antitussives or other mucolytics. Sixty patients were recruited—40 were smokers and 20 'non-smokers'. Twenty smokers received neltenexine tablets in a dose of 37.4 mg twice daily, 20 smokers received placebo tablets twice daily and the 20 non-smokers received neltenexine 37.4 mg twice daily. The duration of treatment appears to have been 20 days followed by discontinuation, but this is not explicitly stated in the paper. Sputum characteristics as well as respiratory symptoms and signs were graded using subjective scores and measured at baseline, on day 10 and at the end of the study period. Spirometry and PaO_2 were measured at baseline and at the end of the study.

The three groups were very well matched for all measured parameters at entry. The patients appeared to describe severe cough (mean of approximately 3.5 on a scale of 0–4) and significant breathlessness at baseline. Symptoms and sputum examination improved significantly in both neltenexine groups as compared with placebo, the effect being observed as early as day 10 and maintained to the end of the study. FEV_1 and PaO_2 also showed a small but significant rise in both neltenexine groups as compared with placebo. Furthermore sputum volume and perceived difficulty of expectoration were significantly improved in the non-smokers taking neltenexine as compared with smokers taking the drug. Neltenexine appears to have been well tolerated. Interestingly the placebo-treated patients had a small but significant fall in sputum volume over the course of the study, and a 40% reduction in perceived dyspnoea.

Even allowing for the marked placebo effect, the results of this trial are very impressive. Neltenexine had an early effect on symptoms and the magnitude of the improvement appeared to increase with time. Unfortunately, however, several issues make accurate interpretation of the data difficult. Perhaps most importantly the smoking status of the patients is not elaborated—one might assume that all 'non-smokers' are *ex*-smokers, but we are given no information on the relative tobacco use of each group. Furthermore, we are told nothing about compliance in the treated groups, and the criteria used to make the original diagnosis of COPD are not explicit. Aside from these more major points the study faces the usual limitations of using multiple subjective criteria, and some of the scoring systems used are poorly explained (for example 'pulmonary auscultation' was graded from 0 [absent] to 4 [severe], but we are not told which auscultatory criteria were used; this parameter improved significantly with the use of neltenexine). It is similarly of some concern that at least one patient aged 37 years is included in the study, in breach of the inclusion criteria. Finally, it seems perhaps a little unusual (though doubtless feasible) that in a trial recruiting 'mild, stable COPD' that perceived dyspnoea and cough severity should have been so high at baseline. Extending this argument it seems potentially incongruous that patients with such notable symptoms were included on the basis that they did not use drugs such as bronchodilators.

These methodological issues, along with the observed placebo effect, detract a little from the impressive results of the study. Certainly the study ought to progress to a rigorous and much larger multicentre trial. This may also afford the benefits of addressing questions inevitably provoked by the study. For example, it would be fascinating to dissect the exact mechanism of action for neltenexine in this context, with particular reference to why the effect is more pronounced in patients who no longer smoke. Similarly, it would be interesting to know whether the drug's efficacy improves further with prolonged use. It would also be useful to know for how long the observed improvements in sputum examination and symptoms are maintained after discontinuation.

In summary, this trial demonstrates effects of neltenexine that may potentially be important for clinical practice. However, firm conclusive evidence of efficacy will require a larger multicentre trial.

Reversal of COPD-associated weight loss using the anabolic agent oxandrolone.
Yeh S-S, DeGuzman B, Kramer T. *Chest* 2002; **122**: 421–8.

BACKGROUND. The association between low body weight and mortality in COPD has already been discussed in this chapter when considering the study by Prescott *et al.*

Traditionally it has proved difficult for patients to regain weight, using diet alone. We need first to demonstrate that weight gain can be safely effected using alternative (or supplementary) methods, and then to demonstrate that the weight gain benefits patients in a meaningful way in terms of end-points like mortality, quality of life, symptoms, exercise tolerance and lung function. The aim of this study was to evaluate whether the oral anabolic steroid oxandrolone could safely stimulate weight gain in patients with COPD and associated weight loss.

INTERPRETATION. In this open-label study, oxandrolone was associated with a mean weight gain of 4.7 lb (around 2.13 kg) at 4 months among the 42% of patients who completed the trial. The weight gain appeared mostly attributable to lean tissue rather than fat. Karnofsky performance status was improved significantly by 4 months of treatment, but mean changes in 6 minute walking distance, symptom scores and spirometry were not significant. Oxandrolone was associated with frequent side-effects.

Comment

This multi-centre community-based study operated for 2 years across 25 American centres. Patients were aged over 40 and had FEV_1 less than 50% predicted with FEV_1/FVC ratio less than 0.7. A history of involuntary weight loss leading to an ideal body weight of 90% or less was required, along with a Karnofsky performance status (a measure of functional abilities) score of 50 or more, and stable COPD over the past month. Patients were excluded if they had any anabolic agent in the previous 6 months or if they had hypercalcaemia, significant renal or hepatic impairment, or (in the case of males) elevated prostate-specific antigen.

Patients were given oxandrolone 10 mg twice daily for 4 months. No specific dietary advice or exercise programme was included in the study. Assessments were performed at baseline, 2 months and 4 months. They included spirometry, 6 minute walking distance, body weight, body composition (using bioelectric impedance analysis), Karnofsky score, and a symptom score.

One hundred and twenty-eight patients participated, with a mean age of 69, FEV_1 34% predicted and BMI 17.8 kg/m². On average, the participants had 79% ideal body weight. It should be noted that the drop-out rate from the study was very high, with only 49 (38%) patients completing the whole study (although another 6 who missed part of the treatment in the middle of the study period were included in the analysis, leading to data on up to 55 patients). The mean weight gain at 2 months ($n = 82$) was 5.1 lb, and at 4 months ($n = 55$) it was 4.7 lb ($P < 0.05$ in each case as compared with baseline). The weight increase was attributable almost exclusively to lean weight and not fat. There was a small but significant improvement in Karnofsky score at 2 months (73.3 vs 70.1, $P < 0.05$) which changed little by 4 months. Mean 6-minute walk distance improved by only 11 metres (we are not told the baseline) at 4 months (not significant), and both maximal inspiratory pressure and FEV_1 fell if anything. Similarly, symptom scores were said not to have changed significantly.

Adverse events were common, in particular oedema (17%) and elevation in transaminases (11.5%). In general the oedema was treatable and the transaminitis self-limiting. Importantly six women were withdrawn because of androgenic effects and one patient taking warfarin died because of over anticoagulation. In total, the authors describe 89 adverse events considered to be possibly or probably associated with oxandrolone. It appears that 22 patients were withdrawn from the study because of drug-related adverse events.

The obvious difficulty in interpreting this pilot study is that it was neither placebo-controlled nor blinded. Furthermore, the patients were not followed up after discontinuation of oxandrolone and so we do not know whether (or for how long) weight gain was maintained. Furthermore, it is not clear whether COPD was the sole cause for weight loss in these patients, and we are told nothing about smoking status (for example, it is conceivable that patients motivated to join a trial may use this as a target date for attempting to stop smoking, which in turn may effect weight gain). The last thing to say is that the drop out rate of 62% is disappointing. If viewed on an intention to treat basis, it would therefore seem that the benefit to the whole study group was relatively small.

Overall, this study confirms that anabolic steroids may potentially increase weight in selected patients with COPD. However, side-effects are common and occasionally serious, and (at least after only 4 months of treatment) no obvious benefits in terms of symptoms, spirometry, maximal inspiratory pressure or exercise tolerance are demonstrable. The authors make the point that subgroups of patients appear to do well with oxandrolone but these groups remain to be defined. Ultimately, the conclusion must be that a randomized, double-blind, placebo-controlled trial is required to evaluate efficacy and safety further. Such a trial is apparently ongoing and the results are awaited with interest.

Home-based neuromuscular electrical stimulation as a new rehabilitative strategy for severely disabled patients with chronic obstructive pulmonary disease (COPD).

Neder JA, Sword D, Ward SA, Mackay E, Cochrane LM, Clark CJ. *Thorax* 2002; **57**: 333–7.

BACKGROUND. Reduced exercise tolerance and skeletal muscle weakness are characteristically associated with advanced COPD. Pulmonary rehabilitation strives to improve these defects, but a proportion of severely incapacitated patients may find active modes of exercise difficult and distressing. The study by Neder and colleagues, therefore, investigated the effect of neuromuscular electrical stimulation (NMES), a form of passive muscle stimulation, on quadriceps muscle function in patients with severe COPD. They also aimed to assess the influence of NMES on exercise capacity and health-related quality of life.

INTERPRETATION. Although this was a small study, NMES was associated with a significant increase in quadriceps muscle strength. Furthermore, use of NMES led to significant improvements in oxygen uptake and endurance capacity during whole body exercise, as assessed using cycle ergometric testing. NMES was also associated with a small but significant reduction in perceived breathlessness.

Comment

Fifteen patients with COPD characterized by an FEV_1 of less than 50% predicted were randomized to receive NMES or no additional treatment for a 6-week period. NMES was performed in the patients' homes after a period of training, and involved application of a portable stimulator to each quadriceps for up to 30 minutes, five times a week. A detailed battery of tests were performed before and after the study period, and included a health-related quality of life questionnaire, assessment of quadriceps strength and endurance, and both maximum incremental and endurance (constant work rate) cardiopulmonary exercise tests.

The two groups were well matched at baseline (although the control group appeared to have higher RV). In both groups baseline quadriceps muscle strength and cycle ergometry tolerance were similar and well below predicted values.

Interestingly, compliance with NMES was assessed using a hidden time monitoring device and was found to be excellent. NMES resulted in both a significant increase in quadriceps function as assessed by maximum isokinetic strength test, and a reduction in fatigue. Similarly, NMES was associated with increased oxygen uptake measured during maximal effort on the cycle ergometer, and with a particularly impressive prolongation of cycling endurance against a fixed work rate (from a mean of 4.5 minutes at baseline to 8.4 minutes after treatment). In general the changes in function in the NMES group were impressive (approaching 50% improvements in several of the parameters tested), with no appreciable differences observed in the control group. In parallel with these changes, a small but significant improvement was noted in the dyspnoea component of the CRDQ (mean improvement of 1.2 on a 7-point scale) in the NMES group, with no change in the control group. NMES did not influence the other three measured components of the questionnaire (fatigue, emotional function and 'mastery').

The principal limitation of this study is the small sample size, a point readily acknowledged by the authors. The nature of the study demands that a larger trial be performed to confirm these observations, and to assess the impact on quality of life more rigorously. It will be fascinating to learn whether exercise capacity can be improved further with longer or more intensive treatments, and indeed, whether exercise capacity can be maintained after withdrawal of NMES (a question not addressed in the current study). A trial comparing NMES with the exercise component of conventional pulmonary rehabilitation programmes would also be fascinating.

While keeping the limitations of small patient groups in mind, however, it is hard not to be impressed by the magnitude of the changes induced by a simple, well-tolerated domiciliary treatment applied over such a short time in patients with such advanced disease. In summary, this new technology appears to have significant potential, particularly as an adjunct to existing rehabilitation services, and future studies are awaited with great interest.

Conclusion

Data relating to patients with COPD continues to cascade from the literature at an increasing rate. What conclusions can be drawn from the collection of papers discussed in this chapter?

First, we must conclude that several groups continue to dissect the most important cellular and chemical targets intrinsic to COPD. The incredibly complex inflammatory process central to COPD has not yet been sufficiently characterized to implicate any single major players, but interesting trends are emerging from the important studies published to date.

Secondly, it seems reasonable to conclude that the treatment of COPD remains sub-optimal. I hope this chapter has demonstrated that we still do not know enough about treatments we regard as established parts of the therapeutic armament for COPD, and that we must strive to tease out the best treatments for individual patients. Thus while in the previous chapter we observed potential hazards for β2-agonists in patients with COPD and ischaemic heart disease, in this chapter we are reminded of the potential detrimental effects of maintenance glucocorticoids in patients with COPD. In contrast, the subgroups of patients in whom inhaled corticosteroids may be useful are beginning to be better defined. We now have excellent information telling us when surgical intervention for COPD will be dangerous, and we have increasing information pointing to the benefits of pulmonary rehabilitation in COPD. We should all stop to think whether the provision for terminal care in this common condition is adequate, and how we might improve our clinical services in this regard.

What is clear is that new, more effective treatments are required for COPD. The emergence of novel pharmacologic agents is driven by increased understanding of pulmonary inflammation, and inevitably is driven to some extent by pharmaceutical industry concerns. The conclusion from this chapter would appear to be that increasingly effective anticholinergic preparations and long-acting β2-agonist preparations are becoming available. In general these have advantages over existing preparations, but we must be mindful of the fact that most of the physiological and symptomatic benefits conferred by these preparations remain relatively small (typically effecting rises in FEV_1 of around 100 ml in the papers discussed here, for example). We have also seen that several new compounds are emerging for the treatment of COPD. In general, the fairest conclusion would appear to be that these are all based on sound scientific principles, but that while most suggest promising results in pilot studies, we need to know much more about these agents before they become part of routine clinical practice. We can confidently anticipate important, large, prospective, randomised, placebo-controlled trials relating to most of the compounds discussed here in the coming years.

A further conclusion from this chapter is that we must not forget the extra-pulmonary manifestations of COPD, which can genuinely be considered a multi-system disorder. The papers discussed here emphasize the insidious rate of depression, osteoporosis, and (to a lesser extent) pulmonary hypertension in patients with COPD.

Finally, I make no apology for making the same ultimate conclusion in this chapter as was made in the previous chapter, namely that smoking prevention/cessation remains the cornerstone of COPD management, and that we remain frustratingly ill-equipped to achieve our aims in this regard. The increasingly scientific approach to the assessment of smoking cessation strategies has been as welcome as it has been important, and should pave the way for identification of strategies with better success rates than we have at present.

References

1. Sakao S, Tatumi K, Igari H, Watanabe R, Shino Y, Shirasawa H, Kuriyama T. Association of tumor necrosis factor-α gene promoter polymorphism with the presence of COPD. *Am J Respir Crit Care Med* 2001; **163**: 420–2.

2. Wilson AG, Symons JA, McDowell TL, McDevitt HO, Duff GW. Effects of a polymorphism in the human tumor necrosis factor α promoter on transcription activation. *Proc Natl Acad Sci USA*. 1997; **94**: 3195–9.

3. American Thoracic Society. Standards for the diagnosis and care of patients with chronic obstructive pulmonary disease. *Am J Respir Crit Care Med* 1995; **152**(5Pt2): S77–121.

4. Higham MA, Pride NB, Alikhan A, Morrell NW. Tumor necrosis factor-α gene promoter polymorphism in chronic obstructive pulmonary disease. *Eur Respir J* 2000; **15**: 281–4.

5. Hurt RD, Sachs DP, Glover ED, Offord KP, Johnston JA, Dale LC, Khayrallah MA, Schroeder DR, Glover PN, Sullivan CR, Croghan IT, Sullivan PM. A comparison of sustained-release bupropion and placebo for smoking cessation. *N Engl J Med* 1997; **337**: 1195–202.

6. Vestbo J, Sorensen T, Lange P, Brix A, Torre P, Viskum K. Long-term effect of inhaled budesonide in mild and moderate chronic obstructive pulmonary disease: a randomized controlled trial. *Lancet* 1999; **353**: 1819–23.

7. Pauwels RA, Lofdahl CG, Laitinen LA, Schouten JP, Postma DS, Pride NB, Ohlsson SV. Long-term treatment with inhaled budesonide in persons with mild chronic obstructive pulmonary disease who continue smoking. European Respiratory Society Study on Chronic Obstructive Pulmonary Disease. *N Engl J Med* 1999; **340**: 1948–53.

8. Burge PS, Calverley PM, Jones PW, Spencer S, Anderson JA, Maslen TK. Randomized, double blind, placebo controlled study of fluticasone propionate in patients with moderate to severe chronic obstructive pulmonary disease: the ISOLDE trial. *BMJ* 2000; **320**: 1297–303.

9. Lung Health Study. Effect of inhaled triamcinolone on the decline in pulmonary function in chronic obstructive pulmonary disease. *N Engl J Med* 2000; **343**: 1902–9.

10. Nocturnal Oxygen Therapy Trial Group. Continuous or nocturnal oxygen therapy in hypoxaemic chronic obstructive lung disease; a clinical trial. *Ann Intern Med* 1980; **93**: 391–8.

11. Medical Research Council Working Party. Long-term domiciliary oxygen therapy in chronic hypoxic cor pulmonale complicating chronic bronchitis and emphysema. *Lancet* 1981; **1**: 681–6.

12. Griffiths TL, Burr ML, Campbell IA, Lewis-Jenkins V, Mullins J, Shiels K, Turner-Lawlor PJ, Payne N, Newcombe RG, Ionescu AA, Thomas J, Tunbridge J, Lonescu AA. Results at 1 year of outpatient multidisciplinary pulmonary rehabilitation: a randomized controlled trial. *Lancet* 2000; **355**: 362–8.

13. Laurell CB, Eriksson S. The electrophoretic α_1-globulin pattern of serum in α_1-antitrypsin deficiency. *Scand J Clin Lab Invest* 1963; **15**: 132–40.

14. Dirksen A, Dijkman JH, Madsen F, Stoel B, Hutchison DCS, Ulrik CS, Skovgaard LT, Kok-Jensen A, Rudolphus A, Seersholm N, Vrooman HA, Reiber JHC, Hansen NC, Heckser T, Viskum K, Stolk J. A randomized clinical trial of α_1-antitrypsin augmentation therapy. *Am J Respir Crit Care Med* 2000; **160**: 1468–72.

15. Massaro GD, Massaro D. Retinoic acid treatment abrogates elastase-induced pulmonary emphysema in rats. *Nat Med* 1997; **3**: 675–7.

11

Exacerbations of COPD and their management

Exacerbations of COPD are responsible for considerable mortality, morbidity and strain on health resources. They may also make a significant contribution to disease progression.

This section will begin by exploring the concept of early supported discharge for those patients considered not to have life-threatening exacerbations, then will move on to consider the central importance of infection to exacerbations.

Thereafter, therapeutic trials in the context of exacerbations will be discussed. It should be noted straight away that the evidence base surrounding the management of exacerbations of COPD is so small precisely because it is so difficult to perform good, ethical trials in patients who are acutely breathless and often in life-threatening respiratory failure. The trials discussed are, therefore, both admirable and immensely important. Finally, we shall assess invaluable data emerging with regard to the outcome of patients with COPD who require invasive mechanical ventilation during exacerbation.

 Supported discharge shortens hospital stay in patients hospitalized because of an exacerbation of COPD.
Sala E, Alegre L, Carrera M, *et al. Eur Respir J* 2001; **17**: 1138–42.

B A C K G R O U N D . Exacerbations of COPD place an enormous burden on hospital resources. Moves to manage exacerbations in the community are, therefore, most welcome in theory, but required to be demonstrably safe and cost-effective. This study aimed to evaluate the effectiveness and safety of a system whereby patients were admitted for a few days prior to early discharge with back up from trained respiratory nurses.

I N T E R P R E T A T I O N . The study allocated patients admitted to hospital with exacerbations of COPD to standard hospital care or early supported discharge. On average, each supported discharge patient spent 2.1 fewer days in hospital. The average duration of home visits was 7.3 days with 4.8 visits per patient. Although selection bias may have influenced the results of the study, early supported discharge significantly reduced in-hospital stay.

Comment

This study ran over one calendar year and involved all patients admitted to hospital with an exacerbation of COPD who responded sufficiently to immediate treatment to allow transfer to a medical ward (as opposed to an intensive care unit). Patients who lived in the hospital city and who were willing to accept supported discharge were allocated to that arm of the study ($n = 105$); those who lived in the city and did not accept supported discharge and all patients living outside the city were allocated to standard care ($n = 100$). During hospital stay both groups received standard treatment for an exacerbation of COPD. The attending specialist decided when discharge was suitable for all patients (i.e. neither patient nor specialist was blinded to the study). The supported discharge patients were visited by a trained nurse the following day and as felt necessary thereafter. Patients could also contact the nurse during working hours on a mobile phone.

The two groups were well matched at baseline, with average age approximately 68, FEV_1 approximately 45% predicted, PaO_2 approximately 57 mmHg and $PaCO_2$ approximately 45 mmHg (breathing room air). Length of hospital stay was 5.9 days in the supported discharge group as opposed to 8 days in the standard care group ($P < 0.001$). The authors' provide data suggesting that this effect had a striking impact with regard to releasing beds for other emergency admissions. The price of the shorter hospital stay equated to an average post-hospital follow up period of 7.3 days, during which nurses visited each patient 4.8 times on average and responded to 2.3 telephone calls per day. Over the course of the study, there were 45 re-admissions, 29 in the early supported discharge group and 16 in the control group, though early readmission was rare. We are told neither the reasons for readmission, nor whether this difference was significant.

The length-of-stay data alone lend persuasive support to early supported discharge. However, a few points should be made before fully endorsing this strategy. First, this trial was neither randomized nor blinded. We learn in the paper that 46 control patients resided in the hospital city, and by definition appear to have declined early supported discharge. It is quite possible, therefore, that the trial compares one group of motivated patients against a group comprised of less motivated city-dwelling patients and patients from outside the city who must have known they were being excluded from the active phase of the trial in the first place. This may well have introduced bias in favour of shorter stay in the early supported discharge group. Second, as the physicians were not blinded to the trial, it is possible that enthusiasm for early supported discharge also introduced bias in favour of reduced length of stay. In this regard, it is interesting that length of stay was so long in the control group, though the authors do point out that this was shorter than in similar patients from the previous calendar year. A limitation of the study, as the authors concede, is that criteria for discharge were not pre-determined, and so bias of the kind mentioned above cannot be excluded.

It would also have been fascinating to know the (presumed) cost savings of the exercise, after accounting for costs of nurse training, nurse visits, provision of extra treatment at home, and the cost of re-admissions attributed to failure of early supported discharge. Similarly, we are told that the nurses made a variety of measurements at home, but we are not told how these influenced management. A critical question for this sort of programme is whether there are parameters that predict safe and effective termination of the contact between nurse and patient.

In summary, this trial contributes to evidence supporting further investigation and use of early supported discharge for patients with acute exacerbations of COPD who improve with immediate treatment in the emergency room. The magnitude of the benefit observed, however, is a little less perhaps than one might have hoped. Further, larger trials are undoubtedly needed and should be randomized, with strictly pre-determined discharge criteria and incorporation of economic evaluation. If possible, they should be blinded at least to the point where potential early discharge criteria are fulfilled. Such trials will be important, as in principle, early supported discharge seems a very attractive use of resource.

Patients' and carers' preferences in two models of care for acute exacerbations of COPD: results of a randomized controlled trial.
Ojoo JC, Moon T, McGlone S, *et al. Thorax* 2002; **57**: 167–9.

BACKGROUND. This study complements the work by Sala and colleagues, considered in the previous discussion. While there is some evidence to suggest that patients favour early discharge over longer hospital stay, virtually nothing is known about the views of patients' main carers. Given the general morbidity and frequency of exacerbations associated with advancing COPD, a significant physical, emotional and economic burden may be placed on carers. This study aimed to assess the attitudes of patients and carers towards early supported discharge.

INTERPRETATION. For the group randomized to receive early supported discharge, 96% of patients and 85% of their carers said they would have preferred this form of care. For the group randomized to conventional hospital management of their exacerbation, 59% of patients and 43% of their carers said they would have preferred early supported discharge. Early supported discharge is, therefore, popular among patients and their carers.

Comment

Patients included in the study had an exacerbation of COPD and were over 18 years of age, with an FEV$_1$/FVC ratio below 0.7, and less than 15% reversibility in baseline FEV$_1$ in response to salbutamol. Exacerbation was defined as worsening of breathlessness with increasing sputum volume and/or increasing sputum purulence. Patients were excluded if they had acidosis or new type II respiratory failure, right heart failure, other significant comorbidity, or acute changes such as pneumonia or cardiac failure on chest X-ray. Importantly, patients could be excluded if they had poor performance status or little home support.

Patients were assessed shortly after admission and randomized to conventional in-patient care or to early supported discharge, which comprised discharge within 48 hours of admission and access to trained respiratory nurses. The nurses monitored treatment daily, provided 'education and reassurance' to patients and carers, and were available by telephone 8 hours a day (the hospital ward took calls in the evening or overnight). For both groups clinical progress and symptom charts were completed daily, and a satisfaction questionnaire completed by patients and carers within 2 weeks of discharge. One of the authors was affiliated to a pharmaceutical company, but it is not clear whether that company provided funding.

Over a 10-month period (which included winter) 328 patients with exacerbations of COPD were screened, of whom 117 were eligible and 60 were randomized ($n = 30$ in each group), with 6 withdrawals during the study, leaving 54 patients for analysis ($n = 27$ in each group). The groups were well matched at baseline with mean age 70, FEV_1 around 0.92 litres, with 9 patients in each group living alone. No significant differences were noted in symptom score, spirometry, or re-admission rates. Importantly the total length of care was not significantly different either (7.4 days for early supported discharge and 5.9 days for hospital care). Health economics were not included in the study but the implication is that early supported discharge must have been far cheaper. Importantly early supported discharge was safe, with if anything fewer associated deaths and re-admissions.

However, 26/27 patients who received early supported discharge and 16/27 patients who received hospital care stated they had a preference for home care ($P = 0.001$). Furthermore, while only 34 carers responded, 17/20 carers from the early supported discharge group and 6/14 carers from the hospital group also said they would have preferred the patient to have had home care ($P = 0.01$).

This study, therefore, provides further support to the argument for early supported discharge. A few comments should be made in trying to tailor these data to clinical practice. First, it is not clear whether the hospital-treated patients and their carers had specific and daily access to a trained nurse providing education and reassurance (though it is implied that they did not). In other words, it would have been interesting to see the results corrected for time exposed to education and reassurance by trained staff as this, rather than location of care, may have been a primary influence on the results. In addition, it is not clear how many previous admissions and how many episodes of early supported discharge patients had received in the past. It is possible that most patients had been in hospital before but that early supported discharge was a new (and welcome) experience for patients in that group. Also, symptom scores were completed by the study nurses who may subconsciously have been more enthusiastic for the newer form of (nurse-led) care, and their enthusiasm may have been conveyed to patients. All of these factors may have biased towards an effect of early supported discharge, though it could equally be argued that each of these factors would be integral to any 'real-life' introduction of early supported discharge schemes.

One final issue relates to the low numbers reaching the trial from original screening. While this trial had rigorous entry criteria, it seems likely that the significant majority of the patients excluded from the trial (for example those with more severe exacerbations) would also necessarily be excluded from routine (i.e. non-trial) early supported discharge services. If this is the case then a disappointingly low proportion of patients with exacerbations may be eligible for this important mode of care. This should not detract, however, from the fact that this study adds significantly to the literature by clearly demonstrating a preference for early supported discharge among patients and their carers. Early supported discharge appears to be effective, safe, relatively cheap, and preferred by patients and carers. On the basis of evidence in this trial, it seems applicable to patients who have non-life threatening exacerbations.

Lower respiratory illnesses promote FEV$_1$ decline in current smokers but not ex-smokers with mild chronic obstructive pulmonary disease.

Kanner RE, Anthonisen NR, Connett JE. *Am J Respir Crit Care Med* 2001; **164**: 356–64.

BACKGROUND. Controversy continues to surround the question of whether exacerbations accelerate the decline in lung function associated with COPD. Whether smoking may independently promote an effect of lower respiratory infection on lung function has not previously been addressed formally. This study (itself set within the framework of the large Lung Health Study |1|) aimed to address this specific question in patients with mild COPD.

INTERPRETATION. Sustained smoking cessation was associated with significantly fewer lower respiratory tract infections. In patients who continued to smoke, the frequency of respiratory infections rose steadily. Among smokers, but not among ex-smokers, a single annual respiratory infection appeared to exert a small but significant acceleration of FEV$_1$ decline. In addition increasing frequency of respiratory infections predicted for accelerated loss of FEV$_1$ in smokers but not in ex-smokers. This study adds a further element of persuasive evidence for smoking cessation in COPD.

Comment

Patients initially recruited to the Lung Health Study (LHS) were young smokers (35–60), with an FEV$_1$ of 55–90% predicted, and no significant comorbidity. LHS patients had annual interview and spirometry. As part of these visits, patients were asked to report episodes of 'bronchitis, pneumonia, influenza or chest colds' resulting in a visit by a doctor in the previous year. The investigators grouped these self-reported symptoms together as lower respiratory illness. As the authors acknowledge, there are potentially important limitations associated with recall and reporting bias in this setting. In addition hospital admissions for infection (apparently rare) and infective symptoms managed at home without a doctor's knowledge (presumably very common) were necessarily excluded, and the multiple individual and social factors influencing consultation rates may, therefore, also have influenced results. However, the impressive size of this multi-centre, randomized study ($n = 5887$ participants) is likely to dilute such confounding factors and distribute their influences evenly among study groups.

For the purposes of the current study, participants were described as continuous smokers (who we shall call *smokers*), intermittent smokers (smoking described on at least one visit), and sustained quitters (who we shall call *ex-smokers*). For some reason the numbers in each group are not stated but the inference is that there were a little fewer than 1000 smokers and many more ex-smokers.

Smokers had a progressive and significant rise in the frequency of respiratory infection over time whereas ex-smokers did not. At 5 years of follow-up, ex-smokers had approximately one-third fewer infections. Importantly, when patients with symptoms compatible with *chronic* bronchitis were removed from the analysis, smokers still had a progressive increase in the rate of intercurrent infection. Among smokers, infection in the past year independently and significantly accelerated the rate of decline of FEV_1, the mean excess attributable to infection being 7 ml/year. The corresponding rate in ex-smokers (2 ml/year) was not significant. Further evidence was presented to demonstrate that in smokers, but not ex-smokers, increasing number of infections correlates with progressive loss of FEV_1. Intriguingly their data also hints that some (but not all) of the loss of FEV_1 in smokers with infection can be recovered if further infection is avoided. Of course, the implication from the other data is that further infection *will* ensue if smoking continues.

In summary, while the limitations of self-reported symptoms must be kept in mind, this study shows that even in mild COPD smoking is a critical determinant of whether infection results in loss of lung function. The overall message may seem predictable to patients and doctors alike, that is we should tell our patients that if they stop smoking they are likely to have fewer infections and that these infections are less likely to cause lasting harm. Conversely, if they continue to smoke they are likely to have more infections that are likely to take a small but cumulative toll on lung function. However, the considerable clinical significance of this study is that we now have critically evaluated evidence with which to back this assertion. This may be particularly important because these data were gathered from relatively asymptomatic patients in whom the perceived requirement for smoking cessation may be less.

New strains of bacteria and exacerbations of chronic obstructive pulmonary disease.

Sethi S, Evans N, Grant BJB, Murphy TF. *N Engl J Med* 2002; **347**: 465–71.

BACKGROUND. The relative contribution of bacteria to exacerbations of COPD remains unclear. The improvement in symptoms when exacerbations of COPD are treated with antibiotics argues for an important role for respiratory pathogens.

However, potential pathogens are commonly isolated from the sputum of patients with stable COPD who remain entirely asymptomatic. Against this background, Sethi *et al.* postulated that exacerbations are associated with acquisition of new strains of bacteria previously unencountered by the immune system.

INTERPRETATION. This study provides clear evidence for an association between exacerbations of COPD and the isolation of new strains of respiratory pathogens.

Comment

This is a large, meticulous and carefully designed study, which makes a significant case for the critical role of bacteria in a proportion of exacerbations of COPD. The study recruited 81 patients with features of chronic bronchitis. Exclusion criteria included significant comorbidity, prescription of immunosuppressant drugs and clinical evidence of asthma or bronchiectasis. Patients were reviewed monthly and whenever they had exacerbations, the follow up period being up to 56 months. Exacerbations were defined using pre-determined criteria describing increases in respiratory symptoms (cough, breathlessness and changes in sputum), and particular efforts were made to exclude pneumonia or cardiac failure as a cause of these. At each visit sputum was collected when possible, and cultured using standard techniques. If *Haemophilus influenzae, Moraxella catarrhalis, Streptococcus pneumoniae, Pseudomonas aeruginosa, Staphylococcus aureus* or assorted Gram-negative rods were isolated they were considered potential pathogens, and isolates of the first four of these species were subjected to detailed molecular typing.

The average age of the patients was 66 years, and the mean FEV_1 was 47% predicted. Data pertaining to 1975 patient visits was collected, and on all but 148 of these, sputum was obtained successfully. The average number of visits per patient was 24, and the average number of exacerbations per patient per year was 2.1.

When considering conventional bacterial isolation, the relative risk of an exacerbation was 1.4 times commoner if a pathogen was isolated ($P < 0.001$). In particular *M. catarrhalis* and *S. pneumoniae* were associated with exacerbations (relative risks 2 and 1.4 respectively) but isolation of *H. influenzae* did not predict for exacerbation. However, when isolates were subjected to molecular typing, a more striking pattern emerged. The emergence of any new strain of pathogen was associated with a greater than 2 fold relative risk of having exacerbation and in this analysis, new strains of *H. influenzae, M. catarrhalis* and *S. pneumoniae* were all associated with a significantly increased risk of exacerbation (Fig. 11.1).

These data greatly strengthen the evidence supporting a role for infection in exacerbations of COPD. As the authors state, a causative role may be inferred but cannot be proven on the basis of these data.

The authors themselves stress that this analysis does not assess the role of viruses (or atypical bacteria), and it remains plausible that these have important roles to play in some exacerbations of COPD. They further acknowledge that the study is critically dependent upon isolates of bacteria from sputum, and that sputum analysis has disappointingly low sensitivity and specificity.

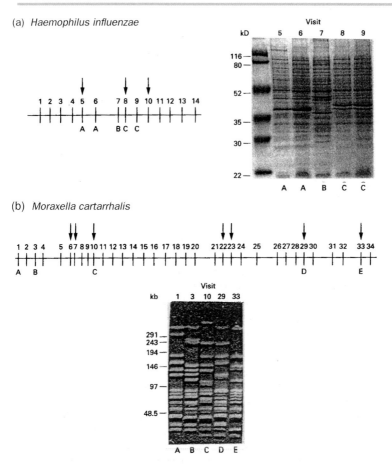

Fig. 11.1 Time lines and molecular typing for two patients. The horizontal lines are time lines, with each number indicating a clinic visit. The arrows indicate exacerbations. Isolates of each bacterial species were assigned types on the basis of banding patterns on gel electrophoresis. The first isolate from each patient was assigned letter A, as were all subsequent isolates with an identical banding pattern. Subsequent isolates with different banding patterns were assigned consecutive letters (B, C, D and so forth). The lettering system was applicable to the individual patient. An isolate labelled A from one patient, for example, was not the same strain as an isolate labelled A from another patient. In (a), each letter under the time line represents a positive sputum culture for *H. influenzae* in one patient. Molecular typing was performed with sodium dodecyl sulfate-polyacrylamide-gel electrophoresis and staining with Coomassie blue. Whole bacterial-cell lysates of isolates recovered at visits 5 through 9 are shown. Three molecular types were identified. In (b), each letter under the time line represents a positive culture for *M. catarrhalis* in another patient. Molecular typing was performed with the use of pulsed-field gel electrophoresis and ethidium bromide staining. *Sma*I-digested DNA from isolates recovered at visits 1, 3, 10, 29 and 33 are shown. Five molecular types were identified. Source: Sethi *et al.* (2002).

A few additional points are worth making. For example, although isolation of new strains of bacteria undoubtedly increased the relative risk of exacerbation being present, it should be noted that in a high proportion of visits where a new strain was isolated there was no clinically apparent exacerbation. Conversely, in many exacerbations no new strain was isolated. These observations may be explained by problems inherent in the culture of sputum. The other possibilities to consider are that new strains often induce inflammatory reactions which are not clinically experienced by the patient as an overt exacerbation, and that a significant proportion of exacerbations of COPD genuinely have little or no link with bacteria.

None of this detracts from the invaluable data in this study, which gives us stronger evidence than ever before to conclude that bacteria are central to (at least a significant proportion of) exacerbations of COPD. The likelihood that other agents contribute in the appropriate setting remains, and in this regard, the specific role of viruses requires clearer definition.

Once daily oral ofloxacin in chronic obstructive pulmonary disease exacerbation requiring mechanical ventilation: a randomized placebo-controlled trial.

Nouira S, Marghli S, Belghith M, Besbes L, Elatrous S, Abroug F.
Lancet 2001; **358**: 2020–5.

BACKGROUND. Whether antibiotics should be used routinely in acute exacerbations of COPD has been fiercely debated for many years. The issue becomes still more difficult when extended to patients with COPD in the intensive therapy unit (ITU). Intuitively it might be expected that infections contribute significantly to airway inflammation in the most severe exacerbations of COPD, lowering the threshold for antibiotics. Alternatively, the ready acquisition of virulent antibiotic-resistant organisms in mechanically ventilated patients, and the association between unselected antibiotic use and ventilator associated pneumonia argues against routine antibiotic prescription. With this background in mind Nouira and colleagues performed a prospective, double-blind, randomized, placebo-controlled trial with the aim of establishing the efficacy of ofloxacin in the management of patients mechanically ventilated with an acute exacerbation of COPD.

INTERPRETATION. Ofloxacin was associated with significant reductions in in-hospital mortality and the requirement for additional antibiotics. Similarly, the risk of nosocomial pneumonia, length of ITU stay and length of hospital admission were significantly reduced in the ofloxacin-treated patients. Ofloxacin appeared to be well tolerated.

Comment

This study screened 213 consecutive patients admitted to two Tunisian ITUs with an exacerbation of COPD in whom mechanical ventilation was required for acute respiratory failure. Crucially, patients were excluded from the study if they had received recent antibiotics and if they had pneumonic infiltrates on chest X-ray.

Indeed 120 patients were excluded, mostly due to co-existent pneumonia or previous antibiotic therapy. As such 93 patients fulfilled entry criteria. It should be noted that wherever possible patients were supported with non-invasive ventilation (NIV), though ultimately all but 12 patients progressed to intubation. Patients were randomized to receive a 10-day course of 400 mg of ofloxacin or placebo (each administered once in the morning for 10 days via the oral/nasogastric/orogastric route as appropriate). Three patients were secondarily excluded on the basis that they recovered with less than 6 hours of NIV and left ITU before starting trial medication. As such 90 patients received ofloxacin or placebo (n = 45 in each group). Sputum (or endotracheal aspirate) was collected for Gram stain and culture before starting treatment. Primary end-points were defined as death in hospital or the clinical requirement for additional antibiotics. Secondary end-points were duration of mechanical ventilation and length of hospital stay. Results were analysed on an intention to treat basis.

The two groups were very well matched at entry. The average age was approximately 66 years, the average FEV_1 around 0.75 litres, and the average arterial blood pH 7.22. For reasons that are not clear the concomitant use of β-2 agonists was below 50% in each group. Positive cultures prior to treatment were obtained from approximately 60% of patients in each group. The majority of these were common organisms associated with COPD but interestingly *Pseudomonas aeruginosa* was isolated on four occasions (three in the group subsequently receiving ofloxacin).

The results of the study were astonishingly impressive (Table 11.1). Ofloxacin was associated with an absolute risk reduction of 17.5% for in-hospital death and 28.4% for additional antibiotic requirement. Ofloxacin reduced the need for mechanical ventilation by 4 days and hospital stay by almost 10 days. It is interesting that ofloxacin caused a significant reduction in pneumonia in the first week, and that all deaths in either group occurred after day 7, with accelerated mortality in the placebo group after day 16. At first glance, it may appear, therefore, that ofloxacin's effect was mediated via direct prevention of nosocomial pneumonia. However, from the available data it appears that nosocomial pneumonia was far from being the only cause of death in the placebo group (we are told that 6 ITU deaths occurred in patients without nosocomial pneumonia). It would have been fascinating to know the detailed cause of death for all 12 patients who died. On balance it appears that ofloxacin has a profound effect on preventing nosocomial pneumonia and that this is likely to explain some (but not all) of the reduction in mortality described. The mechanism of this effect remains to be established.

This trial is both timely and important. Despite being relatively small, the results are surprisingly dramatic. Ideally it would be useful to know more about cause of death as mentioned above, to know how rigorous the original diagnosis of COPD was, and to know how long patients had been in hospital before referral to ITU (i.e. are these data principally applicable to patients who have already been potentially exposed to nosocomial organisms?). However, irrespective of these points this study provides much needed information. Patients with acute severe exacerbations of COPD requiring mechanical ventilation are difficult to manage. With this in mind,

Table 11.1 Outcome measures

	Ofloxacin (n = 47)	Placebo (n = 46)	Absolute risk reduction (95% CI)	P
Primary outcome				
Death				
ICU	2 (4%)	8 (17%)	13.2 (0.8 to 25.6)	0.05
Hospital	2 (4%)	10 (22%)	17.5 (4.3 to 30.7)	0.01
Need for additional antibiotics	3 (6%)	16 (35%)	28.4 (12.9 to 43.9)	0.0006
Combined events	5 (11%)	26 (57%)	45.9 (29.1 to 62.7)	<0.0001
Secondary outcome				
Duration of mechanical ventilation (days)	6.4 (3.1)	10.6 (5.1)	4.2 (2.5 to 5.9)	0.04
Duration of stay (days)				
ICU	9.4 (5.2)	14.5 (6.0)	5.1 (3.9 to 6.3)	0.02
Hospital	14.9 (7.4)	24.5 (8.5)	9.6 (3.4 to 12.8)	0.01
Adverse effects				
Rash	1	0		
Facial oedema	1	0		
Diarrhoea	1	1		
Abnormal serum AST and ALT	2	3		
Total	5 (11%)	4 (9%)	1.9 (−10.0 to 13.8)	0.75

Data are number of patients (%) or mean (SD). ICU = intensive care unit; AST = aspartate aminotransferase; ALT = alanine aminotransferase; Combined events = combination of death in hospital and need for additional antibiotics.

Source: Nouira *et al.* (2001).

and until further information becomes available, it seems pertinent to give 10 days of ofloxacin to the very specific group of patients with severe acute exacerbations of COPD who have a clear chest X-ray at the point that mechanical ventilation is required. As the authors state, routine use of alternative antibiotics in this setting cannot be justified without further trials.

Systemic glucocorticoids in severe exacerbations of COPD.

Sayiner A, Aytemur ZA, Cirit M, Ünsal I. *Chest* 2001; **119**: 726–30.

BACKGROUND. Although systemic corticosteroids are recommended in acute exacerbations, very little evidence exists to indicate the ideal glucocorticoid to use, what dose to give, or how long to give it for. This study, therefore, aimed to compare the efficacy and safety of either 3 or 10 days of intravenous methylprednisolone in exacerbations of COPD.

INTERPRETATION. Ten days of methylprednisolone was associated with significantly higher PaO_2 and FEV_1 at day 10 than was a 3-day course. The exacerbation rate over the next 6 months was similar after either treatment. No obvious differences were observed in adverse events.

Comment

This single-centre randomized, parallel-group, single-blind trial recruited patients with exacerbations severe enough to cause disturbance of sleep and breathlessness preventing minor activities such as dressing. The patients had a PaO_2 of 55 mmHg or less, $PaCO_2$ of 45 mmHg or more, at least a 20 pack-year smoking history, and an FEV_1 of less than 35% predicted. Exclusion criteria included an allergic/atopic tendency, systemic steroids in the preceding month, severe hypertension, poorly controlled diabetes, uncompensated cardiac failure, or requirement for mechanical ventilation. Patients were randomized to receive one of two regimens. The first comprised methylprednisolone 0.5 mg/kg four times a day for 3 days, then 0.5 mg/kg twice daily for 3 days, then 0.5 mg/kg once a day for 4 days, when treatment was discontinued. The second regimen was identical to the first with the exception that saline replaced methylprednisolone on days 4–10 inclusive. Patients remained in hospital throughout the trial. Analyses included spirometry, arterial blood gases (breathing room air) and a locally devised symptom score. Exacerbation rates in the following 6 months were derived from case records. It is unclear how data on adverse events was compiled. Primary outcome measurements were FEV_1 and PaO_2 on days 3 and 10.

From 198 patients screened, the exclusion criteria removed 162, leaving 36 patients ($n = 18$) in each group. One patient in each group was withdrawn due to adverse events (pneumothorax and steroid psychosis) and data was analysed for the remaining 34 patients. The two groups were generally well matched with age around 66, though it should be noted that there were small, non-significant baseline differences in FEV_1 (0.54 versus 0.60 litres in the 3- and 10-day groups respectively), PaO_2 (45 versus 40 mmHg) and $PaCO_2$ (55 versus 58 mmHg).

PaO_2 rose significantly in both groups, but the *change* was significantly greater in the group receiving methylprednisolone for 10 days (Fig. 11.2). Importantly, the change in PaO_2 over days 3–10 was only significant in the group continuing to receive methylprednisolone. Similarly, while FEV_1 rose in both groups, the rise was significantly greater in the 10-day steroid group (FEV_1 0.83 versus 0.61 litres at day 10), with the continued improvement over days 3–10 only being significant in this group. It is worth noting that the rise in FEV_1 and PaO_2 on day 3 was greater in the 10-day steroid group (at a time when both groups had received identical treatment), a point which is developed below. Exacerbation rates over the following 6 months equated to 0.9 and 0.6 per year for the 3- and 10-day steroid groups respectively (no significant difference). The remarkable thing about this statistic is that we are told that the exacerbation rates before the study were 5.2 and 4.9 per year respectively. This anomaly is not explained. Adverse events (other than those

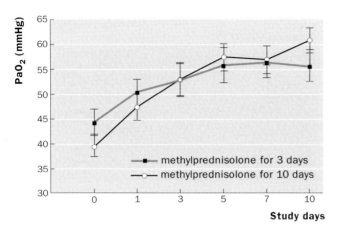

Fig. 11.2 PaO_2 levels in the two study groups (mean $\pm$ SEM). The *change* in PaO_2 was significantly greater in the group receiving methylprednisolone for 10 days, when analysed over the periods 0–10 days ($P = 0.012$) and 3–10 days ($P < 0.01$). Source: Sayiner *et al.* (2001).

mentioned above) were said to be limited to hyperglycaemia in 2 patients from each group.

The potential limitations of this study include the ward staff not being blind to the treatment administered, the fact patients were hospitalized for the duration of the study (i.e. length of hospital stay could not be measured as a discriminator), and the fact that data was not analysed on an intention to treat basis. In addition, while the strict exclusion criteria selected out a pure population of patients with severe COPD (FEV_1 approximately 26% predicted), this did leave the study small and quite removed from 'real life'. Of more concern is the more pronounced improvement in the 10-day steroid group to day 3. This could imply that this group contained patients with inherently more reversible disease—unfortunately, neither bronchodilator nor steroid reversibility appears to have been checked. Furthermore, we are told nothing about which measurements were made, or symptoms ascertained, with regard to adverse events. Finally, the surprisingly low exacerbation rate after discharge could be because exacerbations presented to other hospitals (we are not told about mortality rates), rather than there being a dramatic reduction in illness after the index admission.

While being mindful of these concerns, it seems likely that 10 days of intravenous methylprednisolone was more effective than a 3-day course in this group of patients with severe COPD. It is difficult to extrapolate these data directly to settings in which oral corticosteroids are used routinely in exacerbations. However, this interesting study would appear to emphasize two points, namely that further work is required in larger studies to determine the optimal dose, route, preparation and duration of corticosteroids in COPD, and that courses longer than 3 days appear to give better results.

Comparison of nebulized budesonide and oral prednisolone with placebo in the treatment of acute exacerbations of chronic obstructive pulmonary disease.

Maltais F, Ostinelli J, Bourbeau J, *et al. Am J Respir Crit Care Med* 2002; **165**: 698–703.

BACKGROUND. Systemic corticosteroids have an established place in the management of acute exacerbations of COPD. Because adverse effects such as hyperglycaemia, mood change, insomnia and weight gain can arise in association with short courses of systemic steroids, novel therapies would be welcome. However, any alternative agent would have to demonstrate at least equivalent efficacy and fewer side effects as compared with systemic corticosteroids. The aim of this study was therefore to establish the efficacy and safety of nebulized budesonide in acute exacerbations of COPD.

INTERPRETATION. In this well-designed randomized, placebo-controlled, double-blind, double-dummy, parallel group study, oral prednisolone was significantly more effective in the treatment of acute exacerbations of COPD than was nebulized budesonide, which in turn was significantly more effective than placebo. The profile of adverse effects was similar in each arm of the study.

Comment

Given the difficulties of performing randomized trials in the acutely breathless patient, this is a most impressive study, which incorporated 34 centres in 3 countries. The inclusion of a placebo group adds considerably to interpretation of the data. The authors acknowledge that the manufacturer of budesonide was the sole sponsor of the trial.

Patients were aged over 50 years, fulfilled ATS criteria for COPD and had been admitted to hospital with an exacerbation of the disease. Rigorous exclusion criteria were applied, including systemic corticosteroids in the past month, high dose inhaled corticosteroids (greater than 1500 µg/day of beclomethasone equivalent), arterial pH less than 7.3, $PaCO_2$ above 70 mmHg, PaO_2 less than 50 mmHg on supplemental oxygen, asthma, or an identifiable medical cause for the exacerbation (e.g. pneumonia). Only approximately 10% of screened patients entered the study and were randomized to:

- 3 days of nebulized budesonide (2 mg four times daily) with twice daily placebo tablets, then 7 days of budesonide turbohaler (2 mg twice daily) plus once daily placebo tablets ($n = 71$), or
- 3 days of oral prednisolone (30 mg twice daily) with 4 times daily placebo nebules, then 7 days of once daily prednisolone (40 mg) plus twice daily placebo turbohaler ($n = 62$), or

- days of placebo nebulizer (4 times a day) and tablets (twice a day), then 7 days of placebo tablets (once daily) and turbohaler (twice daily) ($n = 66$).

Inhaled bronchodilators were given after each treatment in the first 3 days. Concomitant antibiotics were given to approximately 80% of patients in each group. Assessments (including spirometry, modified Borg dyspnoea score and arterial blood gases) were performed at 12 hourly intervals initially. The primary end-point was the change in post-bronchodilator FEV_1 72 hours into the admission.

Patients were well matched at baseline, though baseline FEV_1 was a little lower in the placebo group. There is a hint that some of the patients may have had greater than 15% improvement in FEV_1 with nebulized bronchodilator at baseline, but in general, the groups had the characteristics of advanced COPD.

Prednisolone and budesonide effected a significant change in post-bronchodilator FEV_1 at 72 hours as compared with placebo. Change from baseline was approximately 190 ml, 110 ml and 10 ml for prednisolone, budesonide and placebo respectively (Fig. 11.3). Active treatment also effected a small but significant fall in $PaCO_2$. Prednisolone was more effective than budesonide with respect to pre-bronchodilator FEV_1. Active treatment had no significant effect on symptom scores, length of hospital stay, or other blood gas parameters. Adverse effects and withdrawals were similar in all three groups, though hyperglycaemia was notably higher in the prednisolone group.

In summary, this trial provides clear evidence for efficacy and safety of nebulized budesonide in exacerbations of COPD, but there is nothing to suggest that it should

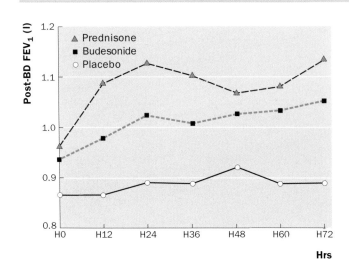

Fig. 11.3 Time-course of post-BD FEV_1 for the three treatment groups from H_0 to H_{72}. BD, bronchodilator. Source: Maltais *et al.* (2002).

replace prednisolone in routine practice. One striking feature of the trial was that prednisolone was very much more effective than budesonide in the first 24 hours with a relative plateau in effect thereafter (Fig. 11.3). This raises the possibility that high dose inhaled steroids might substitute effectively for oral steroids at perhaps 48 hours, thus reducing the risk of systemic side-effects, but only further trials will reveal whether this is the case.

Controlled oxygen therapy and carbon dioxide retention during exacerbations of chronic obstructive pulmonary disease.
Moloney ED, Kiely JL, McNicholas WT. *Lancet* 2001; **357**: 526–8.

BACKGROUND. A proportion of patients with COPD who have chronic carbon dioxide retention develop progressive hypercapnoea and respiratory acidosis in association with high concentrations of oxygen. There is no doubt that if we treated all patients with CO_2-retaining exacerbations with high concentration oxygen some would develop acidosis, of whom some would die; equally there is no doubt that if we treated all hypoxaemic exacerbations of COPD with low concentration oxygen a proportion would develop hypoxia of vital organs, of whom some would die. The vital, unanswered question is whether we can somehow identify those patients in whom delivery of higher concentrations of oxygen can be given safely. Against this background, this study aimed to determine how important the risk of CO_2 retention is in hypoxaemic patients receiving oxygen therapy.

INTERPRETATION. This study demonstrates that significant, progressive hypercapnoea can be avoided in the majority of patients with hypoxaemic, hypercapnic exacerbations of COPD managed with controlled oxygen (FiO_2 0.24–0.4 delivered by Venturi mask, aiming to keep SaO_2 between 91 and 92%). However, if the initial $PaCO_2$ is above 7.5 kPa this observation is much less predictable. Unfortunately, aspects of the data make further interpretation difficult.

Comment

The vexed question of how much oxygen to give the sick patient with COPD who has an exacerbation against a background of CO_2 retention deserves further attention. This study from a group that has made important contributions to this field is, therefore, timely. They apparently assessed 24 consecutive patients presenting to hospital with hypercapnic respiratory failure, and quote entry criteria as PaO_2 less than 8 kPa and $PaCO_2$ at or greater than 6.5 kPa at baseline. Patients then received standard care (bronchodilators, steroids and antibiotics) and oxygen delivered via Venturi mask set to deliver FiO_2 0.24–0.4 to maintain arterial oxygen saturation between 91 and 92%. A second arterial blood gas analysis was performed at 2 hours. The patients had a mean age of 71.5 years and FEV_1 of 37% predicted.

With controlled oxygen therapy, PaO_2 appeared to increase in all patients (mean rise 3.6 kPa from a baseline of 6.2 kPa). $PaCO_2$ increased in most patients but the rise was generally very small and not clinically significant. To my eye, the $PaCO_2$ increased by 1 kPa or more in only 4 patients (the authors say 3). Viewed another way, it appears from the data presented that with an initial $PaCO_2$ of under 7.5 kPa, no patients had a significant further rise in $PaCO_2$, but above this level 50% of patients had a rise in $PaCO_2$ of 0.9 kPa or more.

While this study is well designed to answer such an important question, an unfortunate problem with the paper is that the graphs of data contradict some of the text. Thus, while the entry criteria specify a $PaCO_2$ of 6.5 kPa or above, the plotted initial $PaCO_2$ shows 5 patients to have values *below* 6.5 kPa (Fig. 11.4). Furthermore, the same plot shows 25 patients when only 24 were enrolled (and at least one patient appears to be missing from the graph below). As mentioned above the same plot shows 4 (or perhaps even 5) patients to have increased their $PaCO_2$ by at least 1 kPa, while the text tells us this only occurred in 3 patients. Inevitably, these flaws make the data hard to interpret.

Further issues are that we are not told the arterial pH of the bloods drawn at 2 hours (though the implication is that very few patients developed acidaemia), nor are we told how many patients in the study received an FiO_2 above 0.28 (and whether these patients had increasing hypercapnoea). In addition, an unusually high proportion of patients had an alkalosis at the time of entry to the study, which is not fully explained. Importantly we are not told how many of the study patients when free of exacerbation had CO_2 retention.

Inevitably, the above problems make these data difficult to interpret. My interpretation is that these data provide limited evidence that it is safe to give controlled oxygen up to an FiO_2 of 0.4 (with saturation monitoring) if the initial $PaCO_2$ is less than 7.5 kPa. The 10 patients fulfilling this criterion, and who appear to me to fulfil entry criteria, had minimal changes in $PaCO_2$, while in each case PaO_2 appeared to increase. However, above this level, the change in $PaCO_2$ is unpredictable and an FiO_2 of 0.28 or less would seem preferable, with careful monitoring of $PaCO_2$ if higher concentrations of oxygen are required. The caveat in all of this, as the authors acknowledge, is that much larger studies (and preferably controlled trials) are necessary before clinically applicable conclusions can be drawn. One final point is that if the patients apparently failing to fulfil entry criteria are removed from the graphs in the paper, I estimate that 20–25% of patients had a significant rise in $PaCO_2$ during treatment.

What are the take-home messages? The first is that further, larger studies are required. The second is that I believe the authors make a critical point in emphasizing the need for careful oxygen saturation monitoring in this group of patients. It seems prudent to use the minimum FiO_2 to maintain SaO_2 in the range they quote, with very close monitoring of $PaCO_2$ in patients who require FiO_2 above 0.28 (or in whom initial $PaCO_2$ is of concern). As mentioned later in this chapter, respiratory support, for example with NIV, should be considered for those developing acidosis.

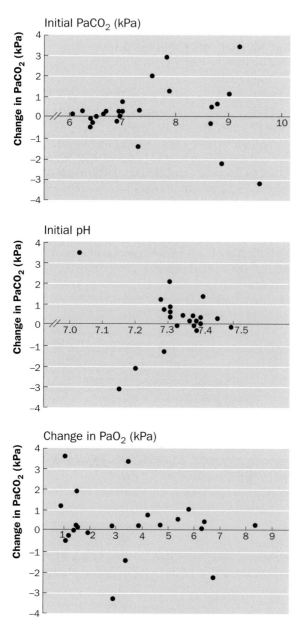

Fig. 11.4 Change in PaCO$_2$ in first 2 hours of oxygen therapy. Source: Moloney *et al.* (2001).

Oxygen therapy for hypercapnic patients with chronic obstructive pulmonary disease and acute respiratory failure: a randomized, controlled pilot study.

Gomersall CD, Joynt GM, Freebairn RC, Lai CKW, Oh TE. *Crit Care Med* 2002; **30**: 113–16.

BACKGROUND. We have already discussed the great dilemma of how much supplemental oxygen is appropriate and safe in exacerbations of COPD. In an undefined proportion of patients, high concentrations of oxygen will accelerate respiratory acidosis, in another, insufficient oxygen will result in critical tissue hypoxia. The present study set out to determine whether outcome differed depending on whether a target PaO_2 of greater than 6.6 kPa or greater than 9 kPa was used in the management of patients with severe, hypoxaemic, hypercapnic exacerbations of COPD.

INTERPRETATION. In the population of patients studied, no significant difference in mortality or requirements for mechanical ventilation was observed in the two groups. Outcome was generally favourable with only 1 death among the 34 patients studied. No patients in the study became comatose or developed arrhythmias because of CO_2 retention. In the absence of clear benefit for either a low or high target PaO_2 it seems reasonable to use the lowest FiO_2 required to maintain adequate oxygenation when patients with hypercapnia have an exacerbation of COPD. In this study the group with 'low' target PaO_2 in fact had a mean PaO_2 of around 9 kPa, and on the basis of this study it seems unnecessary (except under exceptional circumstances) to exceed this level of oxygenation in trying simultaneously to obviate hypercapnic acidosis or significant tissue hypoxia.

Comment

This study recruited patients considered to have an exacerbation of COPD in which arterial blood gases taken breathing room air revealed a PaO_2 less than 6.6 kPa and $PaCO_2$ greater than 6.6 kPa. Exclusion criteria included additional pathology on chest X-ray such as pneumonia or pulmonary oedema, terminal disease, requirement for mechanical ventilation twice or more in the past 6 months, and inability to walk 20 yards on the flat when stable. Patients received nebulized bronchodilators, steroids and antibiotics and were then randomized to two treatment algorithms. One delivered FiO_2 to achieve PaO_2 above 6.6 kPa (on the premise that PaO_2 should be kept low to prevent abolition of hypoxic drive in chronically hypercapnic patients) while the other aimed for PaO_2 above 9 kPa (on the premise that severe hypoxaemia must be avoided). Oxygen was delivered by Venturi mask and was adjusted according to PaO_2 derived from arterial blood samples drawn from an in-dwelling arterial line. Standard treatment for exacerbations was continued. The primary outcome variable was in-hospital death or requirement for mechanical ventilation, and secondary outcome was duration of hospital stay. Spirometry was performed after patients were discharged from hospital.

Thirty-six patients were recruited over a 33-month period. It is not clear whether these were consecutive patients. Two patients were later excluded on the basis that they could not walk 20 yards on the level. Data was analysed for the other 34 patients and as such analysis was not on an intention to treat basis. Baseline characteristics of both groups were similar with mean age approximately 68, PaO_2 5.7 kPa, $PaCO_2$ 9.5 kPa, and (post-recovery) FEV_1 around 0.5 litres. No significant differences in mortality/mechanical ventilation rate were observed. In the low PaO_2 group one patient was mechanically ventilated at 8 hours, while at 2 days one patient died and another was mechanically ventilated. In the high PaO_2 group, no patients died or required mechanical ventilation, but it should be noted that the 2 patients later excluded from the study on the basis of exercise tolerance were both in this group and both were mechanically ventilated. It is not entirely clear why an exercise tolerance of less than 20 yards was specified as an exclusion criterion. No differences were found in length of hospital stay, nor in serial $PaCO_2$ or arterial pH. Overall, the study suggests that relatively high PaO_2 was well tolerated in hypoxaemic, hypercapnic exacerbations of COPD.

The study is a useful contribution to the debate on oxygen administration during exacerbations. As emphasized elsewhere in this chapter, this sort of study is very hard to perform and any such data is valuable. Inevitably, in this setting, a number of questions are generated by the data, for example, throughout the paper the reader expects to see the average (and range of) FiO_2 administered in each group, i.e. how much oxygen can one give to achieve such good outcomes? Frustratingly the answer is not provided, and all we can take away is that either target PaO_2 gave similar outcomes. Interestingly, however, the target PaO_2 seemed to be considerably exceeded in each group, with the mean level in the high and 'low' PaO_2 groups being around 14 and 9 kPa respectively over the first 12 hours. As such, the low PaO_2 group generally achieved the target PaO_2 for the 'high' PaO_2 group, making interpretation of data a little more difficult.

A few other problems arise. First, experience suggests that it is patients with chronic hypercapnia who are driven into acidosis by high FiO_2—unfortunately, we are not told the $PaCO_2$ after recovery. Similarly, we are not told the bronchodilator reversibility of the groups—it is conceivable that those with reversibility would respond more rapidly, thus obviating the risk of acidosis. This leads to a further point which is that, in my experience, it is often sick patients treated with high FiO_2 *before* receiving adequate doses of bronchodilators/steroids (e.g. in the ambulance or immediately upon arrival in the emergency room) who develop respiratory acidosis, and such patients are not included in the study. A slightly more pragmatic point is that of the 24 patients who had spirometry at least 2, and possibly more, had an FEV_1/FVC ratio of greater than 0.7 (the level below which airflow obstruction is considered to be present in several guidelines). This, along with the lack of reversibility data, suggests that the groups may not have comprised pure COPD. The final obvious point is that a study of this size is not powered to detect small differences between groups, as the authors readily acknowledge.

It is hugely reassuring that the patients in this study generally did well. This does not mean that there is not a small and important population of patients who will become acidotic with high FiO_2. We have all seen these patients, and yet still we cannot accurately predict who will respond in this way. In many ways, identifying these patients prospectively remains the big challenge. Until we define this population accurately it seems prudent to monitor patients with acute exacerbations of severe COPD closely, and provide the lowest oxygen concentration giving a PaO_2 (or corresponding saturation) sufficient to prevent tissue hypoxia while obviating further hypercapnia. Oxygen saturation of around 91–92% as incorporated in the study by Moloney and colleagues seems appropriate in this regard. Ironically, however, the mean PaO_2 of around 9 kPa in the 'low' PaO_2 arm of the study by Gomersall and colleagues also appears suited to this aim.

Non-invasive ventilation in acute exacerbations of chronic obstructive pulmonary disease: long-term survival and predictors of in-hospital outcome.

Plant PK, Owen JL, Elliott MW. *Thorax* 2001; **56**: 708–12.

BACKGROUND. These authors previously demonstrated that administration of bi-level NIV in a ward-based setting significantly reduces both the requirement for mechanical ventilation and in-hospital mortality among patients presenting with acute exacerbations of COPD |2|. They subsequently re-analysed the data with the aim of identifying factors predicting treatment failure, as assessed by the requirement for mechanical ventilation. They also assessed long-term survival in the same cohort of patients to determine whether the advantage conferred by NIV in hospital was maintained.

INTERPRETATION. Elevated $PaCO_2$ and H^+ at enrolment were associated with an increased risk of treatment failure. At 4 hours a decrease in H^+ or a decrease in respiratory rate were associated with treatment success. A trend towards improved long-term survival was observed among those patients randomized to NIV during the index admission.

Comment

This study follows on from an important multicentre trial conducted over 23 months in which 236 patients admitted to hospital with an exacerbation of COPD were randomized to receive standard care alone, or standard care with ward-based NIV |2|. Entry criteria included a respiratory rate greater than 23 breaths per minute, arterial blood pH between 7.25 and 7.35, and $PaCO_2$ greater than 6 kPa.

The attempt in the present study to identify parameters predictive of treatment failure was necessarily retrospective. Univariate analysis was used to identify candidate variables for entry into forward stepwise regression analysis. In the multivariate analysis of data collected at the time of enrolment to the study, H^+ and $PaCO_2$ were found to be associated with treatment failure—for H^+ the OR was 1.22 per nmol/l ($P < 0.01$), and for $PaCO_2$ the OR was 1.14 per kPa ($P < 0.01$).

Perhaps not surprisingly, randomization to NIV was found to be protective against treatment failure. Unfortunately, a model based on these three variables gave predictive values for treatment success or failure of only 83% and 67% respectively, and were, therefore, generally unhelpful in assessing the expected response of individual patients.

Changes in the clinical and biochemical variables measured at 1 hour had no appreciable value in predicting treatment outcome. However, this position changed at 4 hours, when a fall in H^+ or a fall in respiratory rate (relative to levels at enrolment) were associated with treatment success. That PaO_2 had no identifiable influence on treatment failure is interesting, but as the authors point out, this is in keeping with previous findings. These collective observations are important in developing our understanding of outcome in COPD, but direct application to the clinical setting should be tempered again by the low predictive value of these parameters for outcome in individual patients. It is also a little disappointing that changes in clinical variables only became potentially important more than 4 hours into admission (assuming an inherent short delay between admission and enrolment). It remains to be seen whether changes in the period between 1 and 4 hours may give an earlier guide to suspected outcome in exacerbations of COPD.

With regard to long-term survival, the authors collected follow-up data on all 236 patients, the one-year survival being 58.4%. The time from enrolment to follow up ranged from 3 months to 26 months. The survival curves for patients treated with or without NIV, diverged to about 3 months from enrolment with a survival advantage for NIV, and then remained approximately parallel (Fig. 11.5). The

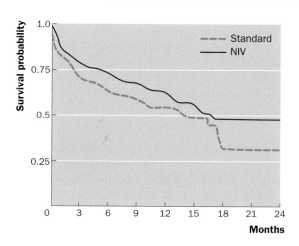

Fig. 11.5 Kaplan–Meier plot of survival from enrolment. Median survival 13.4 months in standard treatment group vs 16.8 months in NIV group ($P = 0.12$). Source: Plant *et al.* (2001).

survival difference was not statistically significant ($P = 0.12$) and interpretation of these data should, therefore, be cautious. This is particularly so when it is considered that there were more women in the NIV-treated group (54% vs 47%). Nevertheless, the implication is that the immediate survival advantage attributed to NIV is maintained at least in the immediate period after treatment.

In summary Plant *et al.* have made a highly significant contribution to the body of evidence demonstrating a place for bi-level NIV in acute exacerbations of COPD associated with acidosis and this study is a further important step towards accurate prediction of outcome in this setting. The data emphasize that high H^+ and $PaCO_2$ early in the admission are bad prognostic features. The challenge now is to develop the *early* identification of those variables that can accurately predict outcome in individual hospitalized patients.

Non-invasive ventilation for acute respiratory failure: a prospective randomized placebo-controlled trial.

Thys F, Roeseler J, Reynaert M, Liistro G, Rodenstein DO. *Eur Respir J* 2002; **20**: 545–55.

B ACKGROUND. One of the intrinsic problems facing trials of NIV in acute exacerbations of COPD characterized by respiratory acidosis is that it is hard to incorporate a placebo arm. With this in mind, Thys *et al.* set out to perform the first placebo-controlled trial of NIV in acute respiratory failure whilst also addressing the question of whether NIV can be effectively administered from the emergency room. It should be noted from the outset that this trial contains a mixture of patients with COPD and acute pulmonary oedema.

I NTERPRETATION. This single-centre, placebo-controlled trial randomized patients being considered for mechanical ventilation to NIV or sham NIV, and was stopped early because of the dramatic difference in the rate of treatment failure (the primary outcome measurement). All 10 patients receiving NIV made a rapid initial recovery, while all 10 patients receiving sham NIV required early intervention in the form of rescue NIV, which was successful in 7 of 10 cases.

Comment

This study employed standard definitions for acute pulmonary oedema and for acute exacerbations of COPD. Patients aged over 18 with either condition were included if they had any three from acute breathlessness, respiratory rate greater than 30 or less than 10 breaths per minute, PaO_2 less than 7.3 kPa breathing room air, or arterial pH less than 7.33. Strict exclusion criteria were applied, principally to ensure that haemodynamically unstable patients were appropriately taken to ITU, and to exclude patients physically unlikely to tolerate a facial mask. Importantly, all patients were given emergency medical treatment for pulmonary oedema or COPD using standard treatment (oxygen, bronchodilators and corticosteroids for COPD).

Only in the absence of benefit did randomization proceed, with medical therapy continuing in all cases. Patients were randomized to bi-level NIV or to bi-level NIV in which holes in the connecting T-piece ensured that the inspiratory and expiratory pressures delivered were zero. The primary end-point was treatment failure as defined by increasing respiratory/heart rate, increasing dyspnoea, and either agitation, haemodynamic compromise or worsening blood gas profiles. The trial had intended to recruit 60 patients, with interim analysis after entry of 20.

Over the 2 years of the trial 187 patients were admitted with pulmonary oedema or exacerbation of COPD, with the investigators informed of 65, of whom only 20 (12 COPD) were eligible or gave informed consent! Although the NIV and placebo groups showed no significant differences at baseline there was a tendency for the placebo group to have lower PaO_2 (64 versus 72 mmHg) and to be more acidotic (pH 7.24 versus 7.28).

The striking finding of the study was that all 10 patients using placebo showed clinical deterioration and stopped the trial at a mean of 30 minutes, while NIV resulted in successful treatment with discontinuation of NIV at 95 minutes (Table 11.2). There were significant improvements in pH and $PaCO_2$ in the NIV group but not the placebo group. Interestingly, 7 of the 10 placebo group patients were then successfully treated with NIV, the remaining 3 patients having apparent complications (acute haemodynamic instability in 2, pneumothorax in the other) and requiring intubation with mechanical ventilation. The dramatic early difference in outcome led to the trial being discontinued at $n = 20$. Interestingly, despite the good early outcome 3 patients in the NIV group (6 in the placebo group) required further NIV later in the admission, 2 patients in the NIV group died in hospital (1 in the placebo group) and no differences were observed in length of stay in the emergency room, intensive care or hospital. Thus, the dramatic improvements conferred by NIV appeared confined to the period of application (in contrast to the study by Plant and colleagues discussed above).

This trial addressed a vital question and further adds to the body of evidence supporting early application of NIV in respiratory failure attributable to COPD. However, by the very nature of this technically difficult trial, there are three main caveats to consider. First, as the authors concede, it was impossible to blind medical

Table 11.2 Main patient outcomes

Protocols	Success	Failure
Active bi-level NPPV	10	0
Placebo NPPV	0	10
Rescue	7	3

Failure: need of endotracheal intubation in the active bi-level non-invasive positive-pressure ventilation (NPPV) arm, and of crossing over to active NPPV (rescue) in the placebo arm.

Source: Thys et al. (2002).

and nursing staff to the treatment being used, and it would be only natural for staff to have a low threshold for discontinuation of placebo (and relative reliance on NIV if it had already been used successfully in that institute). Of equal concern, the patients may not have been blind to the treatment limbs either. For example, if any of the patients had had NIV before and then drew placebo in the trial they would feel the difference, and irrespective of previous use patients on placebo would be likely to sense any anxiety expressed by medical or nursing staff. Thus, while the trial gives us the best placebo control to date, only a truly double-blind trial can answer the initial question categorically. Second, because of the small numbers involved chance has led to more severe disease in the placebo group at baseline. This is more striking when the authors divide the patients by disease. Among the patients with COPD (NIV $n = 7$, placebo $n = 5$) pH, $PaCO_2$ and PaO_2 are 'worse' in the placebo group at baseline (7.24 vs 7.3, 68.8 vs 59.1 mmHg, and 66.2 vs 73.4 mmHg respectively). Indeed, among the patients with COPD PaO_2 falls in the NIV limb and rises in the placebo limb. Disease severity may explain at least some of the dramatic differences in observed effect. It should be noted also that the authors went to great lengths to show that the increased dead space in the placebo mask did not increase work of breathing among healthy volunteers, and while this is encouraging, it cannot be taken to prove that the placebo did not increase work of breathing in sick, distressed patients. Third, and following on from the previous point, it is difficult to make conclusions about COPD specifically given that this was a mixture of 2 diseases in an ultimately small study.

Despite these largely inevitable concerns, this is a most welcome trial. Not only has it tackled the incredibly difficult problems of performing good randomized trials in the emergency room, it has come out with a dramatically significant result which enhances confidence in NIV in the acute setting.

Predictors of outcome for patients with COPD requiring invasive mechanical ventilation.
Nevins ML, Epstein SK. *Chest* 2001; **119**: 1840–9.

BACKGROUND. A significant proportion of patients with COPD are considered for treatment in the ITU. There is a relative paucity of data relating to outcome among such patients. This study, therefore, aimed specifically to determine factors predicting outcome in patients with COPD who received invasive mechanical ventilation.

INTERPRETATION. Overall mortality among intubated and ventilated patients with COPD was 27.7% with a further 6.6% requiring mechanical ventilation or tracheotomy after discharge from ITU. Independent predictors of mortality were invasive mechanical ventilation for over 72 hours, associated comorbidity, high acute physiology score, and associated malignancy. Interestingly, mortality among patients admitted with an *exacerbation* of COPD was significantly lower than in patients with COPD who had an alternative cause for acute respiratory failure (15 versus 31%). Severity of COPD as judged by FEV_1 did not correlate with survival. Overall, this study supports cautious optimism for patients with COPD requiring invasive mechanical ventilation, particularly in the absence of pre-existing comorbidity or malignancy.

Comment

This was a retrospective cohort study based on data prospectively gathered over a 4-year period. Patients were eligible if they required invasive mechanical ventilation and had previous spirometry or a history/clinical findings compatible with COPD. Patients with a tracheotomy or requiring long-term ventilatory support were excluded. The authors studied a wide variety of factors with the potential to influence outcome, including comorbidity defined as 'immunosuppression, cirrhosis, congestive heart failure, and chronic renal failure', as taken from the Acute Physiology and Chronic Health Evaluation (APACHE) II scoring system. Mortality was a primary outcome for the study, while secondary outcomes included duration of weaning from mechanical ventilation. It should be mentioned that NIV was rarely used in the authors' institute over the study period, being administered in only 1% of cases.

One hundred and sixty-six patients were studied. Mean age was 67, mean FEV_1 (measured among 56 patients with spirometric data from the previous 2 years) was 1.24 litres (48% predicted), 17% used domiciliary oxygen, and 12% took maintenance oral corticosteroids. Arterial blood gases on admission ($n = 108$) showed mean pH 7.26 and $PaCO_2$ 69 mmHg. The cause of acute respiratory failure was considered an exacerbation of COPD in 39 cases (23%), pneumonia was present in 70 cases (42%) and cardiac failure in 40 cases (24%). It should be noted that 13% of patients were in a chronic care facility prior to admission.

In total, 46 patients died (27.7%). Median duration of mechanical ventilation was 4.1 days—15 patients were ventilated for more than 21 days, and this subgroup accounted for 22% of all deaths. Median duration of weaning was 1.1 days but the range was huge. When comparing survivors and non-survivors low albumin and low haematocrit were commoner in those who died, while interestingly previous mechanical ventilation was significantly more common among those who survived. However in a logistic regression analysis, the independent factors associated with mortality were malignancy (OR 4.0, 95% CI 2.5–6.4), comorbidity as defined by APACHE II (OR 2.9, 95% CI 1.9–4.4), mechanical ventilation for more than 72 hours (OR 2.6, 95% CI 1.6–4.1), and high acute physiology score (OR 1.1, 95% CI 1.1–1.1). Indeed, in the absence of comorbidity or malignancy, overall mortality was only 16%.

Nineteen per cent of those patients weaned and extubated required re-intubation within 3 days, and this subgroup of patients had significantly higher mortality than those who were extubated only once. Factors predicting failed extubation included low tidal volume and vital capacity.

The subgroup of patients with exacerbation of COPD as the cause for acute respiratory failure deserve particular attention. Exacerbation was defined as increase in breathlessness with or without cough/sputum in the absence of pneumonia, heart failure or another definable process such as adult respiratory distress syndrome. Mortality was significantly lower in this group than in those with an alternative cause for acute respiratory failure. Within the exacerbation group, duration of mechanical ventilation again predicted for mortality (5 versus 26% mortality in those requiring less than 72 hours or more than 72 hours of mechanical ventilation respectively). Unfortunately, however, it was not possible prospectively to predict those patients in whom prolonged ventilation would be required.

The final result to mention relates to the effect of spirometry in predicting outcome. As mentioned above only 56 patients had available spirometry from the previous 2 years, and so data is limited. Nevertheless, mortality was no different among the 14 patients with FEV_1 less than 30% predicted and those with FEV_1 greater than 30% predicted (25 versus 23% respectively).

Whilst these data are both fascinating and important, their interpretation should be coloured by a few points. First, the study is limited by the obvious constraints of retrospective data collection and the general applicability of the data is unclear given both that this was a single-centre experience, and that the centre in question rarely used NIV either with the aim of preventing intubation or assisting weaning. Furthermore, the diagnostic criteria for COPD were not watertight, and a small number of patients may have had an alternative diagnosis. Finally, it is a pity that cause of death was not discussed.

Despite these issues, this large study makes very powerful points that cannot be ignored. In particular, nihilism regarding the prospects of patients with COPD entering ITU can be replaced with cautious optimism, especially in the absence of comorbidity or malignancy, and this would appear to apply particularly to patients with exacerbations of COPD. The observation that disease severity does not predict outcome requires to be confirmed in larger numbers of patients, but suggests that we should not discriminate on the grounds of spirometric severity of COPD. Furthermore, these data largely dispel the myth that previous intubation in patients with COPD predicts for a bad prognosis in ITU—if anything this study suggests the opposite, that previous successful ITU stay selects out a group of patients who tend to do well. The overall conclusion is that patients with COPD appear to do better with invasive mechanical ventilation than had perhaps been thought previously. This is a vitally important message for clinical practice. One challenge ahead is to identify those factors predicting for prolonged ventilation. Another (though extremely difficult) requirement will be to establish and quantify whether survivors of ITU have significantly reduced lung function, exercise tolerance and quality of life (or increased symptoms) because of ITU intervention.

Prognostic factors, clinical course, and hospital outcome of patients with chronic obstructive pulmonary disease admitted to an intensive care unit for acute respiratory failure.

Afessa B, Morales IJ, Scanlon PD, Peters SG. *Crit Care Med* 2002; **30**: 1610–15.

BACKGROUND. In many ways this study follows on nicely from the work by Nevins and Epstein, recognizing a need for further information on the outcome of patients with COPD admitted to the ITU. The present study aimed specifically to determine complications, mortality rates and immediate causes of death among patients with COPD and respiratory failure who were admitted to ITU. One important way in which it differs from the study by Nevins and Epstein is by inclusion of many patients treated with NIV.

INTERPRETATION. In 250 admissions studied, the mortality rate was 15%, against a predicted mortality of 30%. The factors independently associated with increased mortality were multiple organ failure and a high APACHE II score on admission to ITU. In turn, multiple organ failure evolved significantly more often among patients who developed nosocomial sepsis in the ITU. The implication of this study is that patients with COPD have a high chance of surviving an admission to ITU, which may be improved further if sepsis could be reduced.

Comment

Patients with exacerbations of COPD who are considered for ITU tend to be elderly and frail, and to have pre-existing comorbidity. What we require in order to guide clinical practice is good evidence with which to predict the outcome of COPD in the ITU setting, firstly in general terms and secondly with reference to individual patients.

This study gathered data prospectively collected on 250 admissions (relating to 180 patients) to a single ITU for acute respiratory failure associated with COPD over a 3-year period. It is assumed (though not explicitly stated in the paper) that the study covers consecutive admissions over this period. The authors obtained data relating to mechanical ventilation, length of stay, mortality, and organ failure. Definitions of sepsis and organ failure were derived according to standard, pre-determined criteria.

The average age of the patients was 63 years. It should be noted that exacerbation or super-added pneumonia was the reason for admission in just over 80% of patients, with respiratory failure attributed to a cardiac cause in most of the remaining cases. Overall, 37 (21%) of 180 patients died during the study period. Thus death occurred in 15% of admissions (37/250) during the study period. The predicted mortality according to the APACHE II prognostic system was 30%. Death was more common among the 36 patients admitted more than once over the 3-year period.

Differences between the 213 admissions in which patients survived, and the 37 admissions in which patients died were studied in detail. The latter group was found to have significantly lower arterial pH at admission (7.21 versus 7.25), higher APACHE II score at admission (25.6 versus 17.9), higher rates of sepsis developing in ITU (68 versus 24%), increased number of organ failures in ITU (1.87 versus 0.14), greater requirement for mechanical ventilation (100 versus 82%), and increased ITU stay (15.5 versus 7.6 days). However, multiple logistic regression analysis found only APACHE II score at admission and subsequent number of organ failures to be independently associated with mortality. In this regard, it is interesting that sepsis developed in 28% of admissions, and that the likelihood of subsequently developing failure of two or more non-respiratory organs was approximately 10 times higher in those with sepsis (31%) than in those without (3%). Nosocomial pneumonia was by far the commonest source of sepsis, and *Pseudomonas aeruginosa* the most common organism isolated. Cardiac failure was the commonest 'non-respiratory' organ failure observed. It is also interesting to break down deaths by the requirement for invasive mechanical ventilation. One hundred and fifty-three patients were intubated of whom 31 (20%) died; 99 patients required non-invasive mechanical ventilation of whom 53 (54%) improved, 40 were intubated, and 6 died after refusing intubation.

Overall, this study suggests that patients with COPD have lower than expected mortality, with 85% of patients surviving ITU admission. Additionally, it appears that prevention of sepsis (and in particular nosocomial pneumonia) could improve this figure further. Several points are worth making with regard to the wider applicability of these specific data however. First, this is a single-centre study. Second, the study is necessarily observational and, therefore, criteria for intubation were not pre-determined. Third, it must be remembered that ITUs differ from country to country. For example, no mechanical ventilation support was used in 38 patients in this study and a further 59 patients had non-invasive mechanical ventilation; in the UK a very high proportion of such patients would be managed in a high dependency unit close to, but not part of, the hospital ITU. This may explain why the cohort of patients in this study has less severe disease (PaCO$_2$ around 59 mmHg, pH around 7.24) than might be expected in, for example, British series.

Furthermore, as the authors point out, we know nothing about the level of function or respiratory status of the patients either before or after ITU, and strictly speaking, there is no hard evidence to confirm that all patients had COPD. Finally, it must be recalled that a significant minority of patients in this study were admitted with a 'non-respiratory' reason for respiratory failure (principally cardiac failure) or with a clear super-added complication of COPD such as pneumonia or pneumothorax. It would have been very useful to learn about outcome specifically in the group of patients with 'exacerbations of COPD' ($n = 144$) – in the meantime these data apply to 'all-comers' with COPD.

In summary, this important paper contributes to literature suggesting cautious but increasing optimism for patients admitted to ITU with COPD, while emphasizing the potential advantages of NIV and the need to develop strategies to obviate nosocomial infection in invasively ventilated patients.

Conclusion

Several important conclusions can be drawn from this chapter, the most important being that despite the inherent difficulties in conducting rigorous studies in patients with exacerbations, an increasing number of elegant and informative papers have emerged.

With regard to early supported discharge from hospital, increasing evidence suggests that this is efficacious. This has enormous implications for health care provision, and for the costs associated with hospital medicine.

A further important conclusion emerges from studies of the role of infection in exacerbations of COPD. It seems reasonable to conclude that infection can now be clearly identified as being the cause of exacerbation in a large proportion of patients with COPD (but not all), and that in smokers, at least, infective exacerbations may leave a lasting effect on lung function.

The vexed question of how much oxygen to give patients with chronic hypercapnoea who present with exacerbations of COPD remains. The studies discussed here appear to add weight to the argument that the lowest concentration of oxygen effecting an oxygen saturation of at least 91–92% should be used, and that increasing oxygen requirements demand closer monitoring of gas exchange.

Finally, the papers discussed here suggest that we should carefully re-evaluate attitudes towards the anticipated outcome for patients with COPD who require respiratory support in the ITU. The emerging picture is that non-invasive ventilation has a striking impact on outcome in a large number of patients with exacerbations of COPD and respiratory failure. However, if non-invasive ventilation fails, then – especially in the absence of significant comorbidity – patients with COPD appear to have a better prognosis with intubation and mechanical ventilation in the ITU than may have been traditionally expected. This message will become increasingly important given the anticipated increase in hospital workload associated with COPD in the coming years.

References

1. Connett J, Kusek J, Bailey W, O'Hara P, Wu M. Design of the Lung Health Study: a randomized clinical trial of early intervention for chronic obstructive pulmonary disease. *Controlled Clin Trials* 1993; 14(2S): 3–19.

2. Plant PK, Owen JL, Elliott MW. Early use of non-invasive ventilation for acute exacerbations of chronic obstructive pulmonary disease on general respiratory wards: a multicentre randomized controlled trial. *Lancet* 2000; 355: 1931–5.

Part III

Respiratory infection

Respiratory infection

Introduction

The section on respiratory infection for the *Year in Respiratory Medicine 2003* includes 50 key articles selected from 2001 and 2002. The articles selected are of clinical relevance and aid in the investigation and management of patients with respiratory infection. Areas covered include the investigation and management of patients with tuberculosis, patients with community and ventilator associated pneumonia, and patients with bronchiectasis.

12

Tuberculosis

The chapter starts with tuberculosis and addresses the investigation and management of patients with latent tuberculosis infection, discusses management strategies for the treatment of active tuberculosis, and discusses treatment strategies for
multi-drug resistant tuberculosis and Mycobacteria other than tuberculosis.

Tuberculosis accounts for more than 2 million deaths per year in the world and
the World Health Organisation estimates one third of the world's population is
infected with Mycobacterium tuberculosis. The first paper highlights that the
newer immunosuppressants (tumour necrosis factor alpha-blockers) used for the
treatment in refractory cases of conditions such as rheumatoid arthritis and inflammatory bowel disease are not without risk and are associated with an increase in
tuberculosis.

Tuberculosis associated with Infliximab, a tumour necrosis factor alpha-neutralizing agent.
Keane J, Gershon S, Wise RP, *et al. N Engl J Med* 2001; **345**(15): 1098–104.

BACKGROUND. **Infliximab is a humanized antibody against tumour necrosis factor alpha that is used in the treatment of refractory cases of Crohn's disease and rheumatoid arthritis. There have been concerns about tuberculosis reactivating with treatment with Infliximab therapy. This study analysed all reports of tuberculosis after Infliximab therapy that had been received as of 29 May 2001 (from 1998), through the MedWatch spontaneous reporting system of the Food and Drug Administration.**

INTERPRETATION. Approximately 147 000 people throughout the world have received treatment with Infliximab during this period. There were 70 reported cases of tuberculosis, with a median age of 57 years (interquartile range [IQR] 39–67). Cases presented after a median treatment with Infliximab for 12 weeks (IQR 8–22 weeks) and developed after three or fewer infusions in 69%. Of all patients, 79% were using concomitant immunosuppressant treatment and no information was available in the other 21%. Of the 70 reports, 91% were from countries with a low incidence of tuberculosis. Thirty-one per cent had pulmonary tuberculosis, 57% had extrapulmonary tuberculosis and 11% were not reported. Of the 40 patients that had extrapulmonary disease, 17 had disseminated disease, 11 lymph node disease, 4 peritoneal disease, 2 pleural disease, and 1 each meningeal, enteric, paravertebral, bone, genital, and bladder disease. After tuberculosis was diagnosed, Infliximab therapy treatment ceased and patients received anti-tuberculosis treatment. Seventeen per cent died, and at least 33%

of the deaths were attributable to tuberculosis. In conclusion, active tuberculosis may develop soon after the initiation of treatment with Infliximab therapy.

Comment

The reported frequency of tuberculosis in association with Infliximab therapy was much higher than the reported frequency of other opportunistic infections associated with this drug. In addition, the rate of reported cases of tuberculosis among patients treated with Infliximab was higher than the available background rates. The estimated rate of tuberculosis among US patients with rheumatoid arthritis who received Infliximab therapy within the previous year was 24.4 cases per 100 000 per year compared with the background rate of tuberculosis of 6.2 cases per 100 000 per year in US patients with rheumatoid arthritis that had not received Infliximab therapy.

The majority of tuberculosis (around 80%) in HIV-negative patients are pulmonary, approximately 18% are manifested as extrapulmonary disease and disseminated disease accounts for <2%. In contrast, the tuberculosis occurring in patients that were treated with Infliximab therapy presented differently where 57% presented with extrapulmonary tuberculosis and 24% had disseminated disease.

The treatment of Infliximab therapy is reserved for patients that are refractory to standard immunosuppressant therapies. As expected, therefore, the majority of patients using Infliximab therapy are on concomitant immunosuppressant treatments, which will likely potentiate the risk of tuberculosis reactivating. Before prescribing Infliximab drug, it is recommended that physicians screen patients for latent tuberculosis infection. The next section discusses the detection of latent tuberculosis infection.

Detection of latent Mycobacterial tuberculosis infection

Latent tuberculosis infection is defined as evidence of Mycobacterium tuberculosis infection (patients with a strongly positive tuberculin skin test) without evidence of active tuberculosis. The identification and treatment of latent infection is central to tuberculosis elimination because the development of active tuberculosis in these persons can effectively be prevented with treatment, thereby stopping further spread of disease. The tuberculin skin test using purified protein derivative as the antigen is currently the international gold standard for diagnosing latent Mycobacterial tuberculosis infection and can aid the diagnosis of disease due to Mycobacterium tuberculosis. The skin test, however, can be influenced by environmental Mycobacteria, high Mycobacterial load, concomitant infections, prior BCG vaccination, immunosuppression – in particular HIV infection – and is prone to errors both in the placement and in the reading of results. Because of these inaccuracies, there remains concern about the specificity of the tuberculin skin test.

The discovery of the role of T lymphocytes and interferon gamma in the immune response has led to the development of *in vitro* assays for the cell-mediated immune reaction to Mycobacterium tuberculosis that is hoped to be superior to the conventional tuberculin skin test. The next two papers compared the whole blood interferon gamma assay (using purified protein derivative as the common antigen) with the tuberculin skin test.

Comparison of a whole-blood interferon gamma assay with tuberculin skin testing for detecting latent Mycobacterium tuberculosis infection.

Mazurek GH, LoBue PA, Daley CL, *et al. JAMA* 2001; **286**: 1740–7.

BACKGROUND. The aim of this study was to compare the whole-blood interferon gamma assay with the tuberculin skin test for detecting latent Mycobacterial tuberculosis infection and to identify factors associated with discordance between the tests. This multi-centred US study compared the interferon gamma assay (using purified protein derivative from both Mycobacterium tuberculosis and Mycobacterium avium complex as the antigens) with the tuberculin skin test in 1226 adults (all ≥18 years old, mean age 39 years) with varying risks of Mycobacterial tuberculosis infection (Table 12.1).

INTERPRETATION. The authors indicate that overall reasonable agreement between the interferon gamma assay and the tuberculin skin test was 83% (Kappa = 0.60). Despite this, the agreement with a positive skin test and a positive interferon gamma assay varied from 50–79% and a negative skin test and a negative interferon gamma assay from 79–100% (Table 12.1). Multivariate analysis was carried out in Groups 1 and

Table 12.1 The whole blood interferon gamma assay and the tuberculin skin test were compared

Group*	1	2	3	4	Overall
Number	98	947	94	87	1226
Per cent agreement with a positive skin test	50%	65%	79%	68%	68%
Per cent agreement with a negative skin test	93%	90%	79%	100%	90%
Per cent with negative skin tests but positive interferon gamma assay	7%	8%	3%	0%	7%
Per cent with positive skin tests but negative interferon gamma assay	1%	8%	18%	31%	10%

*Group 1 were thought to be at low risk of latent mycobacterial tuberculosis infection (LTBI) e.g. pre-employment; Group 2 was thought to be at high risk of LTBI e.g. tuberculosis contacts; Group 3 were suspected of having active tuberculosis (received <6 weeks anti-tuberculosis treatment) and Group 4 were subjects who had finished treatment for culture confirmed tuberculosis in the past 2 years.

Table 12.2 Factors associated with a positive skin test but negative interferon gamma assay in Groups 1 and 2 (the groups normally screened for LTBI. Data presented as odds ratio (OR) with 95% confidence intervals (CI)

	OR (95% CI)	*P* value
Prior BCG vaccination	6.92 (3.56–13.43)	<0.001
Mycobacterium avium complex	2.64 (1.28–5.42)	0.01
Asian race	2.33 (1.05–5.21)	0.04

2, the groups conventionally screened for latent mycobacterial infection (Table 12.1), and the odds of having a positive tuberculin skin test but negative interferon gamma assay were increased by prior BCG vaccination, atypical Mycobacterial infection (Mycobacterium avium complex) and Asian race (Table 12.2). The interferon gamma assay provided evidence that among unvaccinated persons with a positive tuberculin skin test result but negative interferon gamma assay result, 21% were responding to mycobacteria other than Mycobacterium tuberculosis. The authors concluded that the interferon gamma assay was comparable with the tuberculin skin test to detect LMTI. It was also less affected by prior BCG vaccination, discriminated responses to environmental Mycobacteria, and it avoided the variability and subjectivity associated with the placing and reading of the tuberculin skin test.

Evaluation of a whole-blood interferon gamma release assay for the detection of Mycobacterium tuberculosis infection in 2 study populations.

Bellete B, Coberly J, Barnes GL, *et al. Clin Infect Dis* 2002; **34**: 1449–56.

BACKGROUND. This study evaluated the potential of the interferon gamma assay from whole blood using purified protein derivative as the antigen to replace the tuberculin skin test for detecting Mycobacterium tuberculosis infection. This study used a population in which tuberculosis is highly endemic (253 volunteers from Ethiopia) and another population representative of an urban US population (175 volunteers from Baltimore) and compared the interferon gamma assay from peripheral blood with the tuberculin skin test in the diagnosis of Mycobacterium tuberculosis infection.

INTERPRETATION. The agreement between the two tests was 68% among subjects from Baltimore and only 35% among those from Ethiopia. The interferon gamma assay had a sensitivity of 71% compared with 95% sensitivity for the tuberculin skin test among 21 subjects who had finished treatment for culture confirmed tuberculosis within the previous two years. The specificity was 85% for the interferon gamma assay and 96% for tuberculin skin test among the 52 low-risk subjects with no known history of exposure to tuberculosis from Baltimore. The sensitivities and specificities were similar to the previous larger US study (Table 12.3).

Table 12.3 Sensitivities and specificities for the last two studies comparing the interferon gamma assay with the tuberculin skin test

	Mazurek et al. Interferon gamma assay	Mazurek et al. Tuberculin skin test	Bellete et al. Interferon gamma assay	Bellete et al. Tuberculin skin test
Sensitivity	64%	95%	71%	95%
Specificity	92%	98%	85%	96%

Comment

Despite the optimism of the interferon gamma assays using purified protein derivative as the antigen being less influenced by prior BCG vaccination and exposure to environmental mycobacteria, the latter two studies demonstrated poorer sensitivity and specificity of the interferon gamma assays compared with the tuberculin skin test. There may be improved results with the interferon gamma assay utilizing antigens that are more specific, such as early secretory antigenic target (ESAT-6), which is restricted to Mycobacterium tuberculosis complex, Mycobacterium kansassi, marinum, flavescens, and szulgai. It is, therefore, absent from all strains of Mycobacterium bovis BCG and the majority of environmental bacteria. The next five studies utilized the more specific antigen ESAT-6 in both low and high tuberculosis endemic countries.

Rapid detection of Mycobacterium tuberculosis infection by enumeration of antigen-specific T cells.
Lalvani A, Pathan AA, McShane H, et al. Am J Respir Crit Care Med 2001; **163**(4): 824–8.

BACKGROUND. This study utilized the more specific antigen ESAT-6 in four groups of individuals to determine whether ESAT-6 was a reliable means for the detection of infection with Mycobacterium tuberculosis. This was a small UK study carried out in a low tuberculosis endemic country (prevalence around 10/100 000). The groups consisted of 47 cases of bacteriological confirmed tuberculosis with 47 controls, 26 healthy household tuberculosis contacts of smear positive pulmonary tuberculosis cases and 26 healthy unexposed controls (all had prior BCG vaccination).

INTERPRETATION. Forty-five of 47 patients (mean age 35 years) with bacteriological confirmed tuberculosis had ESAT-6-specific interferon gamma-secreting T-cells, compared with 4 of 47 patients with non-tuberculosis illnesses (mean age 39 years), indicating that these T-cells are an accurate marker of Mycobacterium tuberculosis infection. This assay thus has a sensitivity of 96% (95% CI 92–100) for detecting Mycobacterium tuberculosis infection in this patient population. By comparison, of 26 patients with bacteriological confirmed tuberculosis who had a diagnostic tuberculin skin test, only 18 (69%) were tuberculin skin test positive, indicating the tuberculin skin test had poorer sensitivity ($P = 0.003$). Twenty-two of 26 (85%) tuberculin skin test positive (grade 3 or 4 Heaf tests) exposed household contacts had ESAT-6-specific T-cells suggesting latent infection whereas 0 of 26 healthy unexposed controls responded. This indicated that the interferon gamma assay using ESAT-6 as the antigen is highly specific for Mycobacterium tuberculosis and not influenced by prior BCG vaccination. In summary, in this small study in a low tuberculosis endemic country, the interferon gamma assay using ESAT-6 had a higher sensitivity than the tuberculin skin test in patients with bacteriological confirmed cases of tuberculosis. In addition, the interferon gamma assay successfully distinguished between Mycobacterial tuberculosis infection and prior BCG vaccination.

Enhanced contact tracing and spatial tracking of Mycobacterium tuberculosis infection by enumeration of antigen-specific T cells.

Lalvani A, Pathan AA, Durkan H, *et al. Lancet* 2001; **357**: 2017–21.

BACKGROUND. The study assessed and compared the efficacy of the interferon gamma assay from blood using ESAT-6 as the antigen with the conventional tuberculin skin test for the detection of symptomless infected individuals, by correlation of test results with the degree of exposure to an infectious index case with tuberculosis. This was a prospective UK study of 50 healthy contacts, with varying but well-defined degrees of exposure to Mycobacterium tuberculosis, who attended an urban contact tracing clinic.

INTERPRETATION. The ESAT-6 interferon gamma assay results had a strong positive relation with increasing intensity of exposure (OR 9.0 per unit increase in level of exposure, 95% CI 2.6–31.6, $P = 0.001$), whereas the tuberculin skin test results had a weaker relation with exposure (OR 1.9, 95% CI 1.0–3.5, $P = 0.05$). By contrast, the interferon gamma assay did not correlate with BCG vaccination status ($P = 0.7$), whereas the tuberculin skin test results were significantly more likely to be positive in BCG-vaccinated contacts (OR 12.1, 95% CI 1.3–115.7, $P = 0.03$). In summary, in this small UK study in a low tuberculosis endemic country, there was a strong relationship between the interferon gamma assay using ESAT-6 and Mycobacterium tuberculosis exposure and a lack of relationship with prior BCG vaccination.

Enumeration of T-cells specific for RD1-encoded antigens suggests a high prevalence of latent Mycobacterium tuberculosis infection in healthy urban Indians.

Lalvani A, Nagvenkar P, Udwadia Z, *et al. J Infect Dis* 2001; **183**: 469–77.

BACKGROUND. This study examined 100 prospectively recruited healthy adults (mean age 47 years) in Bombay, India for latent Mycobacterial tuberculosis infection utilizing the interferon-gamma-secreting T cells specific for peptides derived from ESAT-6 and a second RD1 gene product, CFP10. The adults recruited were corporate executives who were sent for a medical examination for their health insurance. None had self-referred with symptoms, none had features of HIV infection, and all had normal chest radiographs.

INTERPRETATION. Eighty per cent responded to ≥1 antigen. In contrast, in 40 United Kingdom resident healthy adults (most had received prior BCG vaccination) none responded to either antigen. In conclusion this study shows a high prevalence (80%) of latent Mycobacterium tuberculosis infection in urban India.

Tuberculosis contacts but not patients have higher gamma interferon responses to ESAT-6 than do community controls in The Gambia.

Vekemans J, Lienhardt C, Sillah JS, *et al. Infect Immun* 2001; **69**(10): 6554–7.

BACKGROUND. This study investigated whether tuberculosis patients and contacts have higher interferon gamma responses to ESAT-6 than do community controls in a tuberculosis endemic country (The Gambia). This study compared the interferon gamma induced by ESAT-6 in 30 patients with smear positive pulmonary tuberculosis (blood samples were taken prior to commencement and at the end of anti-tuberculosis treatment) with 28 healthy household contacts and 30 community controls. All were HIV negative in this study.

INTERPRETATION. In The Gambia, the incidence of tuberculosis is high, there is believed to be widespread exposure to environmental mycobacteria, and BCG vaccination is >90%. Thirty-eight per cent of the community controls had a positive skin test to tuberculin, which could be due to prior BCG vaccination, exposure to environmental bacteria or infection with Mycobacterium tuberculosis. Thirty per cent of the community controls had positive responses to ESAT-6 suggesting that a significant proportion of the community controls had latent Mycobacterium tuberculosis infection. There were a higher proportion of responders to *in vitro* stimulation with ESAT-6 and to the tuberculin skin test among household contacts than community controls (Table 12.4). Prior to the commencement of tuberculosis treatment, the concentrations of interferon gamma were similar to community controls whereas the tuberculin skin test was positive in 93% of patients (Table 12.4). The interferon gamma concentrations were

Table 12.4 Proportion of individuals with a positive interferon gamma response to ESAT-6 and positive tuberculin skin tests (≥10 mm with 2 units of intradermal tuberculin)

	Community controls (%)	Household contacts (%)	Tuberculosis patients pre-treatment (%)
Tuberculin skin test	11/29 (38)	24/28 (86)	27/29 (93)
ESAT-6 assay	9/30 (30)	20/28 (71)	13/30 (43)

higher at the end of anti-tuberculosis treatment (mean [95% CI] post-treatment 525 pg/ml [187–1477] and pre-treatment 238 pg/ml [81–697], $P = 0.05$). In summary, in this high tuberculosis endemic country, a significant percentage (30%) of community controls and, as expected, a higher percentage (71%) of household contacts had evidence of latent Mycobacteria tuberculosis infection utilizing the interferon gamma assay with ESAT-6. Active tuberculosis was associated with a decreased interferon gamma production that improved following anti-tuberculosis therapy (the current study carried out the assay prior to the commencement and at the end of anti-tuberculosis treatment). This immune suppression associated with active tuberculosis may prevent the use of this interferon gamma assay in the diagnosis of tuberculosis. In active tuberculosis there were, however, a high proportion of tuberculin skin test responders suggesting that skin responses to mycobacterial antigens may be relatively resistant to the immunosuppression associated with active tuberculosis.

Immune responses to the Mycobacterium tuberculosis-specific antigen ESAT-6 signal subclinical infection among contacts of tuberculosis patients.

Doherty TM, Demissie A, Olobo J, *et al*. *J Clin Microbiol* 2002; **40**: 704–6.

BACKGROUND. This was a 2-year prospective Ethiopian study of 24 healthy household contacts of sputum smear positive patients who all had baseline interferon gamma responses using ESAT-6 as the antigen. All patients were HIV negative and at baseline active tuberculosis was excluded (clinical and radiological examination, and by sputum microscopy and tuberculosis culture). No patients received anti-tuberculosis chemoprophylaxis.

INTERPRETATION. Seven of the 24 contacts (29%) developed active tuberculosis during the 2-year study period. Nine contacts had positive ESAT-6 responses and 15 contacts had negative responses to ESAT-6 at baseline. Six of the 9 positive responders (67%) and only 1 of the 15 negative responders (7%) to ESAT-6 developed active tuberculosis during this 2-year study. This is in contrast to 3/17 (18%) of contacts who did not develop tuberculosis and had responded to ESAT-6. In conclusion, this small study shows that a significant proportion of ESAT-6 positive household contacts subsequently developed active tuberculosis during a 2-year follow up period, if left untreated.

Comment

The conventional tuberculin skin test has a lack of specificity due to being influenced by environmental mycobacteria, high mycobacterial load, concomitant infections, prior BCG vaccination, immunosuppression (in particular HIV infection) and is prone to errors both in the placement and reading of results. In light of this, there has been an increased interest in the whole blood interferon gamma assays.

The above studies have examined the role of the interferon gamma assay from blood using both the purified protein derivative and ESAT-6 as the antigens. Despite the optimism of the interferon gamma assays using purified protein derivative as the antigen being less influenced by prior BCG vaccination and exposure to environmental mycobacteria, the studies utilizing the interferon gamma assay using purified protein derivative had less sensitivity and specificity compared with the tuberculin skin test. In view of this, there has been increased interest in the more specific antigens for Mycobacterium tuberculosis.

ESAT-6 is a more specific antigen for Mycobacterium tuberculosis and less influenced by prior BCG vaccination and exposure to environmental mycobacteria. The first 2 UK studies utilizing ESAT-6 were carried out in a low tuberculosis endemic country. From these studies, ESAT-6 had both a high sensitivity and specificity and ESAT-6 correlated well with tuberculosis exposure and was not influenced by prior BCG vaccination. Therefore, in low tuberculosis endemic countries, this assay may be of use in contact tracing and aid in the diagnosis of active tuberculosis. These were, however, small studies and need confirmation from larger multi-centre studies.

The next two studies were in high tuberculosis endemic countries. Unlike the UK studies, there were a high proportion of healthy controls with latent Mycobacterial tuberculosis infection, which may limit its use in contact tracing to detect recent infection with Mycobacterium tuberculosis. In addition, low sensitivities were found in patients with bacteriological confirmed cases of tuberculosis. Therefore, in high tuberculosis endemic countries this assay may be of limited use in both contact tracing and in the detection of active tuberculosis. There are discrepancies between the UK and The Gambia study in the use of ESAT-6 in the diagnosis of active tuberculosis and further studies are required to determine its role.

The last small study was a 2-year prospective study and demonstrated that many ESAT-6 positive contacts, if left untreated, subsequently develop active tuberculosis. This reinforces the importance of tuberculosis contact tracing and the need for chemoprophylaxis in patients suspected of being recently infected.

Overall, this interferon gamma assay utilizing ESAT-6 promises to be more specific compared with the conventional tuberculin skin test. The conventional tuberculin skin test will likely continue until there are larger multi-centre studies in both low and high tuberculosis endemic countries comparing the conventional tuberculin skin test with both the interferon gamma assay and skin test using ESAT-6 and/or other Mycobacteria tuberculosis specific antigens for the diagnosis of latent infection and active tuberculosis.

The next section covers treatment aspects of latent Mycobacterial tuberculosis infection.

Treatment of latent Mycobacterial infection

Latent Mycobacterial tuberculosis infection is predominantly identified through tuberculosis contact tracing, although it can be detected by other routes, for example, immigrant screening, pre-employment screening or as part of the BCG vaccination programme. To reduce the probability of developing active tuberculosis, a variety of regimens is recommended internationally to treat latent Mycobacterial tuberculosis infection. Some of the available regimens include 6–9 months Isoniazid therapy, 4 months Rifampicin therapy, 3 months combination of Rifampicin and Isoniazid therapy and 2 months combination therapy with Rifampicin and Pyrazinamide. The first two studies investigated the safety of the shorter 2-month regimen (in patients with and without HIV infection) and the study following investigated the efficacy of Isoniazid chemoprophylaxis in patients with systemic lupus erythematosis (SLE).

Short-course Rifampicin and Pyrazinamide compared with Isoniazid for latent tuberculosis infection: a multi-centre clinical trial.

Jasmer RM, Saukkonen JJ, Blumberg HM, *et al.* Short-Course Rifampicin and Pyrazinamide for Tuberculosis Infection (SCRIPT) Study Investigators. *Ann Intern Med* 2002; **137**(8): 640–7.

BACKGROUND. This multi-centre US study compared the safety and tolerance of a 2-month regimen of Rifampicin and Pyrazinamide with that of a 6-month regimen of Isoniazid for treatment of latent Mycobacterial tuberculosis infection in 589 non-HIV infected adults. Patients were assigned to receive Rifampicin and Pyrazinamide daily for 2 months ($n = 307$) or Isoniazid daily for 6 months ($n = 282$). The primary end-points were hepatotoxicity, other adverse events, and the percentage of patients who completed treatment.

INTERPRETATION. Results are shown in Table 12.5. Of the patients assigned to Rifampicin and Pyrazinamide, 7.7% developed ≥grade 3 hepatotoxicity (serum ALT >250 U/L or >5 times normal) compared with 1% of patients assigned to Isoniazid (OR 8.46, 95% CI 1.9–76.5, $P = 0.001$). In addition the Rifampicin plus Pyrazinamide regimen was more likely than the Isoniazid regimen to be discontinued because

Table 12.5 Outcomes for the two groups were compared—patients taking Rifampicin + Pyrazinamide with patients taking Isoniazid alone

	Rifampicin + Pyrazinamide	Isoniazid alone
Number	307	282
≥Grade 3 hepatotoxicity	7.7%***	1%
Discontinuation because of hepatotoxicity	5.8%*	1%
Non-hepatotoxic adverse events	20%	16%
Skin rash	6%**	2%
Completed treatment	61%	57%

*$P < 0.05$, **$P < 0.01$ and ***$P < 0.005$.

of hepatotoxicity (OR 5.19, 95% CI 1.11–49.1, $P = 0.033$). The overall percentage of non-hepatotoxic adverse events in the Rifampicin and Pyrazinamide group (20%) was similar to the Isoniazid group (16%) although skin rash was more frequent ($P = 0.007$) in the Rifampicin and Pyrazinamide group. The proportion of patients who completed the study treatment was similar with either treatment regimen (61% and 57% respectively). In conclusion the 2-month regimen of Rifampicin and Pyrazinamide was associated with an increased risk for grade 3 or 4 hepatotoxicity compared with a 6-month regimen of Isoniazid and did not improve compliance.

Comment

The shorter regimen of Rifampicin and Pyrazinamide has the attraction of being shorter, which should improve compliance. It is interesting, however, that those completion rates did not differ with the two arms of the study and were only approximately 60%, showing that compliance remains sub-optimal. The increase in hepatotoxicity with the Rifampicin and Pyrazinamide regimen remains a concern and if the regimen were used, then it would be advisable to monitor liver function tests before and during treatment to screen for hepatotoxicity.

Short-course Rifamycin and Pyrazinamide treatment for latent tuberculosis infection in patients with HIV infection: the 2-year experience of a comprehensive community-based program in Broward County, Florida.
Narita M, Kellman M, Franchini DL, McMillan ME, Hollender ES, Ashkin D.
Chest 2002; **122**(4): 1292–8.

BACKGROUND. This study assessed the completion rates and tolerability of the short-course Rifamycin and Pyrazinamide treatment for latent tuberculosis infection in HIV-infected patients through a comprehensive community-based programme.

Rifampicin was used when patients were not receiving a protease inhibitor or a non-nucleoside reverse transcriptase inhibitor whereas patients used Rifabutin if on a protease inhibitor or a non-nucleoside reverse transcriptase inhibitor. Of 3118 patients with HIV infection screened for latent tuberculosis infection between February 1999 and March 2001, 135 patients were placed on Rifamycin and Pyrazinamide for 2 months under directly observed therapy and were compared to a historical group comprised of 93 HIV-infected patients who were placed on self-administered treatment of Isoniazid for 12 months between 1996 and 1998.

INTERPRETATION. The results are shown in Table 12.6. Of the 135 patients receiving Rifamycin and Pyrazinamide, 93% completed treatment but 5 patients (4%) had to discontinue treatment due to side-effects (allergic skin reactions [$n = 4$] and hepatitis [$n = 1$]). The completion rate of the historical group who received Isoniazid therapy was 61% (57 of 93 patients; $P < 0.001$) and none of those who received Isoniazid experienced significant side-effects. This was a non-randomized controlled study, but suggested a higher adherence in HIV patients with the shorter 2-month regimen of Rifamycin and Pyrazinamide than that of the 12 months Isoniazid therapy. Four per cent of patients treated with Rifamycin and Pyrazinamide had side-effects that led to its discontinuation whereas there was no discontinuation of therapy in patients treated with Isoniazid.

Comment

As in the previous study, shorter regimens have the attraction of decreasing length of treatment, which are likely to improve compliance. Compliance rates were better in the latter study and the patient group may explain this. As many patients with HIV infection are already on a cocktail of different therapies, shorter regimens would likely be welcome and improve compliance. As in the previous study, however, there were more side-effects with the Rifamycin and Pyrazinamide combination compared with the Isoniazid monotherapy. Multi-centre randomized controlled trials assessing the safety, efficacy and tolerability of Rifamycin and Pyrazinamide in HIV patients would be the key before its uptake into routine clinical practice.

Table 12.6 Demographics and outcome comparing Rifamycin + Pyrazinamide with Isoniazid treatment regimens

	Rifamycin + Pyrazinamide	Isoniazid alone
Number	135	93
Mean age $\pm$ SD	41.7 $\pm$ 9.1 years	38.2 $\pm$ 10.0 years*
Completed treatment	93%	61%**

*$P < 0.01$ and **$P < 0.001$.

Efficacy of Isoniazid prophylaxis in patients with systemic lupus erythematosis receiving long-term steroid treatment.

Gaitonde S, Pathan E, Sule A, Mittal G, Joshi VR. *Ann Rheum Dis* 2002; **61**(3): 251–3.

BACKGROUND. This study carried out in India evaluated the efficacy of Isoniazid chemoprophylaxis in patients with SLE receiving long-term glucocorticosteroid treatment (97% being on >0.25 mg/kg/day of steroids and 49% on concurrent cytotoxic agents). In this high tuberculosis endemic country, an 80% prevalence of latent tuberculosis has been shown (see earlier study by Lalvani A *et al. J Infect Dis* 2001; 183: 469–97). The authors have previously reported a 12% prevalence over a 5-year period of active tuberculosis rates in 146 patients with SLE receiving long-term steroids. Treatment with Isoniazid (5 mg/kg/day, max 300 mg/day) together with Pyridoxine 10 mg/day for 1 year was started in all patients with SLE seen between January 1994 and December 1999 and followed up thereafter. Clinical examination and chest radiography were carried out in all patients before the start of Isoniazid treatment. A liver profile was obtained only if liver toxicity was suspected. Only the data of those patients who completed the Isoniazid treatment or who were withdrawn owing to toxicity have been analysed. This was compared with the results of an earlier study of the prevalence of tuberculosis in patients with SLE not receiving Isoniazid.

INTERPRETATION. Ninety-seven patients were included, of whom 95 completed 1 year of treatment with Isoniazid. Treatment was discontinued in 2 patients owing to toxicity (1 due to hepatitis and 1 due to peripheral neuropathy at 8 and 10 months respectively). One patient developed tuberculosis within 1 month of starting Isoniazid. Seventy patients were followed up further for at least 1 year (mean 26.4 months, range 12–60 months) after completion of the Isoniazid treatment. During this period 1 patient developed tuberculosis after 1 month. No deaths due to tuberculosis or hepatitis occurred. In comparison with the earlier series, the prevalence of tuberculosis decreased from 12 to 2%, a reduction of 82%. The authors concluded from this non-randomized controlled study that 1 year of treatment with Isoniazid was safe and effective in reducing the prevalence of developing active tuberculosis in patients with SLE.

Comment

This was not a randomized controlled trial, but results were compared to their historical controls. The authors found that Isoniazid was safe and reduced the prevalence of active tuberculosis in patients with SLE on long-term oral steroids. The blind approach of treating all SLE patients on long-term oral steroids with Isoniazid chemoprophylaxis may be appropriate in this high tuberculosis endemic setting but may be inappropriate in low tuberculosis endemic countries. In low tuberculosis endemic countries, it may be more appropriate to treat patients with evidence of latent tuberculosis infection or previously untreated tuberculosis.

The authors treated their patients with 12 months of chemoprophylaxis. There is increasing evidence from international guidelines that shorter regimens suffice, and currently for immunosuppressed patients a 9-month regimen with Isoniazid would be recommended.

The next section discusses treatment strategies for tuberculosis, including multidrug resistant tuberculosis and mycobacteria other than tuberculosis.

Directly observed therapy

Internationally it is recognized that up to 50% of patients do not complete their treatment for tuberculosis. Incomplete treatment can lead to prolonged infectiousness, drug resistance, relapse of tuberculosis and death and therefore poses a problem to both the individual and the community. Strategies to improve adherence to treatment regimens are therefore important. It is currently believed that directly observed therapy would improve compliance and treatment outcomes. Such patients have supervised treatment either two or three times on a weekly basis depending on the regimen used. The supervised treatment is conventionally carried out by a health care worker, usually a health visitor or a district nurse. It is, however, difficult to institute directly observed therapy with current resources internationally and there has been increased interest in using family members to supervise treatment. Two papers are presented on direct observed therapy, a randomized controlled trial and a Cochrane review that compared the effectiveness of directly observed therapy (by health workers or a family member) with self-administered treatment for patients being treated for tuberculosis.

Effectiveness of the direct observation component of DOTS for tuberculosis: a randomized controlled trial in Pakistan.
Walley JD, Khan MA, Newell JN, Khan MH. *Lancet* 2001; **357**(9257): 664–9.

B ACKGROUND . **This randomized controlled study compared the effectiveness of directly observed therapy with self-administered treatment for patients being treated for tuberculosis. Four hundred and ninety-seven adults with new sputum positive pulmonary tuberculosis were enrolled. One hundred and seventy were assigned with direct observation of treatment by health workers, 165 were assigned with direct observation of treatment by family members, and 162 were assigned self-administered treatment. A standard daily short course regimen was used (2 months of Isoniazid, Rifampicin, Pyrazinamide, and Ethambutol, followed by 6 months of Isoniazid and Ethambutol). The main outcome measures were cure and treatment completion. Treatment failure was defined as being smear positive at $\geq$5 months.**

Table 12.7 There was no significant difference in the outcomes comparing self-administered treatment with direct observed therapy from both a family member and a health care worker

	Direct observed therapy Health worker	Direct observed therapy Family member	Self-administered treatment
Number	170	165	162
Cured	64%	55%	62%
Cured and/or completed treatment	67%	62%	65%
Treatment failure	0	0	0
Defaulted	27%	32%	33%
Transferred out	2%	1%	1%
Died	4%	4%	2%

INTERPRETATION. The health worker directly observed therapy, family member directly observed therapy, and self-administered treatment strategies gave very similar outcomes, with cure rates of 64, 55, and 62%, respectively, and cure or treatment completed rates of 67, 62, and 65%, respectively (Table 12.7). In summary, a significant percentage of patients defaulted from tuberculosis treatment and direct observed therapy did not improve default rates. In addition, compared with self-administered treatment, direct observation of treatment did not give any additional improvement in cure rates. Finally directly observed therapy by a family member was equally as effective as direct observed therapy by a health care worker.

Directly observed therapy for treating tuberculosis.
Volmink J, Garner P. *The Cochrane Library* 2002; **2**: 1–18.

Background. The Cochrane review assessed the effects of directly observed therapy by an appointed agent (health worker, community volunteer or family member) on cure and treatment completion in people on treatment for tuberculosis.

INTERPRETATION. There were four randomized controlled studies ($n = 1603$ participants) from 1966–2001 conducted in South Africa, Thailand and Pakistan. There was no significant difference detected between direct observation and self-treatment for cure (RR 1.06, 95% CI 0.98–1.14) and for cure plus treatment completion (RR 1.06, 95% CI 1.00–1.13). A stratified analysis by the appointed agent (health professional, lay health worker or family/community member) did not reveal any important differences. One study conducted in an optimal setting in which patients were given a choice of supervisor did show modest benefit: cure (RR 1.13, 95% CI 1.04–1.24) and cure plus treatment completion (RR 1.11, 95% CI 1.03–1.18) but this patient-centred approach may have influenced the results. In conclusion these randomized controlled trials provide no evidence that directly observed therapy in low- and middle-income country settings improves cure or treatment completion rates in patients with tuberculosis.

Comment

Although there are potential benefits with direct observed therapy in that patients are closely monitored and social process with peer pressure may improve adherence, there are also pitfalls. These include patient autonomy, resource implications, and may make adherence worse if patients are required to travel long distances. These randomized controlled trials provided no evidence that directly observed therapy improved cure or treatment completion rates but did provide evidence that a family member providing supervision was as effective as a health care worker. It would thus seem advisable to target direct observed therapy to patients thought to be at high risk of non-adherence to treatment. Utilizing suitable family members, if available, would facilitate the provision of directly observed therapy. Finally there is a need for newer simpler regimens to improve completion rates and facilitate the provision of directly observed therapy (there is currently a once weekly Rifapentine regimen which is discussed later).

Role of Mycobacterium vaccae as an adjunct to treatment in tuberculosis

There has been much controversy over whether the addition of heat-killed Mycobacterium vaccae to standard tuberculosis treatment can improve the outcome in patients with tuberculosis, including patients with multi-drug resistant tuberculosis (MDRTB). The precise mechanism for Mycobacterium vaccae is unknown but is thought to allow immune recognition of antigens common to all mycobacteria, thought to direct T lymphocyte responses towards a type 1 (Th1), and thought to enable the host to destroy organisms and achieve a more rapid cure of infection. Three papers are presented. The first two papers include a Cochrane review and a randomized controlled trial on the role of a single dosage of Mycobacterium vaccae as an adjunct to standard tuberculosis treatment, and the third paper discusses the role of multiple doses of Mycobacterium vaccae in patients with MDRTB.

Mycobacterium vaccae immunotherapy for treating tuberculosis.

de Bruyn G, Garner P. *The Cochrane Library* 2002; **2**: 1–17.

BACKGROUND. This review assessed the effects of a single dose of whole, killed Mycobacterium vaccae as an adjunct to treatment for treating tuberculosis.

INTERPRETATION. There were six randomized controlled trials (898 patients), 70% were males and age ranged from 15–80. In five trials, patients were undergoing treatment for the first episode of pulmonary tuberculosis. There was no significant effect on mortality (three trials, OR 1.01, 95% CI 0.51–1.99), no consistent effect of sputum negativity on sputum culture, and a high level of adverse reactions. Most immunotherapy recipients experienced local adverse reactions (two trials, OR 18, 95% CI 9–37). These included redness and swelling, some of which progressed to ulceration and scarring. The conclusion of this Cochrane review was that immunotherapy with single dose Mycobacterium vaccae does not appear to confer additional benefit in patients being treated for pulmonary tuberculosis.

Mycobacterium vaccae (SRL172) immunotherapy as an adjunct to standard anti-tuberculosis treatment in HIV-infected adults with pulmonary tuberculosis: a randomized placebo-controlled trial.

Mwinga A, Nunn A, Ngwira B, *et al. Lancet* 2002; **360**(9339): 1050–5.

BACKGROUND. This randomized controlled study investigated the efficacy of immunotherapy with single-dose heat-killed Mycobacterium vaccae (SRL172) added to standard anti-tuberculosis treatment in HIV patients with pulmonary tuberculosis. This double-blind trial enrolled 1229 patients aged 18–60 years, who had never received anti-retroviral treatment and who presented with newly diagnosed, sputum smear-positive pulmonary tuberculosis to referral centres in Lusaka, Zambia, and Karonga, Malawi. Both HIV-positive and HIV-negative patients were enrolled, to avoid stigmatization. Participants were randomly assigned a single injection of SRL172 or matching placebo within 2 weeks of starting 8 months of anti-tuberculosis treatment and followed up for at least 12 months. The primary end-point was time to death in the HIV-infected population. Analyses were based on 760 HIV-positive patients after exclusion of 84 patients with errors in storage of the injection, no bacteriological confirmation, or no HIV result.

INTERPRETATION. Of 760 HIV-infected patients, 374 received SRL172 and 386 received placebo. The follow up rate was 88% at 12 months in both groups. There were three reports (<1%) of adverse events at the injected site, which only occurred in the patients that received SRL 172. Two patients reported pain at the injection site and one patient reported discharging pus from the injection site at week 12. SRL172, however, did not cause any serious adverse events. Mycobacterium vaccae conferred no improvement in mortality rates in HIV-positive or HIV-negative patients with tuberculosis (Table 12.8). In conclusion immunotherapy with single-dose heat-killed Mycobacterium vaccae as an adjunct to standard anti-tuberculosis treatment in HIV-positive and -negative adults with pulmonary tuberculosis had no significant effect on survival, though the treatment was safe and well tolerated.

Table 12.8 Mycobacterium vaccae (M. vaccae) conferred no additional benefit in patients with tuberculosis with and without HIV infection

	HIV +ve M. vaccae	HIV +ve placebo	HIV –ve M. vaccae	HIV –ve placebo
Number	374	386	185	200
Mean (SD) age years	30.8 (8.0)	31.0 (8.0)	29.9 (10.1)	29.6 (10.8)
Mortality at 12 months	20%	18%	1%	1%
Deaths rate per 100 person years (95% CI)	19.5 (16.0–23.6)	19.3 (15.8–23.3)	2.1 (0.9–4.4)	2.0 (0.8–4.1)

Does immunotherapy with heat-killed Mycobacterium vaccae offer hope for the treatment of multi-drug resistant pulmonary tuberculosis?

Stanford JL, Stanford CA, Grange JM, Lan NN, Etemadi. A. *Respir Med* 2001; **95**(6): 444–7.

BACKGROUND. Most previous studies have been of single doses of immunotherapy with Mycobacterium vaccae given early in the course of treatment. This observational international study evaluated whether multiple doses of heat-killed Mycobacterium vaccae (NCTC 11659), as an adjunct to the available treatment, improved the outcome in patients with MDRTB who had not been cured by treatment alone. Initially, single doses of Mycobacterium vaccae were given but subsequently up to 12 doses at 2-month intervals were given. Treatment varied from Isoniazid alone to drugs selected according to susceptibility tests. Most patients had failed to respond to repeat courses of treatment and the majority were expected to die from their disease. Results were assessed by sputum smear and culture and by clinical observations.

INTERPRETATION. There were 337 patients grouped according to the length of their histories of disease: less than or greater than 2 years' duration. Eighteen of 22 (82%) patients with disease for less than 2 years had bacteriological cure with one or two doses of Mycobacterium vaccae. Among 315 chronic patients (disease >2 years duration), 8% had bacteriological cure after one dose, 38% after seven doses and 42% after 12 doses. Twenty-one per cent of the chronic patients were lost to follow-up, or died, during the multi-dose regimens. The best outcome was obtained in 65 patients who received Mycobacterium vaccae as an adjunct to treatment tailored to their drug susceptibility patterns. A total of 18.5% achieved bacteriological cure rates after one injection and 58% after multiple injections with Mycobacterium vaccae (*P* <0.005). This study has several weaknesses being an observational non-placebo controlled study, having non-standardized treatment regimens, and patients receiving a variable number of injections of Mycobacterium vaccae. The data, however, provided preliminary evidence that the addition of multiple doses of immunotherapy with Mycobacterium vaccae as an adjunct to treatment may improve the rate of cure of MDRTB. Randomized placebo controlled studies with standardized multiple doses of immunotherapy with Mycobacterium vaccae, as an adjunct to standardized regimens containing at least three susceptible drugs in MDRTB, are required.

Comment

From data to date there is little evidence that the addition of single dose Mycobacterium vaccae confers any additional benefit as an adjunct to standard tuberculosis treatment in patients with non-MDRTB. This is independent of the presence or absence of HIV infection. Although the last study is not a randomized controlled study, it is of potential interest as patients with multi-drug resistant pulmonary tuberculosis in whom treatment has failed are expected to have a poor outcome with an associated high mortality rate. The addition of >1 dose of Mycobacterium vaccae seemed to confer additional benefit and some patients managed sputum conversion. This needs confirmation with randomized controlled trials to investigate whether multiple doses of Mycobacterium vaccae truly influence the outcome.

Management of tuberculosis

The next four papers look at the clinical management of tuberculosis. The majority of patients respond to the internationally accepted first line anti-tuberculosis regimens (assuming the Mycobacterium tuberculosis is sensitive to the conventional first line drugs Rifampicin, Isoniazid, Pyrazinamide and Ethambutol). A small number of patients do not respond to these standard regimens; the next paper suggests measuring Rifampicin blood levels in such patients, and if subtherapeutic, to increase the Rifampicin dosages till therapeutic levels are achieved. The following paper investigated when to start antiretroviral therapy in patients with concomitant HIV infection and tuberculosis. The final papers in this section investigated whether the once weekly Rifapentine regimens were as successful as standard regimens in the continuation phase in the management of patients with tuberculosis.

Utility of Rifampicin blood levels in the treatment and follow-up of active pulmonary tuberculosis in patients who were slow to respond to routine directly observed therapy.

Mehta JB, Shantaveerapa H, Byrd RP Jr, Morton SE, Fountain F, Roy TM. *Chest* 2001; **120**(5): 1520–4.

BACKGROUND. The standard daily dose of Rifampicin in directly observed treatment of Mycobacterium tuberculosis is 600 mg taken orally. The purpose of this study was to assess the efficacy of standard dose Rifampicin therapy in patients who were slow to respond to routine directly observed therapy. Patients with non-drug resistant pulmonary tuberculosis who were receiving 600 mg of oral Rifampicin by direct observed therapy were eligible for inclusion. Patients were deemed slow to respond if their sputum smears and cultures remained positive for Mycobacterium tuberculosis and if the patient's condition did not improve clinically or radiographically after 3 months of treatment. Serum Rifampicin levels were ascertained to determine the adequacy of the standard Rifampicin dosing (normal Rifampicin levels were 8–24 μg/ml). Patients with subtherapeutic blood levels had their Rifampicin dose increased to 900 mg and Rifampicin levels were repeated. Rifampicin dosage was increased again if blood levels were still subtherapeutic. No new anti-tuberculosis medications were added to the treatment regimen. The total weekly dose of the other standard treatment drugs was not increased.

INTERPRETATION. Of 124 new patients with active pulmonary tuberculosis, 6 patients were identified as slow to respond to the standard anti-tuberculosis regimen. All 6 patients had subtherapeutic serum Rifampicin levels. All six patients responded clinically, radiographically and microbiologically after an increase in Rifampicin dosage to reach target drug blood level. In summary, standard dosing with Rifampicin resulted in a poor clinical response in 5% of patients, all of which had subtherapeutic serum Rifampicin levels. Increasing the dosage of Rifampicin improved the outcome without additional side-effects.

Comment

This small study suggests that in the small number of patients that do not clinically improve, an inadequate dose of Rifampicin should be suspected and that increasing the dose will lead to clinical improvements.

There were, however, limitations with this study. As it was not a randomized controlled study, it is not known whether the outcome would have been the same had the Rifampicin dose not been increased. The serum Rifampicin levels were only carried out in the non-responders and, therefore, it is not known how many other patients had serum Rifampicin concentrations below the therapeutic range, in patients that were clinically responding. Another limitation with the study was that the serum levels of the other anti-tuberculosis drugs were not determined. Larger cohort studies measuring the serum concentrations of all the anti-tuberculosis drugs would be required to determine whether the authors' conclusions are valid.

Treatment of tuberculosis in HIV-infected persons in the era of highly active antiretroviral therapy.
Dean GL, Edwards SG, Ives NJ, et al. AIDS 2002; **16**(1): 75–83.

BACKGROUND. This retrospective UK study (January 1996 to June 1999) assessed the risks and benefits of administering highly active antiretroviral therapy (HAART) during the treatment of culture proven tuberculosis in HIV-infected patients.

INTERPRETATION. Patients ($n = 188$) were severely immunocompromised with a median CD4 cell count at tuberculosis diagnosis of 90×10^6 cells/l (IQR 30–180) and had a median age of 34 years (range 21–70). Fifty-four per cent were not prescribed HAART during their tuberculosis therapy. Eighteen per cent were taking HAART when tuberculosis was diagnosed and 27% commenced HAART during tuberculosis treatment after a median of 2 months (range 0–14). Treatment with HAART was associated with significant reductions in viral load (Table 12.9) and subsequent AIDS-defining illness (ADI) (3.5 versus 24.5%; $P < 0.001$). Nine of 91 (10%) patients with a CD4 count $>100 \times 10^6$ cells/l at tuberculosis diagnosis experienced a further ADI, whereas 39% of patients with a CD4 count $<100 \times 10^6$ cells/l who did not receive antiretrovirals developed this complication. Adverse events occurred in 54% of patients, which led to 34% changing or interrupting HIV and/or tuberculosis medication. The majority of adverse events occurred within the first 2 months and patients on antiretroviral therapy and tuberculosis therapy concomitantly had a greater likelihood of adverse events (OR 1.88, 95% CI 1.03–3.42). Peripheral neuropathy (21%), rash (17%), gastrointestinal upset (10%), neurological side-effects other than peripheral neuropathy (7%) and hepatitis (6%) were the most frequent adverse events. In summary, adverse effects are common in HIV patients concomitantly treated with anti-tuberculosis treatment and antiretroviral therapy. Commencing HAART, however, improved the viral load and patients had less subsequent ADI.

Comment

Many physicians delay HAART in patients presenting with tuberculosis because of pill burden, drug interactions and toxicity. Although the use of HAART led to significant reductions in viral load and subsequent ADI, co-infected patients commonly experienced adverse events leading to interruptions in tuberculosis/HIV therapy, particularly within the first 2 months. The authors recommended starting HAART early for patients with advanced HIV disease (CD4 $<100 \times 10^6$ cells/l) and deferring HAART until the continuation phase of tuberculosis therapy (after 2 months initiation therapy) for patients who are clinically stable (CD4 $>100 \times 10^6$ cells/l).

This study is relevant to patients presenting with tuberculosis who are co-infected with newly diagnosed HIV infection or in patients with known HIV disease not currently treated with HAART. This study, however, does have limitations, as it was a retrospective study only. Prospective randomized controlled studies are required to explore the risks and benefits of concomitant treatment with anti-

Table 12.9 The viral load fell significantly following commencement of HAART. Data presented as median (95% CI)

	Baseline	12 months	P value
Log_{10} viral load	5.12 (95% CI 4.83–5.41)	2.61 (2.07–3.15)	0.005

tuberculosis treatment and HAART, and to determine when HAART should be commenced.

Rifapentine and Isoniazid once a week versus Rifampicin and Isoniazid twice a week for treatment of drug-susceptible pulmonary tuberculosis in HIV-negative patients: a randomized clinical trial.

Benator D, Bhattacharya M, Bozeman L, *et al.* The Tuberculosis Trials Consortium. *Lancet* 2002; **360**(9332): 528–34.

BACKGROUND. **To improve compliance with anti-tuberculosis treatment, there has been increased interest in a once-weekly regimen. Rifapentine has a long half-life in serum, which offers a possible once-weekly treatment for tuberculosis. This study compared the efficacy and tolerability of Rifapentine and Isoniazid once a week with Rifampicin and Isoniazid twice a week. This randomized, multi-centre, open-label trial in the USA and Canada comprised of HIV-negative people with drug susceptible pulmonary tuberculosis who had completed the initial 2 months of a 6-month treatment regimen. Patients were then randomly allocated directly observed treatment with either 600 mg Rifapentine plus 15 mg/kg (maximum 900 mg) Isoniazid once a week or 10 mg/kg (maximum 600 mg) Rifampicin plus 15 mg/kg (maximum 900 mg) Isoniazid twice a week. Follow-up was for 2 years following the cessation of the study treatment. Primary outcome was failure/relapse.**

INTERPRETATION. The results are shown in Table 12.10. One thousand and four patients were enrolled (502 per treatment group). Nine hundred and twenty-eight successfully completed treatment, and 803 completed the 2-year 4-month study. Failure and relapse was defined as the following: sputum culture positive at 4 months after starting initial treatment for tuberculosis; clinical failure, that is progressive tuberculosis

Table 12.10 Demographics and outcomes comparing once weekly Rifapentine and Isoniazid with the standard twice weekly direct observed therapy regimen

	Rifapentine + Isoniazid Once weekly treatment	Rifampicin + Isoniazid Twice weekly treatment
Number	502	502
Age (mean ± SD) years	45 ± 15	45 ± 15
Follow up post-treatment (mean ± SD)	20.4 ± 6.4 months	20.3 ± 6.3 months
Study drugs permanently discontinued	3%	3%
Failed to complete treatment	6%	9%
Failure and/or relapse	9.2%	5.6%*
Failure and/or relapse if no cavitation on the chest radiograph	2.5%	2.9%
Mortality during study treatment	1%	1%

*$P < 0.05$.

Table 12.11 Multivariate analysis showing variables associated with failure/relapse

Variable	OR (95% CI)	P value
Cavitation on the chest radiograph*	3.0 (1.5–5.8)	0.001
Bilateral pulmonary involvement*	1.8 (1.0–3.2)	0.05
Sputum culture positive*	2.8 (1.7–4.7)	<0.001
Underweight (>10% below ideal body weight)*	2.8 (1.7–4.7)	<0.001
Non-Hispanic white person	1.8 (1.1–3.0)	0.02

*At randomization (after completion of the standard 2 months initiation treatment).

after 8 weeks of study therapy; defaulters with subsequent relapse with culture positive tuberculosis; relapse with culture positive tuberculosis following completion of treatment; and clinical relapse following cessation of treatment. The crude rates of failure/relapse were 9.2% in those on Rifapentine once a week, and 5.6% in those given Rifampicin twice a week (RR 1.64, 95% CI 1.04–2.58, $P = 0.04$). By proportional hazards regression, five characteristics were independently associated with increased risk of failure/relapse: sputum culture positive, cavitation on the chest radiograph, bilateral pulmonary involvement, and being underweight at randomization (after completion of the standard 2 months initiation treatment), and being a non-Hispanic white person (Table 12.11). Of the participants without cavitation on the chest radiograph (at randomization), rates of failure/relapse were 2.9% in the once-a-week Rifapentine group and 2.5% in the standard twice-weekly treatment group (RR 1.15, 95% CI 0.38–3.50, $P = 0.81$). The rates of adverse events and death were similar in the two treatment groups (Table 12.10). In summary Rifapentine once a week is safe and effective for the treatment of pulmonary tuberculosis in the continuous phase in HIV-negative patients, without cavitation on the chest radiograph after 2 months' initiation therapy. Clinical, radiographic, and microbiological data help to identify patients with tuberculosis who are at increased risk of failure or relapse when treated with either regimen.

A prospective, randomized, double-blind study of the tolerability of Rifapentine 600, 900 and 1200 mg plus Isoniazid in the continuation phase of tuberculosis treatment.

Bock NN, Sterling TR, Hamilton CD, et al., The Tuberculosis Trials Consortium, Centers For Disease Control Prevention, Atlanta, Georgia. *Am J Respir Crit Care Med* 2002; **165**: 1526–30.

BACKGROUND. Once-weekly Rifapentine 600 mg plus Isoniazid during the continuation phase treatment of tuberculosis is associated with a relapse rate higher than that of twice-weekly Rifampicin plus Isoniazid. This prospective randomized

double-blind trial assessed the safety and tolerability of Rifapentine at three doses (600, 900 and 1200 mg) plus Isoniazid 15 mg/kg once weekly in the continuation phase (16 weeks) treatment of culture positive tuberculosis in 150 HIV-negative adults. Outcome measures were discontinuation of therapy for any reason and adverse events on therapy.

INTERPRETATION. There were 23 adverse events, but only 4 were possibly related to study treatment. There were deranged liver function tests in 3 patients (1 in the Rifapentine 900 mg arm and 2 in the Rifapentine 1200 mg arm). In the Rifapentine 1200 mg arm, 1 of the patients had to discontinue Rifapentine due to hepatotoxicity. The other adverse event in the Rifapentine 1200 mg arm was a first trimester abortion thought possibly related to the study treatment. There was a trend towards more adverse events possibly associated with study therapy in the highest-dose arms ($P = 0.051$). Overall treatment was discontinued in 3/52 (6%), 2/51 (4%), and 3/47 (6%) in the Rifapentine 600 mg, 900 mg, and 1200 mg treatment arms respectively. Only one discontinuation in the Rifapentine 1200 mg arm was due to an adverse event possibly associated with study therapy (hepatotoxicity). In summary Rifapentine 900 mg once-weekly dosing appears to be safe and well tolerated but further evaluation of the safety and tolerability of Rifapentine 1200 mg is warranted. As compliance is essential for tuberculosis treatment, once-weekly regimens may improve compliance and be easier for the implementation of direct observed therapy regimens. Trials comparing these higher dose regimens with standard treatment regimens for tuberculosis are required.

Comment

The creation of simpler regimens will likely improve compliance, which will subsequently improve long-term outcomes. It will also allow easier implementation for direct observed therapy regimens. The drawbacks with these shortened regimens can be increased drug toxicity and the shortened regimens may be less efficacious.

The study by Benator *et al.* investigated the efficacy of the once-weekly Rifapentine therapy in the continuation phase of tuberculosis treatment. Standardly, patients in the initiation phase receive 3 or 4 drugs (Rifampicin + Isoniazid + Pyrazinamide ± Ethambutol) for the first 2 months. Following this, patients enter the continuation phase (4 months if the combination of Rifampicin and Isoniazid is used). The regimen described assumes no drug resistance. In the study by Benator *et al.*, there was no increased drug toxicity but Rifapentine was less efficacious, with an increased failure/relapse rate. The once-weekly Rifapentine regimen was, however, as effective as the standard twice-weekly therapy in patients that have responded well to the initial 2 months' initiation therapy with no cavitation on the chest radiograph and being sputum culture negative for tuberculosis. Thus, this newer regimen (600 mg Rifapentine plus 15 mg/kg [maximum 900 mg] Isoniazid once a week) can be considered for such patients that have responded well to the initial 2 months' initiation therapy. In other cases, it seems sensible at this stage to continue with the standard regimens.

Multi-drug resistant tuberculosis

MDRTB is defined as resistance to Rifampicin and Isoniazid and frequently others. MDRTB remains a global threat internationally and the first paper highlights this. The papers following looked at the outcomes of MDRTB in the UK and in Turkey. The final papers explored the outcomes of a standardized MDRTB regimen and examined the benefits and risks of surgery as an adjunct to medical treatment.

Global trends in resistance to anti-tuberculosis drugs. World Health Organization—International Union against Tuberculosis and Lung Disease Working Group on Anti-Tuberculosis Drug Resistance Surveillance.

Espinal MA, Laszlo A, Simonsen L, *et al. N Engl J Med* 2001; **344**(17): 1294–303.

BACKGROUND. This study assessed resistance to anti-tuberculosis drugs in countries on six continents. This study obtained data from 1996–1999 using standard protocols from ongoing surveillance or from surveys of representative samples of all patients with tuberculosis.

INTERPRETATION. Between 1996 and 1999, patients in 58 geographic sites were surveyed. The median prevalence of multi-drug resistance among new cases of tuberculosis for all countries was 1.0% (95% CI 0.3–2.4) but was higher for patients who had prior treatment for tuberculosis with a median of 9.3% (95% CI 3.5–19.2). The prevalence of MDRTB is highly variable throughout the world and the table below (Table 12.12) highlights a few countries to illustrate this variance. MDRTB remains a global threat internationally.

Table 12.12 Percentage of patients (95% CI) with MDRTB occurring in new TB cases and in patients with prior TB treatment

		New TB cases	Prior TB treatment
America	US	1.2 (1.0–1.4)	5.6 (3.9–7.7)
	Peru	3.0 (2.3–3.9)	12.3 (8.6–16.9)
Europe	England & Wales	0.8 (0.5–1.2)	13.2 (8.7–18.9)
	Russia province	9.0 (5.6–13.6)	25.9 (14.9–39.6)
	Latvia	9.0 (7.1–11.2)	23.7 (18.2–29.7)
	Estonia	14.1 (10.7–17.9)	37.8 (27.3–49.1)
Africa	Botswana	0.5 (0.1–1.4)	9.0 (4.9–14.8)
Asia	Singapore	0.3 (0.1–0.9)	4.0 (1.5–8.4)
	Iran	5.0 (3.4–6.9)	48.2 (34.6–61.9)
	China province	10.8 (8.5–13.5)	34.4 (30.9–38.0)

Comment

This study highlights the variance of the threat of MDRTB internationally. As expected, there is an increased risk of MDRTB if there has been prior tuberculosis treatment, and prior inadequate or incomplete treatment will be important factors. MDRTB remains a global problem and it should be tackled internationally. Patients should ideally be treated with directly observed therapy in centres with experience in the management of MDRTB. The studies following looked at the outcomes of MDRTB in the UK and in Turkey.

A national study of clinical and laboratory factors affecting the survival of patients with multiple-drug resistant tuberculosis in the UK.

Drobniewski F, Eltringham I, Graham C, Magee JG, Smith EG, Watt B.
Thorax 2002; **57**(9): 810–16.

BACKGROUND. This study aimed to describe the clinical, microbiological and treatment details of MDRTB cases in the UK, and to determine factors associated with survival. Ninety MDRTB cases were identified from 1 January 1996 to 30 June 1997. The date of diagnosis was determined and data were collated on key demographic factors, clinical, radiological and treatment details. Variables associated with survival were included in a Cox proportional hazards model.

INTERPRETATION. The demographics are shown in Table 12.13 below. Eighty-two per cent of cases received at least three drugs to which the bacterial isolate was sensitive on *in vitro* drug susceptibility analysis. Radiological improvement was seen in 60.8% of cases, 50.7% had three negative sputum smears and 54.9% had at least one negative culture. The median survival was influenced by immune status, treatment with ≥3 susceptible drugs and age. The overall median survival time was 3.78 years, 2.35 years in immunocompromised individuals and 4.26 years in immunocompetent cases. The median survival in patients treated with at least three drugs to which the bacterium was susceptible on *in vitro* testing was 5.66 years whereas those treated with <3 susceptible drugs survival was 1.64 years (Table 12.14). There was an increased

Table 12.13 Demographics of the patients with MDRTB

Number	90
Per cent male	72.4%
Per cent born outside the UK	57.1%
Per cent non-UK residents that came to live in the UK within the past 5 years	38.1%
Per cent white ethnic group	46.5%
Per cent that had prior TB	48.7%
Per cent HIV positive	29.1%
Per cent smear positive	83.3%

Table 12.14 The overall median survival (95% CI) is shown with survival figures given for both immunocompetent and immunocompromised patients and whether treatment was given with ≥3 susceptible drugs

Overall	3.78 years (3.66–6.89)
Immunocompetent patients	4.26 years (3.66–5.66)
Immunocompromised patients	2.35 years (1.45–6.89)
Patients treated with ≥3 susceptible drugs	5.66 years (3.66–6.89)
Patients treated with <3 susceptible drugs	1.64 years (0.52–2.65)

risk of death with increasing age: for every 10-year increase in age the risk almost doubled (RR 2.08, 95% CI 1.27–3.42). In summary, the overall survival was lower than that reported in previous studies and immunocompromised status, failure to apply appropriate three drug treatment, and age were significant factors in mortality.

The treatment of multi-drug resistant tuberculosis in Turkey.

Tahaoglu K, Torun T, Sevim T, *et al. N Engl J Med* 2001; **345**(3): 170–4.

BACKGROUND. **This Istanbul study evaluated the results of treatment in 158 consecutive patients with MDRTB between March 1992 and October 1999. There were 21 female patients and 137 male patients (age range 15–68 years) and all were HIV negative. The patients were infected with organisms that were resistant to a mean of 4.4 drugs (all resistant to both Isoniazid and Rifampicin). All patients received at least three drugs thought to be active; the treatment was continued for at least 18 months after the conversion to a negative culture and for at least 24 months in the absence of first-line drugs.**

INTERPRETATION. The mean number of drugs given during the study was 5.5 (range 3–9). Surgical resection was performed in 23% after a mean of 5.9 months (range 3–10 months) anti-tuberculosis treatment and in this group, 89% were suspected to have been cured. Adverse effects led to discontinuation of one or more drugs in 39%. Cultures became negative in 95% after a mean of 1.9 months (range 1–9). The outcomes are shown in Table 12.15. The patients with unsuccessful outcomes were older than those with successful outcomes, had received a larger number of drugs previously, were more likely to have been treated previously with Ofloxacin, and were less likely to have received Ofloxacin as part of the study protocol (Table 12.16). Thirty-eight per cent of the patients with unsuccessful outcomes were resistant to more than five drugs. In a step-down logistic-regression analysis, a successful outcome was independently associated with a younger age ($P = 0.013$) and the absence of previous treatment with Ofloxacin ($P = 0.005$). In summary, a significant percentage of patients (about 75%) can be cured if patients can be treated with ≥3 susceptible drugs, for at least 18 months after the conversion to a negative culture and for at least 24 months in the absence of first-line drugs.

Table 12.15 Outcomes for the 158 cases with MDRTB. Suspected cure is defined as negative smears and culture for >6 months throughout treatment, and treatment failure is defined as persistence of positive smears or cultures despite treatment for at least 18 or 24 months

Suspected cure	Treatment failure	Not completed treatment regime	Died
77%	8%	11%	4%

Table 12.16 Factors associated with a poor outcome defined as treatment failure, incomplete treatment or death

	Poor outcome	Successful outcome	P value
Mean age ± SD years	42 ± 11	36 ± 12	0.008
Median number of drugs used previously	6	5	0.048
Previous Ofloxacin use	57%	30%	0.004
Frequency Ofloxacin use in study protocol	65%	84%	0.018
Resistance to ≥5 drugs	38%	12%	0.001

Comment

The first UK study was smaller than the latter study and included almost 30% of patients that were HIV positive. The latter study was a larger cohort that were all HIV negative. Overall the prognosis for MDRTB is variable but successful outcomes can be achieved in around 75% if HIV negative and if patients can be treated with ≥3 (preferably ≥5) susceptible drugs, from *in vitro* drug testing, for at least 18 months after conversion to a negative sputum culture. Important indicators of poor outcome appear to be increasing age, compromised immune status and the inability to use ≥3 susceptible drugs. Treatment regimens can be complex and are often associated with a significant side-effect profile. It is recommended that patients should ideally be treated with a directly observed therapy regimen in centres with experience in the management of MDRTB. This recommended regimen is not always feasible internationally and the next study investigated the efficacy of a standardized regimen in Peru which is independent of susceptibility testing.

Feasibility and cost-effectiveness of standardized second-line drug treatment for chronic tuberculosis patients: a national cohort study in Peru.

Suarez PG, Floyd K, Portocarrero J, *et al. Lancet* 2002; **359**(9322): 1980–9.

BACKGROUND. This study assessed the feasibility and cost-effectiveness of using a standard second-line drug regimen to treat patients with chronic tuberculosis, many of whom are infected with multi-drug resistant strains of Mycobacterium tuberculosis. Patients with chronic tuberculosis are defined as patients who have failed both standard and a re-treatment regimen (Table 12.17). A national programme to treat chronic tuberculosis patients with a directly observed standardized 18-month daily regimen was established in Peru in 1997 (second-line treatment regimen, Table 12.17). Compliance and treatment outcomes were analysed for the cohort started on treatment between October 1997, and March 1999. Total and average costs were assessed and cost-effectiveness was estimated as the cost per disability adjusted life year (DALY) gained.

INTERPRETATION. Four hundred and sixty-six patients were enrolled; 344 were tested for drug susceptibility and 97% were resistant to ≥1 drug and 87% had MDRTB. The outcome for the whole group and patients with MDRTB is shown in Table 12.18. Among multi-drug resistant patients, resistance to five or more drugs was significantly

Table 12.17 Re-treatment regimen was given either to patients failing to respond to the standard regimen, patients that default with the standard regimen, or patients initially cured but who later relapsed. Second-line treatment regimens were available for patients that remained smear positive after completing the fully supervised re-treatment regimen or patients that were defined as exceptions, e.g. prior treatment not under direct observed therapy

	Initiation phase	Continuation phase	Total treatment
Standard regimen	Oral R H E Z 2 months	Oral R H 4 months	6 months
Re-treatment regimen	Oral R H E Z + injectable S 3 months (2 months for S)	Oral R H F 5 months	8 months
Second-line treatment regimen	Oral Ciprofloxacin 1 g, Ethionamide 750 mg, Pyrazinamide 1500 mg, and Ethambutol 1200 mg + injectable Kanamycin 1 g for first 3 months only		18 months

R = Rifampicin, H = Isoniazid, E = Ethambutol, Z = pyrazinamide, and S = Streptomycin.

Table 12.18 Outcome at 18 months for all the patients grouped together and separately analysed for patients with MDRTB. In the multi-drug resistant group, a worse outcome was found with patients with resistance to ≥5 drugs (OR 3.37, 95% CI 1.32–8.60)

	Number	Cured	No response to treatment	Defaulted	Died
Overall	466	48%	28%	11%	12%
MDRTB	298	46%	32%	11%	11%

associated with an unfavourable outcome (death, non-response to treatment, or default; OR 3.37, 95% CI 1.32–8.60; $P = 0.01$). The programme cost was US $0.6 million per year, which was 8% of the National Tuberculosis Programme budget, and US $2381 per patient for those who completed treatment. The mean cost per DALY gained was $211 ($165 at drug prices projected for 2002). In summary, treating chronic tuberculosis patients with high levels of multi-drug resistance with a standardized second-line drug regimen can be feasible and cost-effective in middle-income countries, provided a strong tuberculosis control programme is in place.

Comment

This standardized regimen was found to be feasible and cost-effective. The cure rate (46%) for MDRTB was, however, much lower than the previous study (77%). It is possible that there would be improved outcomes with individually tailored therapies according to susceptibility tests. This may not be feasible in certain regions and this standardized regimen used in Peru may be applicable in these circumstances.

Surgery can be an effective adjunct to medical treatment in patients with MDRTB. It is normally considered in patients with localized disease whose medical treatment has failed or for whom treatment failure seems likely. The next three retrospective studies investigated the outcomes of surgery as an adjunct to medical treatment in such patients.

Pulmonary resection in the treatment of patients with pulmonary multi-drug resistant tuberculosis in Taiwan.

Chiang CY, Yu MC, Bai KJ, Suo J, Lin TP, Lee YC. *Int J Tuberc Lung Dis* 2001; **5**(3): 272–7.

BACKGROUND. This retrospective Taiwan study evaluated the role of pulmonary resection in the treatment of pulmonary tuberculosis resistant to Isoniazid and Rifampicin (MDRTB).

INTERPRETATION. Twenty-seven MDRTB patients (mean ± SD age of 44.3 ± 11.6 years) who underwent pulmonary resection between December 1990 and March 1999 were reviewed. Surgery was performed for selected patients, essentially those: (1) whose medical treatment had failed, or for whom treatment failure seemed highly likely, or for whom post-treatment relapse seemed likely; (2) with predominantly localized disease; (3) with adequate cardiopulmonary reserve; and (4) whose treatment regimen had been composed of at least two effective drugs to diminish the mycobacterial burden. Surgery was carried out after a mean of 10 months' anti-tuberculosis treatment (range 2–33 months) and anti-tuberculosis treatment was continued post-surgery for a mean of 15 months (range 8–24 months). Thirty-seven per cent had a pneumonectomy, 48% had a lobectomy and 15% had a segmentectomy and/or wedge resection. There were 11% of patients that developed complications and there was one peri-operative death (4%). Ninety-two per cent of patients demonstrated sputum conversion and/or remained negative after surgery. Eight-five per cent of patients have already completed treatment, and during a mean ± SD of 42 ± 18 follow-up months (range 15–80 months), one patient (4%) relapsed. This patient was disease-free after another course of treatment. The results are summarized in Table 12.19.

A retrospective study for the outcome of pulmonary resection in 49 patients with multi-drug resistant tuberculosis.

Park SK, Lee CM, Heu JP, Song SD. *Int J Tuberc Lung Dis* 2002; **6**(2): 143–9.

BACKGROUND. This retrospective study examined 49 patients with MDRTB who underwent pulmonary resection for pulmonary tuberculosis between January 1995 and December 1999 in Korea (12 pneumonectomies, 28 lobectomies, 7 lobectomies with segmentectomies or wedge resections, one wedge resection and one cavernoplasty).

INTERPRETATION. The mean SD number of drugs to which the patients were resistant was 4.5 ± 2.0. Patients had a mean age of 35 ± 13 years, cavitating lesions on plain chest X-rays were shown in 88%, and 63% had positive sputum cultures for tuberculosis pre-operatively. Surgery was carried out within 6 months of starting anti-tuberculosis treatment and treatment was continued for 18–24 months following surgery. The sputum conversion rate was 94% with continuous post-operative treatment. There were no deaths after surgery. Post-operative complications that developed were 6 cases (12%) of air leakage over a week, 1 (2%) of post-operative bleeding and 1 (2%) of wound infection. The relapse rate was 6% after a mean follow up of 20 months (range 6–36) (Table 12.19).

Pulmonary resection for multi-drug resistant tuberculosis.
Pomerantz BJ, Cleveland JC Jr, Olson HK, Pomerantz M. *J Thorac Cardiovasc Surg* 2001; **121**(3): 448–53.

BACKGROUND. This retrospective US study reported the authors' experience with surgical intervention for MDRTB. All patients had MDRTB, and had a minimum of 3 months of medical therapy before surgery and had post-operative anti-tuberculosis treatment for 2 years.

INTERPRETATION. During a 17-year period, 172 patients underwent 180 pulmonary resections (98 lobectomies and 82 pneumonectomies). Operative mortality was 3.3% (3 died of respiratory failure, 2 died of a cerebrovascular accident, and 1 died of a myocardial infarct). Late mortality was 6.8% and significant morbidity was 12%. Half (91) of the patients were smear positive at the time of surgery. After the operation, the sputum remained positive in only 4/91 (4%) patients. Two per cent relapsed after a mean follow-up of 7.6 years (range 4–204 months). The results are summarized in Table 12.19.

Comment

The key to successful treatment regimens for MDRTB is to commence patients by direct observed therapy on at least three anti-tuberculosis drugs to which the patient has *in vitro* sensitivities and to continue for 18 months after conversion to a negative sputum culture. The latter three retrospective studies highlight that surgery can be a useful adjunct to medical therapy in selected patients with MDRTB allowing sputum conversion from smear positive to negative and ultimately leading to cure. Surgery is not without risks with morbidity rates of 11–16% and mortality rates in this selected series from 0–4%. Surgery should be considered for patients with MDRTB in the setting of localized disease, persistent sputum positivity, failure or patient intolerance of medical therapy and patients with few co-morbidities and adequate cardio-pulmonary reserve. The studies highlight the importance of treating patients with anti-tuberculosis treatment prior to surgery to reduce the

Table 12.19 Summary of the outcomes from surgery in patients with MDRTB

Study	Number	30-day mortality	Morbidity	Sputum conversion	Recurrence of MDRTB	Mean follow-up
Chiang *et al.*	27	4%	11%	92%	4%	42 months
Park *et al.*	49	0*	16%	94%	6%	20 months
Pomerantz *et al.*	172	3%	12%	96%	2%	7.6 years

*30-day mortality not reported but there were no operative deaths in this study.

mycobacterial load and to continue anti-tuberculosis treatment post-surgery for around 18 months assuming a conversion to a negative sputum culture.

Treatment of mycobacteria other than tuberculosis

The treatment of pulmonary disease caused by opportunist mycobacteria is controversial and it is uncertain whether *in vitro* sensitivity testing predicts clinical response. The literature suggests that the combination of Rifampicin (R) and Ethambutol (E) is important whereas Isoniazid (H) may not be. The next two papers include a randomized controlled study comparing different treatment regimens and a retrospective study investigating surgery as an adjunct to medical therapy.

First randomized trial of treatments for pulmonary disease caused by Mycobacterium avium intracellulare, Mycobacterium malmoense and Mycobacterium xenopi in HIV-negative patients: Rifampicin, Ethambutol and Isoniazid versus Rifampicin and Ethambutol.

Research Committee of the British Thoracic Society. *Thorax* 2001; **56**(3): 167–72.

B ACKGROUND . **The British Thoracic Society conducted a randomized study of two regimens in HIV-negative patients with pulmonary disease caused by Mycobacterium avium intracellulare (MAC), Mycobacterium malmoense and Mycobacterium xenopi. When the Mycobacterium Reference Laboratories for England, Wales and Scotland confirmed two positive cultures, the co-ordinating physician invited the patient's physician to enrol the patient. Patients were also recruited from Scandinavia. Randomization to 2 years of treatment with RE or REH was performed from lists held in the co-ordinator's office. Clinical, bacteriological and radiological progress was monitored for 3 years after the end of treatment.**

I NTERPRETATION . From October 1987 to December 1992, 141 physicians entered 223 patients (106 with Mycobacterium malmoense, 75 with MAC, 42 with Mycobacterium xenopi) from Britain and Scandinavia. At entry the RE and REH groups were comparable over a range of demographic and clinical features (mean age 61.3 years; 59% had previous lung disease; 14% having reduced immunity but HIV negative; 58% were sputum smear positive and 71% had cavitation on the chest radiograph). For each species there was no significant difference between RE and REH in the number of deaths, but when the three species were combined there were fewer deaths from the mycobacterial disease with RE (1% for RE and 8% for REH, $P = 0.018$, OR 0.10, 95% CI 0.00–0.76) (Table 12.20). For Mycobacterium malmoense the failure of treatment/relapse rates did not differ appreciably between the regimens, but for MAC there were fewer failures of treatment/relapses with REH (16% for REH and 41% for RE, $P = 0.03$). With M xenopi there was a non-significant trend in the same direction (5% for REH and 18% for RE, $P = 0.41$) and when all three species were combined there was a significant

Table 12.20 Outcome comparing the regimens RE and REH

	RE	REH
Number	112	111
Total deaths	29%	38%
Deaths due to mycobacteria	1%	8%*
Completed treatment and cured at 5 years	31%	35%

*$P = 0.02$.

Table 12.21 Comparisons in outcome at 5 years comparing Mycobacterium malmoense, Mycobacterium avium complex (MAC) and Mycobacterium xenopi

	Mycobacterium malmoense	MAC	Mycobacterium xenopi	P value
Total deaths	25%	31%	57%	0.001
Deaths due to mycobacteria	4%	4%	7%	0.65
Failure of treatment or relapse	10%	28%	12%	0.004
Alive and cured	42%	31%	17%	0.015

difference in favour of REH (11% for REH and 22% for RE, $P = 0.03$). There was no correlation between failure of treatment/relapse and *in vitro* resistance. The differences between species are shown in Table 12.21: Mycobacterium xenopi was associated with the greatest mortality (57% at 5 years), MAC was the most difficult to eradicate, and Mycobacterium malmoense had the most favourable outlook (42% known to be alive and cured at 5 years). In summary the results of susceptibility tests performed by the modal resistance method do not correlate with the patient's response to treatment. Treatment of Mycobacterium malmoense with RE for 2 years is preferable to REH. The addition of Isoniazid reduces the failure of treatment/relapse rates for MAC and has a tendency to do so also for Mycobacterium xenopi, but there is a suggestion that REH is associated with higher death rates overall.

Surgery for Mycobacterium avium complex lung disease in the Clarithromycin era.
Shiraishi Y, Nakajima Y, Takasuna K, Hanaoka T, Katsuragi N, Konno H.
Eur J Cardiothorac Surg 2002; **21**(2): 314–18.

BACKGROUND. This study examined whether surgery can still play an important role in the management of MAC lung disease. Between April 1993 and January 2001, 21

patients (**11 men and 10 women**) underwent a pulmonary resection for MAC infection.
The median age of the patients was 56 years (range 27–67 years) and none were
immunocompromised. Regimens employing Clarithromycin were initiated pre-
operatively in all patients. The indications for surgery were failure of drug therapy in
19 patients and discontinuation of treatment because of drug toxicity in 2 patients.
The pulmonary resections (19 right lung, 2 left lung) performed included lobectomy in
16 patients, pneumonectomy in three, bilobectomy in one, and lobectomy plus
segmentectomy in one.

INTERPRETATION. The results are shown in Table 12.22. All of the patients survived
the surgery. Six major post-operative complications occurred (29%) and these included
two bronchopleural fistulas after right pneumonectomy, two space problems, one
prolonged air leak, and one case of interstitial pneumonia. All post-operative
complications were manageable, and four of these were treated surgically. All patients
had sputum smear negative status after their operation. Relapse occurred in two
patients (10%) at six months and two years post-operative, respectively. The first patient,
who originally had a right upper lobectomy, underwent a left upper lobectomy during the
follow-up period, attaining sputum conversion. The second patient underwent a right
pneumonectomy and then died of respiratory failure four years post-operatively. This one
late death was the only fatality. Although surgery is associated with a high morbidity,
surgery provided a high sputum conversion rate for patients whose MAC disease
responded poorly to drug therapy.

Comment

The British Thoracic Society study gives physicians the evidence base for the treatment of mycobacteria other than tuberculosis. Standard regimens can be used
independent of sensitivity testing which is clearly different to the regimens used for
patients with Mycobacterium tuberculosis. In addition it allows physicians to give
patients clearer ideas of response rates and prognosis. The current cure rates with
the regimes with RE and REH are disappointing and we await the results from
the multi-centre study from the research committee of the British Thoracic Society
assessing the value of the addition of Clarithromycin, Ciprofloxacin and Mycobacterium vaccae. In this study patients were randomized with a regimen of 2 years
Rifampicin, Ethambutol and Clarithromycin versus Rifampicin, Ethambutol and
Ciprofloxacin. In addition there was an optional arm where patients could be
further randomized to receive immunotherapy with Mycobacterium vaccae (SRL
172).

Table 12.22 Outcome for surgery in 21 patients with MAC disease

Study	Number	30-day mortality	Morbidity	Sputum conversion	Recurrence at 2 years
Shiraishi et al.	21	0%	29%	100%	10%

The next retrospective study showed that surgery may be a useful adjunct when MAC lung disease had not been successfully eradicated by drug treatment alone or drug treatment was not tolerated. It is not without risk, and the study was associated with significant morbidity. Patients should be carefully selected, with patients having localized disease, no comorbidities, a good performance status and in patients with failure or intolerance with medical therapy.

13

Community acquired pneumonia

This section covers the investigation and management of patients with community acquired pneumonia. This first two articles are based on the guidelines issued by the British and American Thoracic Societies. It starts with the epidemiology and aetiology for community acquired pneumonia treated in the community, in hospital and in the intensive care unit (ICU). After this there is discussion where patients should be treated (at home, in hospital or in an ICU) and then the antibiotic regimens advocated by the two societies are summarized. Following this there are papers on the management in specific patient groups including the elderly, patients admitted from a nursing home and patients that are pregnant. Following this there are specific articles on the risk factors and outcomes for patients with community acquired pneumonia due to Gram-negative bacteria, the role of pressure support ventilation in severe pneumonia, the indications and outcome for patients admitted to an ICU and finally the impact of early hospital discharge.

British Thoracic Society guidelines for the management of community acquired pneumonia in adults.
Pneumonia guidelines committee of BTS Standards of Care Committee.
Thorax 2001; **56**(Suppl 4): 1–64.

Guidelines for the management of adults with a community acquired pneumonia.
American Thoracic Society. *Am J Respir Crit Care Med* 2001; **163**(7): 1730–54.

BACKGROUND. Community acquired pneumonia in adults is a common problem both for General Practitioners and hospital physicians. The annual incidence in the community is 5–11 per 1000 adult population (from the UK, Finland and North American studies) and rises with age. The incidence for patients requiring hospital admission varies between 1 and 4 per 1000 population (from European, Canadian and

US studies). In the UK between 22 and 42% are admitted to hospital, of which 5% are managed in an ICU. The mortality rates vary from <1% for patients managed in the community, between 5.7 and 12% for patients admitted to hospital, and can be >50% for patients admitted to an ICU.

INTERPRETATION. Tables 13.1–13.3 show the pathogens identified in studies of community acquired pneumonia conducted in the community, in hospital, and in the ICU. Understanding the aetiology helps in the preparation of guidelines for antimicrobial therapy. The studies highlight that *Streptococcus pneumoniae* remains an important pathogen, but that in a large percentage of cases no aetiological agent can be found.

Which patients can be treated at home?

Patients with community acquired pneumonia with no adverse risk factors have a good prognosis and mortality rates are low. Treatment of such patients is feasible at home assuming social circumstances permit and patients' progress can be monitored in the community.

Table 13.1 Studies of CAP conducted in the community

	UK (1 study, *n* = 236)		Rest of Europe (6 studies, *n* = 654)		North America (1 study, *n* = 149)	
	Mean (%)	95% CI	Mean (%)	95% CI	Mean (%)	95% CI
S pneumoniae	36.0	29.9 to 42.1	8.4	6.4 to 10.8	?	?
H influenzae	10.2	6.3 to 14.0	1.1	0.4 to 2.2	?	?
Legionella spp	0.4	0.01 to 2.3	2.8	1.6 to 4.3	0.7	0.01 to 3.7
S aureus	0.8	0.1 to 3.0	0	0.0 to 0.7	?	?
M catarrhalis	?		0	0.0 to 0.6	?	
Gram negative enteric bacilli	1.3	0.3 to 3.7	0.2	0.0 to 1.0	?	?
M pneumoniae	1.3	0.3 to 3.7	13.3	10.7 to 15.9	26.2	19.3 to 34.0
C pneumoniae	?	?	8.7	6.5 to 11.3	14.8	9.5 to 21.5
C psittaci	?	?	2.0	1.1 to 3.4	14.8	9.5 to 21.5
C burnetii	0	0 to 1.6	0.8	0.3 to 1.9	2.7	0.7 to 6.7
All viruses	13.1	8.8 to 17.4	12.4	9.9 to 14.9	8.1	4.2 to 13.6
Influenza A & B	8.1	4.9 to 12.3	6.3	4.5 to 8.4	6.0	2.8 to 11.2
Mixed	11.0	7.0 to 15.0	4.7	2.8 to 7.3	4.7	1.9 to 9.4
Other	1.7	0.5 to 4.3	2.0	1.1 to 3.4	0	0 to 2.5
None	45.3	39.0 to 51.7	53.7	49.8 to 57.5	50.3	42.0 to 58.6

Source: Pneumonia Guidelines Committee of BTS Standards of Care Committee (2001).

Table 13.2 Studies of CAP conducted in hospital

	UK (5 studies, n = 1137)		Rest of Europe (23 studies, n = 6026)		Australia & New Zealand (3 studies, n = 453)		North America (4 studies, n = 1306)	
	Mean (%)	95% CI	Mean (%)	95% CI	Mean (%)	95% CI	Mean (%)	95% CI
S pneumoniae	39	36.1 to 41.8	19.4	18.4 to 20.4	38.4	33.9 to 42.9	11.3	9.5 to 13.0
H influenzae	5.2	4.0 to 6.6	3.9	3.4 to 4.4	9.5	7 to 12.6	6.3	5.0 to 7.7
Legionella spp	3.6	2.6 to 4.9	5.1	4.6 to 5.7	7.5	5.3 to 10.3	4.8	3.7 to 6.0
M catarrhalis	1.9	0.6 to 4.3	1.2	1.0 to 1.5	3.1	1.4 to 6.1	1.2	0.5 to 2.5
S aureus	1.9	1.2 to 2.9	0.8	0.5 to 1.1	2.9	1.5 to 4.9	3.8	2.0 to 5.0
Gram negative enteric bacilli	1	0.5 to 1.7	3.3	2.8 to 3.7	4.6	2.9 to 7	5.3	4.1 to 6.6
M pneumoniae	10.8	9.0 to 12.6	6	5.4 to 6.6	14.6	11.3 to 17.8	4.1	3.1 to 5.3
C pneumoniae	13.1	9.1 to 17.2	6.3	5.5 to 7.3	3.1	1.4 to 6.1	5.9	4.3 to 7.8
C psittaci	2.6	1.7 to 3.6	1.4	1.1 to 1.8	1.4	0.5 to 3.2	0.1	0 to 0.7
C burnetii	1.2	0.7 to 2.1	0.9	0.6 to 1.1	0	0 to 3.4	2.3	1.5 to 3.7
All viruses	12.8	10.8 to 14.7	9.5	8.6 to 10.3	10.6	7.8 to 13.4	8.9	7.4 to 10.6
Influenza A & B	10.7	8.9 to 12.5	5.3	4.6 to 6.1	6.4	4.3 to 9.1	5.9	4.5 to 7.6
Mixed	14.2	12.2 to 16.3	6.3	5.5 to 7.1	19.6	16 to 23.3	8.5	7.0 to 10.3
Other	2	1.3 to 3	2	1.7 to 2.4	4	2.4 to 6.2	8.0	6.6 to 9.7
None	30.8	28.1 to 33.5	50.7	49.5 to 52.0	31.6	27.3 to 35.8	40.7	38.1 to 43.4

Source: Pneumonia Guidelines Committee of BTS Standards of Care Committee (2001).

Table 13.3 Studies of CAP conducted in the ICU

	UK (4 studies, *n* = 185)		Rest of Europe (10 studies, *n* = 1148)	
	Mean (%)	95% CI	Mean (%)	95% CI
S pneumoniae	21.6	15.9 to 28.3	21.8	19.4 to 24.2
H influenzae	3.8	1.5 to 7.6	5.3	4.1 to 6.8
Legionella spp	17.8	12.6 to 24.1	5.5	4.2 to 7.2
S aureus	8.7	5.0 to 13.7	7.0	5.6 to 8.6
M catarrhalis	?	?	3.8	2.4 to 5.9
Gram negative enteric bacilli	1.6	0.3 to 4.7	8.6	7.1 to 10.4
M pneumoniae	2.7	0.9 to 6.2	2.0	1.3 to 3.0
C pneumoniae	?	?	6.6	2.5 to 13.8
C psittaci	2.2	0.6 to 5.4	0.9	0.4 to 1.9
C burnetii	0	0 to 2.0	0.7	0.3 to 1.4
Viruses	9.7	5.9 to 14.9	4.0	2.7 to 5.6
Influenza A & B	5.4	2.6 to 9.7	2.3	1.1 to 4.2
Mixed	6.0	3.0 to 10.4	5.0	2.4 to 9.1
Other	4.9	2.3 to 9.0	8.4	6.8 to 10.1
None	32.4	25.7 to 39.7	43.3	40.4 to 46.2

Source: Pneumonia Guidelines Committee of BTS Standards of Care Committee (2001).

Adverse risk factors include the following:

1. Age ≥50.
2. Co-morbid illness e.g. congestive cardiac failure; ischaemic heart disease; cerebrovascular disease; diabetes; chronic lung disease; carcinoma.
3. New mental confusion.
4. Physical findings including respiratory rate ≥30/minute, pulse ≥125/min, low blood pressure (systolic <90 mmHg and/or diastolic ≤60 mmHg), and temperature <35 or ≥ 40°C.
5. Laboratory findings with blood urea >7 mmol/l, white blood cell count <4 × 10^9/l or >20 × 10^9/l or an absolute neutrophil count below 1 × 10^9/l, and hypoxaemia. The British Thoracic Society guidelines define hypoxaemia as SaO_2 <92% or PaO_2 <8 kPa regardless of inspired oxygen concentration whereas the American Thoracic Society guidelines define it as PaO_2/FiO_2 <250.
6. Bilateral or multi-lobe involvement of the chest radiograph.

Which patients should be treated in hospital?

It is not always clear-cut whether to treat patients with community acquired pneumonia at home or in hospital and such cases should be decided by an experienced clinician taking into account the social and community back up. Patients with ≥2 of the following (new mental confusion, blood urea >7 mmol/l, respiratory rate ≥30/minute and low blood pressure [systolic <90 mmHg and/or diastolic ≤60 mmHg]) should be regarded as having a *severe pneumonia* and should be managed in hospital.

Which patients should be treated in an intensive care unit?

Patients with *severe pneumonia* who do not respond to medical treatment should ideally be transferred to a high dependency unit or an ICU. In particular assisted ventilation should be considered for patients with persistent hypoxia with PaO_2 <8 kPa despite maximal oxygen therapy, progressive hypercapnia, severe acidosis (pH <7.26), shock or depressed consciousness.

How long should antibiotics be given?

For patients managed in the community, 7 days of antibiotics is recommended. In patients admitted to hospital 7 days is recommended for patients with non-severe uncomplicated pneumonia and 10 days for patients with severe microbiologically undefined pneumonia. This should be extended to 14–21 days where legionella, staphylococcal or Gram-negative enteric bacilli pneumonia are suspected or confirmed.

What antibiotic regimen should be prescribed?

The regimens in Table 13.4 below recommended by the British Thoracic Society may be applicable to other countries but local regimens are likely to be driven by local aetiology, antibiotic availability, microbial sensitivity and resistance patterns, and cost.

The American Thoracic Society recommendations for antibiotic therapy are based on the assessment of place of therapy (outpatient, in-patient ward and ICU), the presence of cardiopulmonary disease and the presence of 'modifying factors' including risk factors for drug resistant *Streptococcus pneumoniae*, enteric Gram-negatives, and *Pseudomonas aeruginosa*. The American Thoracic Society in their community acquired pneumonia guidelines highlight the risk factors for penicillin resistant and drug resistant pneumococci, Gram-negative organisms, and *Pseudomonas aeruginosa*. The risk factors for penicillin resistant and drug resistant pneumococci are age >65, β lactam therapy within the past 3 months, alcoholism, immune suppressive illness or therapy, multiple medical comorbidities, and exposure to a child in a day care centre. The risk factors for enteric Gram-negatives include residence in a nursing home, underlying cardiopulmonary disease, multiple medical comorbidies and recent antibiotic therapy, and finally the risk factors for *P. aeruginosa* include bronchiectasis, broad spectrum antibiotic therapy >7 days within the past month, malnutrition and chronic corticosteroid therapy >10 mg/day.

Prompt antibiotic therapy is recommended within 8 hours of arrival at the hospital and it is desirable to give as narrow a spectrum as possible to limit drug

Table 13.4 The British Thoracic Society antibiotic guidelines are based on the severity of the community acquired pneumonia and whether treatment is based in the community or in hospital

	Severity	Drug	Dose	Frequency per day	Route
Community–standard	Non-severe	Amoxicillin	500 mg–1 g	Three	Oral
Community–alternatives	Non-severe	Erythromycin *or*	500 mg	Four	Oral
		Clarithromycin	500 mg	Twice	Oral
Hospital–standard	Non-severe	Amoxicillin	500 mg–1 g	Three	Oral
		+			
		Erythromycin *or*	500 mg	Four	Oral
		Clarithromycin	500 mg	Twice	Oral
Hospital–alternative	Non-severe	Levofloxacin	500 mg	Once	Oral
Hospital–standard	Non-severe	Ampicillin *or*	500 mg	Four	IV
		Benzylpenicillin	1.2 g	Four	IV
		+			
		Erythromycin *or*	500 mg	Four	IV
		Clarithromycin	500 mg	Twice	IV
Hospital–alternative	Non-severe	Levofloxacin	500 mg	Once	IV
Hospital–standard	Severe	Co-amoxiclav *or*	1.2 g	Three	IV
		Cefuroxime *or*	1.5 g	Three	IV
		Cefotaxime *or*	1 g	Three	IV
		Ceftriaxone	2 g	Once	IV
		+			
		Erythromycin *or*	500 mg	Four	IV
		Clarithromycin	500 mg	Twice	IV
		±			
		Rifampicin	600 mg	Once or twice	IV
Hospital–alternative	Severe	Levofloxacin	500 mg	Twice	IV
		+			
		Benzylpenicillin	1.2 g	Four	IV

resistance. The American Thoracic Society recommends that atypical pathogens (*Chlamydia pneumoniae, Mycoplasma pneumoniae* and Legionella species) be routinely covered for all cases of community acquired pneumonia. Intravenous treatment is recommended in the initial management of patients with *severe pneumonia*, or in patients with impaired consciousness, loss of swallowing reflex, or functional or anatomical reasons for malabsorption.

The treatment regimens recommended by the British and American Thoracic Societies are summarized in Tables 13.4 and 13.5 respectively.

Table 13.5 The American Thoracic Society recommendations for antibiotic therapy are based on the assessment of place of therapy (outpatient, in-patient ward, intensive care unit), the presence of cardiopulmonary disease and the presence of 'modifying factors' including risk factors for drug resistant *Streptococcus pneumoniae*, enteric Gram-negatives, and *Pseudomonas aeruginosa*

	Recommendation	Alternative
Outpatients with no cardiopulmonary disease and no modifying risk factors	Advanced generation Macrolide (Azithromycin or Clarithromycin)	Doxycycline
Outpatients with cardiopulmonary disease and/or modifying risk factors	β lactam (oral Cefpodoxime or Cefuroxime or high dose Amoxicillin or Amoxicillin/Clavulanate; or parenteral Ceftriaxone followed by oral Cefpodoxime) + Macrolide or Doxycycline	Antipneumococcal Quinolone e.g. Levofloxacin
In-patients not in an ICU with no cardiopulmonary disease and no modifying risk factors	Intravenous Azithromycin	β lactam (Cefotaxime or Ceftriaxone or Ampicillin/Sulbactam or high dose Ampicillin) + Doxycycline OR Monotherapy with an antipneumococcal Quinolone
In-patients not in an ICU with cardiopulmonary disease and/or modifying risk factors	Intravenous β lactam* + Intravenous or oral Macrolide or Doxycycline	Intravenous monotherapy with an antipneumococcal Quinolone
ICU with no risks for *Pseudomonas aeruginosa*	Intravenous β lactam (Cefotaxime, Ceftriaxone) + Intravenous Macrolide (Azithromycin)	Intravenous β lactam (Cefotaxime, Ceftriaxone) + Intravenous Fluoroquinolone
ICU with risks for *Pseudomonas aeruginosa*	Intravenous antipseudomonal β lactam (Cefepime or Imipenum or Meropenum or Piperacillin/Tazobactam) + Intravenous anti-pseudomonal Quinolone (Ciprofloxacin)	Intravenous anti-pseudomonal β lactam + Intravenous aminoglycoside + either intravenous Macrolide or intravenous non-pseudomonal Fluoroquinolone

*Only use anti-pseudomonal drugs if risk factors for *Pseudomonas aeruginosa*.

The next section includes specific articles on the management of community acquired pneumonia in the elderly, the management of patients admitted from a nursing home and patients that are pregnant, and the risk factors and outcomes of community acquired pneumonia due to Gram-negative bacteria. The role of non-invasive positive pressure ventilation is now well established for the management of acute exacerbations of chronic obstructive pulmonary disease and hypercapnic respiratory failure but not for community acquired pneumonia. Two studies are presented of the use of non-invasive positive pressure ventilation in patients with community acquired pneumonia. Finally, in this section, the indications and outcome for patients admitted to an ICU with community acquired pneumonia and the implications of early hospital discharge are discussed.

Hospitalized community acquired pneumonia in the elderly: age- and sex-related patterns of care and outcome in the United States.

Kaplan V, Angus DC, Griffin MF, Clermont G, Scott Watson R, Linde-Zwirble WT. *Am J Respir Crit Care Med* 2002; **165**(6): 766–72.

BACKGROUND. **Community acquired pneumonia is a frequent cause of hospital admission and death among elderly patients. In this elderly cohort there is little information on age- and sex-specific incidence, patterns of care (ICU admission and mechanical ventilation), resource use (length of stay and hospital costs), and outcome (mortality). This was an observational cohort study of all Medicare recipients, aged 65 years or older, hospitalized in non-federal US hospitals in 1997 with community acquired pneumonia.**

INTERPRETATION. There were 623 718 hospital admissions for community acquired pneumonia (18.3 per 1000 population ≥65 years), of which 4.3% were from nursing homes and of which 10.6% died. The incidence rose 5-fold and mortality doubled as age increased from 65–69 to older than 90 years (Table 13.6). Factors associated with increased mortality were increasing age, male sex, admissions from nursing homes, patients with co-morbid illness, patients who had a complex course (requiring admission to the ICU or requiring mechanical ventilation), and patients who developed acute organ dysfunction (Table 13.7). In addition, there was an increased mortality in patients with a microbiologic aetiology with either *Staphylococcus species* (OR 1.85, 95% CI 1.77–1.92), enteric Gram-negatives (OR 1.21, 95% CI 1.18–1.25) or *Pseudomonas*

Table 13.6 Increased incidence and mortality rates for the cohorts age >90 compared with the cohort age 65–69 years

	Age 65–69	Age >90
Incidence	8.4 per 1000	48.5 per 1000*
Mortality rates	7.8%	15.4%*

*P <0.001.

species (OR 1.47, 95% CI 1.41–1.52). There are sex differences noted with an increased incidence, more complex cases, and increased mortality rates in males (Table 13.8). There was an increased length of hospital stay and associated costs with patients that required admission to the ICU and mechanical ventilation (Table 13.9). The overall hospital costs were $4.4 billion (6.3% of the expenditure in the elderly for acute hospital care) of which $2.1 billion was incurred by cases managed in ICUs.

Table 13.7 Increased mortality rates in patients admitted from a nursing home, male patients, patients with co-morbid illness, patients having a complex course (requiring admission to the ICU or requiring mechanical ventilation) or developing acute organ dysfunction

Mortality rates

Admission from a nursing home	17.6%*	Community admission	10.3%
Male sex	11.6%*	Females	9.8%
Co-morbid illness	11.9%*	No co-morbid illness	7.6%
Complex course	22.5%*	Non-complex course	7.1%
Acute organ dysfunction	23.2%*	No organ dysfunction	9.9%

*$P < 0.001$.

Table 13.8 Males had an increased incidence of community acquired pneumonia, a greater per cent of complex cases and had higher mortality rates

	Male	Female
Incidence	19.4 per 1000*	15.6 per 1000
Per cent complex cases	24.4%*	20.8%
Mortality rates	11.6%*	9.8%

*$P < 0.001$.

Table 13.9 Overall mean length of stay and costs in US$. Sub-set data available for patients requiring ICU services and mechanical ventilation, which accounted for 22.4% and 7.2% of patients respectively. There are increased lengths of stay and associated costs for patients requiring admission to the ICU and/or receiving mechanical ventilation

	Mean length of stay	Mean cost $
Overall	7.6 days	6949
22.4% of admissions were to the ICU	11.3 days	14 294
7.2% received mechanical ventilation	15.7 days	23 961

Comment

In this US study, where elderly patients were admitted with community acquired pneumonia, it was a common and frequently fatal disease (mortality rates ranging from approximately 7–23%). Patients often required ICU admission (around 22%) and mechanical ventilation (around 7%), and consumed considerable health care resources. The increased mortality associated with increasing age, admissions from nursing homes, patients with co-morbid illness, patients who had a complex course and patients who developed acute organ dysfunction is expected. The sex differences are of concern and require further investigation (increased incidence, more complex cases and increased mortality rates in males).

A prospective comparison of nursing home acquired pneumonia with community acquired pneumonia.

Lim WS, Macfarlane JT. *Eur Respir J* 2001; **18**(2): 362–8.

BACKGROUND. This prospective study compared the clinical and microbiological aspects of nursing home acquired pneumonia with community acquired pneumonia. This was an 18-month prospective UK study of 437 patients admitted to hospital with community acquired pneumonia, 40 (9%) of whom came from nursing homes. Detailed microbiological tests were performed in a small sub-set of patients (66) over 12 months.

INTERPRETATION. Patients with nursing home acquired pneumonia were less likely to have a productive cough (OR 0.4, 95% CI 0.2–0.9, $P = 0.02$), pleuritic pain (OR 0.1, 95% CI 0.01–0.8, $P = 0.03$) but more likely to be confused (OR 3.9, 95% CI 1.9–7.9, $P < 0.001$) than patients admitted with community acquired pneumonia. In addition patients with nursing home acquired pneumonia had poorer functional status ($P < 0.001$), more severe disease ($P = 0.03$) and higher mortality (53% for nursing home patients versus 13% for the control group). The increased mortality in nursing home acquired pneumonia was mainly explained by prior functional status. Pathogens were identified in 68% of 22 nursing home acquired pneumonia and 80% of 44 matched community acquired pneumonia control patients. *Streptococcus pneumoniae* was the most common pathogen identified (found in 55% in nursing home acquired pneumonia and 43% in community acquired pneumonia control patients) and atypical pathogens, enteric Gram-negative bacilli and *Staphylococcus aureus* were uncommon. In summary the poor functional status of patients admitted with nursing home acquired pneumonia accounted for the high mortality. From the small sub-set of patients that had microbiological assessment, the pathogens implicated were similar to control patients and *Streptococcus pneumoniae* remains the main aetiological pathogen.

Comment

This small study investigated patients that were admitted with community acquired pneumonia from nursing homes. The increased mortality in nursing home acquired pneumonia due to poor functional status is not a surprise, which clearly reflects the patients that are often admitted to nursing homes with multiple co-morbidities. In this study, the microbiology aetiology of community acquired pneumonia was similar for nursing home residents and non-nursing home patients. Other studies have found that nursing home residents have an increased incidence of community acquired pneumonia due to enteric Gram-negative bacteria and *Staphylococcus aureus*. The sample size for microbiological assessment in the study by Lim and colleagues was very small and needs confirmation with larger studies.

Pneumonia and pregnancy.
Lim WS, Macfarlane JT, Colthorpe CL. *Thorax* 2001; **56**: 398–405.

BACKGROUND. **Studies suggest the incidence of community acquired pneumonia in pregnancy varies between 0.2 and 2.7 per 1000 deliveries, which does not differ significantly from community acquired pneumonia in young non-pregnant adults. Mortality rates vary from 0–4% which are similar to the mortality from community acquired pneumonia in hospitalized non-pregnant adults. Pre-term delivery and infants of lower birth rates are more common in pregnant women who have had community acquired pneumonia.**

INTERPRETATION. In about 60% of cases, no aetiological agent is identified. As in community acquired pneumonia in non-pregnant women, *Streptococcus pneumoniae* (17%) is the commonest pathogen implicated. Other pathogens implicated include *Haemophilus influenzae* (5.5%), *Mycoplasma pneumoniae* (3%), and Legionella species, *Staphylococcus aureus* and Influenza A virus at 1.2% each. There is a good safety profile with the Penicillins, Cephalosporins and Macrolide group of antibiotics in pregnancy. In the Macrolide group, there is a greater safety data for Erythromycin than Clarithromycin or Azithromycin. It is recommended that classes including the Quinolones, Tetracyclines, Chloramphenicol and Sulpha-compounds be contraindicated in pregnancy. The treatment of Amoxil and Erythromycin seems a safe treatment for community acquired pneumonia in pregnant women.

Comment
This article was a review of community acquired pneumonia occurring in pregnancy. There were no major differences in community acquired pneumonia arising in pregnancy than in non-pregnant women. Similar management strategies developed for non-pregnant adults can be applied to the pregnant women but with modifications to take into account the issues of toxicity to the fetus.

Community acquired pneumonia due to Gram-negative bacteria and *Pseudomonas aeruginosa*: incidence, risk and prognosis.

Arancibia F, Bauer TT, Ewig S, *et al. Arch Intern Med* 2002; **162**(16): 1849–58.

BACKGROUND. *Streptococcus pneumoniae* **is the most frequent aetiological factor in community acquired pneumonia. This Spanish study determined the incidence, prognosis and risk factors for community acquired pneumonia due to Gram-negative bacteria, including *Pseudomonas aeruginosa*. Patients were prospectively collected from a Spanish university teaching hospital.**

INTERPRETATION. From 1 January 1997 to 31 December 1998, 559 hospitalized patients with community acquired pneumonia were included. The demographics are shown in Table 13.10. Eleven per cent had community acquired pneumonia due to Gram-negative bacteria. This was predominantly due to *Pseudomonas aeruginosa* in 65% and *Escherichia coli* in 20%. Independent risk factors for community acquired pneumonia due to Gram-negative bacteria were probable aspiration, previous hospital admission or antimicrobial treatment within 30 days prior to admission, and the presence of pulmonary comorbidity with bronchiectasis (Table 13.11). In addition the frequency of community acquired pneumonia due to Gram-negative bacteria increased with the number of risk factors; 2.5% chance if no risk factors versus 50% if $\geq$3 risk factors ($P <$0.001). In a subgroup analysis of pneumonia due to *Pseudomonas aeruginosa*, risk factors were pulmonary comorbidity (OR 5.8, 95% CI 2.2–15.3, $P <$0.001) and previous hospital admission within the previous 30 days (OR 3.8, 95% CI 1.8–8.3, $P =$ 0.02). Infection with Gram-negative bacteria was independently associated with death (RR 3.4, 95% CI 1.6–7.4, $P =$ 0.002) (Table 13.10). The other risk factors associated with a poor outcome are shown in Table 13.12.

Comment

This Spanish study highlights the incidence, risk and prognosis of community acquired pneumonia due to Gram-negative bacteria. Gram-negative bacteria were implicated in 11% of community acquired pneumonia patients and was associated

Table 13.10 Demographic and mortality data in patients with community acquired pneumonia due to Gram-negative bacteria and other pathogens

	Others	Gram-negative
Number	499	60
Mean age $\pm$ SD	69 $\pm$ 18 years	72 $\pm$ 13 years
Mortality rates	9%	32%*

*P value <0.001.

Table 13.11 Multivariate analysis identifying the risk factors for community acquired pneumonia due to Gram-negative bacteria

	OR (95% CI)	P value
Suspected aspiration	2.3 (1.02–5.2)	0.04
Previous hospital admission (8–30 days before this episode)	3.5 (1.7–7.1)	<0.001
Use of antibiotics during the 30 days prior to admission	1.9 (1.01–3.7)	0.049
Pulmonary co-morbid illness	2.8 (1.5–5.5)	0.02

Table 13.12 Multivariate analysis identifying factors associated with a poor outcome

	OR (95% CI)	P value
Suspected aspiration	3.3 (1.5–7.5)	0.004
Acute respiratory failure on admission	4.1 (1.0–11.3)	0.005
Severe sepsis or septic shock on admission	9.2 (4.6–18.3)	<0.001
Gram-negative bacteria	3.4 (1.6–7.4)	0.002

with a higher mortality rate than other pathogens. Independent risk factors for Gram-negative bacteria were probable aspiration, previous hospitalization or antimicrobial treatment within the past 30 days, and pulmonary co-morbidity with bronchiectasis. In addition, the risk for Gram-negative bacteria increased with the number of risk factors. The American Thoracic guidelines take these risk factors on board in deciding empirical therapy for patients with community acquired pneumonia (see Table 13.5).

The next two papers discuss the management of community acquired pneumonia, and investigate whether nasal intermittent positive pressure ventilation (NIV) has a role to play in the management of severe pneumonia. NIV is now well established for the treatment of chronic obstructive pulmonary disease exacerbations that develop hypercapnic respiratory failure and has been shown to improve outcomes, including a reduced need for mechanical ventilation, reduced length of hospital stay and improved mortality rates. There has been recent interest as to whether this is applicable in patients with pneumonia although it is uncertain whether continuous positive airways pressure or NIV should be used. The next two studies used NIV. The first study was an observational study of the use of NIV in patients with severe community acquired pneumonia and the next study was a randomized controlled study using NIV in immunosuppressed patients with pulmonary infiltrates, fever and acute respiratory failure.

Non-invasive pressure support ventilation in severe community acquired pneumonia.

Jolliet P, Abajo B, Pasquina P, Chevrolet JC. *Intensive Care Med* 2001; **27**(5): 812–21.

B ACKGROUND . This prospective observational Swiss study explored the use of NIV in an intensive care setting in 24 patients with acute respiratory failure due to severe community acquired pneumonia. The indications for NIV were at least one of the following, including respiratory rate ≥25/minute, arterial CO$_2$ ≥45 mmHg and PaO$_2$/FiO$_2$ <300. Patients had an initial 30-minute NIV trial and NIV was subsequently used if tolerated.

I NTERPRETATION . The demographics for the 24 patients are shown in Table 13.13. The pressure settings for NIV were a mean ± SD inspired positive airways pressure of 17 ± 4 cm H$_2$0 and expired positive airways pressure of 4 ± 2 cm H$_2$0. During the initial 30 minutes NIV trial respiratory rate decreased, arterial oxygenation improved while PaCO$_2$ and pH remained unchanged (Table 13.14). Subsequently, 133 NIV trials were performed (median duration 55 min, range 30–540 min) over 1–7 days. Despite NIV, 16 patients needed to be intubated (66%) and 33% died (all in the intubated group). In summary despite an initial improvement following 30 minutes NIV, a large percentage (66%) needed mechanical ventilation.

Table 13.13 The baseline data are shown for the patients with community acquired pneumonia that used NIV

Age (years)	49 ± 17
pH	7.4 ± 0.1
PaO$_2$/FiO$_2$	104 ± 48
Arterial CO$_2$ mmHg	40 ± 9

Data presented as mean ± SD.

Table 13.14 Respiratory rate and arterial blood gas data before and 30 minutes post-NIV

	Pre-NIV	Post-30 minutes NIV
Respiratory rate (breaths/minute)	34 ± 7	28 ± 10*
pH	7.40 ± 0.08	7.42 ± 0.06
Arterial CO$_2$ mmHg	40 ± 9	38 ± 7
PaO$_2$/FiO$_2$	104 ± 48	153 ± 49*

Data presented as mean ± SD; *P value <0.001.

Comment

This small observational study does not answer whether NIV has a beneficial role in community acquired pneumonia. Large randomized controlled studies are needed to evaluate whether NIV reduces the need for intubation, length of hospital stay and mortality.

Non-invasive ventilation in immunosuppressed patients with pulmonary infiltrates, fever and acute respiratory failure.

Hilbert G, Gruson D, Vargas F, *et al*. *N Engl J Med* 2001; **344**(7): 481–7.

BACKGROUND. This French prospective randomized controlled trial compared NIV with standard treatment with supplemental oxygen and no ventilatory support, in 52 immunosuppressed patients with pulmonary infiltrates, fever (>38.3ºC), and an early stage of hypoxaemic acute respiratory failure (PaO$_2$:FiO$_2$ <200). Periods of NIV were delivered through a facemask and alternated every three hours with periods of spontaneous breathing with supplemental oxygen. The ventilation periods lasted at least 45 minutes (Table 13.15). Decisions to intubate were made according to standard criteria (failure with standard or NIV treatment or failure to tolerate NIV; failure to maintain a PaO$_2$:FiO$_2$ >85; airways needing protection; development of copious secretions; increase PaCO$_2$ with pH ≤7.3; agitation necessitating sedation; haemodynamic instability (systolic blood pressure <70 mmHg or ischaemia on the electrocardiograph or significant ventricular arrhythmias).

INTERPRETATION. The baseline characteristics of the two groups were similar (Table 13.16). Each group of 26 patients included 15 patients with haematologic cancer and neutropenia. There was a high mortality in immunosuppressed patients with pneumonia and hypoxaemic respiratory failure. Fewer patients in the NIV group than in the standard-treatment group, however, required endotracheal intubation and fewer died in the ICU or in hospital (Table 13.16). In summary the early introduction of NIV in this small study was associated with significant reductions in the rates of endotracheal intubation and improved the likelihood of survival to hospital discharge.

Table 13.15 Details of the use of nasal intermittent positive pressure ventilation for this study

Inspired positive airways pressure	15 ± 2 cm H$_2$0
Expired positive airways pressure	6 ± 1 cm H$_2$0
Use in first 24 hours	9 ± 3 hours
Use subsequently	7 ± 3 hours
Duration NIV used	4 ± 2 days

Data is presented as mean ± SD.

Table 13.16 The baseline characteristics and outcome are shown for the groups comparing NIV and standard treatment. Fewer patients receiving NIV required mechanical ventilation, died in the intensive care unit or died in hospital

	NIV	Standard treatment
Number	26	26
Mean ± SD age (years)	48 ± 14	50 ± 12
Mean ± SD baseline respiratory rate/minute	35 ± 3	36 ± 3
Mean ± SD baseline arterial pH	7.45 ± 0.04	7.43 ± 0.04
Mean ± SD baseline $PaCO_2$ mmHg	37 ± 4	38 ± 5
Mean ± SD baseline PaO_2:FiO_2	141 ± 24	136 ± 23
Per cent patients with a sustained improvement in PaO_2:FiO_2 without intubation	50%	19%*
Need for intubation	46%	77%*
Mean ± SD duration in the ICU	7 ± 3 days	9 ± 4 days
Death in the ICU	38%	69%*
Hospital mortality rate	50%	81%*

*P value <0.05.

Comment

The latter randomized controlled study supports that NIV can reduce the need for mechanical ventilation and improve mortality rates in immunosuppressed patients with pulmonary infiltrates, fever and acute respiratory failure. Further specific randomized controlled studies are needed to assess the role of pressure support ventilation in patients with severe community acquired pneumonia (in non-immunosuppressed patients). In addition, further studies are needed to decide whether continuous positive airways pressure or nasal intermittent positive pressure ventilation should be the method used in patients with pneumonia.

The next two studies change tack and assess the use and outcomes of mechanical ventilation in community acquired pneumonia and the last paper discusses the implications of early hospital discharge.

Severe community acquired pneumonia: use of intensive care services and evaluation of American and British Thoracic Society Diagnostic criteria.

Angus DC, Marrie TJ, Obrosky DS, *et al. Am J Respir Crit Care Med* 2002; **166**(5): 717–23.

B A C K G R O U N D . This US and Canadian study compared the characteristics, course and outcome of in-patients who did ($n = 170$) and did not ($n = 1169$) receive ICU care in the Pneumonia Patient Outcomes Research Team prospective cohort.

INTERPRETATION. Patients admitted to the ICU were more likely to be admitted from home and had more co-morbid conditions. The reasons for ICU admission included respiratory failure (57%), haemodynamic monitoring (32%) and shock (16%). Patients admitted to the ICU incurred longer hospital stays, higher hospital costs and higher hospital mortality (Table 13.17). ICU patients were more likely to be discharged to a nursing home or institutional care, and had a lower proportion that returned to their usual activities or work by 30 days (Table 13.17). The definitions of severe pneumonia by both the American Thoracic Society and British Thoracic Society (Table 13.18) had poor positive predictive values for ICU admission (26.4 and 20.2%) respectively. This indicated that many patients who met the criteria for severe community acquired pneumonia by the American Thoracic Society and British Thoracic Society did not require ICU support.

Comment

In this US and Canadian study, ICU use for community acquired pneumonia was common, and was associated with an increased length of hospital stay, an increased mortality, was expensive, and resulted in a greater percentage of patients requiring discharge to a nursing home or other institutional care. In addition, patients discharged home took longer to recover functionally. Although the American and British Thoracic Society guidelines for community acquired pneumonia guide us to predicting the severity of the pneumonia, they do not adequately predict the need for ventilation.

This highlights that many patients with severe community acquired pneumonia do not need formal mechanical ventilation. The British and American Thoracic Society guidelines do, however, help us stratify patients with severe pneumonia. Such patients should receive aggressive medical therapy and be monitored more intensely, preferably in a high dependency unit or an ICU. Patients that deteriorate despite aggressive medical therapy should be considered for mechanical ventila-

Table 13.17 Outcomes for patients admitted with community acquired pneumonia

	ICU care	No ICU care
Number	170	1169
Mean age (years)	63.2	64.5
Per cent males	14%*	10.3%
Mean $\pm$ SD length of stay (days)	23.2 $\pm$ 26.5**	9.1 $\pm$ 9.3
Hospital mortality rate	18.2%**	5.0%
Median cost ($)	$21 144**	5785
Discharge to a nursing home/institution (per cent of hospital survivors)	29%**	17.0%
Return to usual activities at 30 days	38.3%**	65.0%
Return to work at 30 days (those who worked before the pneumonia %)	25.9%*	70.5%

*P value <0.05 and **P value <0.001.

Table 13.18 Definition of severe pneumonia from the British and American Thoracic Society guidelines

American Thoracic Society	
1 of 2 major Or 2 of 3 minor	**MAJOR** • Need for mechanical ventilation • Septic shock **MINOR** • Systolic blood pressure ≤90 mmHg • Multilobar disease • PaO_2/FiO_2 <250
British Thoracic Society Any 2 risk factors	• New mental confusion • Serum urea >7mmol/l • Respiratory rate ≥30/minute • Systolic blood pressure <90 mmHg or diastolic blood pressure ≤60 mmHg

tion. In light of the morbidity and mortality associated with mechanical ventilation, the decision to ventilate can often be difficult. The decision to ventilate is usually decided in conjunction with the physicians, anaesthetists/intensivists, patient and/ or family and information from the general practitioner/family physician. Many factors will be needed to help in this decision including the patients' expected prognosis, co-morbid illness, number of systems failure, and patients' and families' wishes.

Instability on hospital discharge and the risk of adverse outcomes in patients with pneumonia.
Halm EA, Fine MJ, Kapoor WN, Singer DE, Marrie TJ, Siu AL. *Arch Intern Med* 2002; **162**(11): 1278–84.

BACKGROUND. Increasingly there is pressure on hospital beds, and there are claims that patients are being sent home from the hospital 'quicker and sicker'. This prospective multi-centre US study collected information on daily vital signs and clinical status in the 24 hours prior to discharge. Unstable factors were temperature greater than 37.8°C, heart rate greater than 100/min, respiratory rate greater than 24/min, systolic blood pressure lower than 90 mmHg, oxygen saturation lower than 90%, inability to maintain oral intake, and abnormal mental status. Outcomes were deaths, re-admissions, and failure to return to usual activities within 30 days of discharge.

INTERPRETATION. There were 680 patients in this study with a mean age ± SD of 58 ± 19 years. The median (interquartile range) length of stay was 7 days (5–10) and 19% left the hospital with ≥1 instabilities. At 30 days post-discharge, 10% of patients with no instabilities on discharge died or were readmitted compared with 14% of those with 1 instability and 46% of those with ≥2 instabilities (*P* <0.003) (Table 13.19).

Instability on discharge (≥1 unstable factor) was associated with higher risk-adjusted rates of death or readmission (OR 1.6, 95% CI 1.0–2.8, $P<0.01$) and failure to return to usual activities (OR 1.5, 95% CI 1.0–2.4, $P<0.01$). Patients with two or more instabilities had 5-fold greater risk-adjusted odds of death or readmission (OR 5.4, 95% CI 1.6–18.4, $P<0.001$). In summary instability on discharge led to an increased risk of hospital readmission and mortality. Local guidelines and pathways should include objective criteria for judging stability on discharge to ensure that efforts to shorten length of hospital stay do not jeopardize patient safety.

Comment

This study investigated the outcome of sending patients home too early with community acquired pneumonia. It highlights the dangers of early discharge if patients are not clinically stable, and physicians should ensure patients are stable at discharge. If patients insist on early discharge, it is recommended that there should be close community follow up.

Table 13.19 Outcomes at 30 days comparing no instabilities at discharge to 1 and ≥2 instabilities at discharge

	No instability	1 instability	≥2 instabilities	P
Mortality rate	2.6%	3.4%	38.6%	<0.001
Mortality rate or readmission	10.5%	13.7%	46.2%	<0.001

14

Ventilator associated pneumonia

The next section covers ventilator associated pneumonia (VAP) and discusses the prevention, diagnosis and management strategies. The conventional definition of VAP is pneumonia developing more than 48 hours after endotracheal intubation and ventilation (although it is recognized that patients may develop it sooner). It affects 8–28% of patients receiving mechanical ventilation and is associated with a high mortality rate ranging from 24–76%. There are multiple risk factors for the development of VAP, some of which include intubation, re-intubation, naso-tracheal intubation, supine body position, pharmacological paralysis and daily change of ventilator circuits. The prevention of VAP may have a major impact on the patients' outcome and two studies are presented. The first study investigated the role of oral decontamination and the second study examined the role of continuous sub-glottic secretion drainage in the prevention of VAP.

The diagnosis of VAP can be difficult and there is much debate about the role of tracheal aspirates, protective specimen brushes and broncho-alveolar lavage by bronchoscopy. Many believe that the protective specimen brushings and broncho-alveolar lavage remain the gold standard. An interesting preliminary study is presented that evaluated the role of serum and alveolar procalcitonin as an aid for both the diagnosis and prognosis in patients with VAP.

Finally, it is well recognized that instituting early antimicrobial therapy is important in the management of VAP and a paper by Iregui *et al.* investigated the effect of delayed antimicrobial therapy.

Prevention of ventilator associated pneumonia by oral decontamination: a prospective, randomized, double-blind, placebo-controlled study.
Bergmans DC, Bonten MJ, Gaillard CA, *et al. Am J Respir Crit Care Med* 2001; **164**(3): 382–8.

BACKGROUND. Colonization of the intestinal tract is thought to be important in the pathogenesis of VAP, but relative impacts of oropharyngeal, gastric or intestinal colonization have not been elucidated. This prospective randomized placebo-controlled double-blind intensive care unit (ICU) study from the Netherlands aimed to prevent VAP by modulation of oropharyngeal colonization, without influencing gastric and intestinal colonization and without systemic prophylaxis. **Eighty-seven patients received topical antimicrobial prophylaxis (Gentamicin/Colistin/Vancomycin 2% in Orabase, every 6 h) in the oropharynx, and 139 patients, divided over two control groups, received placebo (78 patients were studied in the presence of patients receiving topical prophylaxis [control Group A] and 61 patients were studied in an ICU where no topical prophylaxis was used [control Group B]). Eradication of colonization was defined as the disappearance of micro-organisms in ≥2 consecutive cultures from a body site colonized on admission, and is expressed as the proportion of colonized patients in whom eradication occurred. Acquired colonization was defined as colonization >24 hours after ICU admission, in patients without colonization on admission.**

INTERPRETATION. Baseline characteristics were comparable in all three groups. Topical prophylaxis significantly eradicated colonization present on admission in the oropharynx and in the trachea (Table 14.1). Moreover, topical prophylaxis prevented acquired oropharyngeal and possibly tracheal colonization whereas colonization rates in the stomach and intestine were not affected (Table 14.1). The incidence of VAP in the patients that received topical prophylaxis (10%) was lower than the placebo arms of the study (31% in Group A and 23% in Group B patients; $P = 0.001$ and $P = 0.04$ respectively). This was not associated with shorter duration of ventilation, ICU stay or better survival (Table 14.1). In summary this study demonstrated the importance of oropharyngeal colonization in the pathogenesis of VAP and that 5 patients need to be treated to prevent one episode of VAP. This study demonstrated that a targeted

Table 14.1 Outcomes comparing oral decontamination versus no oral decontamination. Group A was the placebo arm in ICUs where oral decontamination takes place. Group B was also the placebo arm but in ICUs where oral decontamination does not takes place

	Oral decontamination arm	Group A: placebo	Group B: placebo
Number	87	78	61
Mean age ± SD (years)	56.6 ± 19	58.1 ± 16.4	58.7 ± 16.7
Per cent eradication in oropharyngeal colonization	75%	0***	9%***
Per cent acquisition of oropharyngeal colonization	10%	59%***	63%***
Per cent eradication in tracheal colonization	52%	22%*	7%**
Per cent acquisition of tracheal colonization	36%	50% γ	43%
Incidence VAP	10%	31%***	23%*
Median (range) duration ICU	13 (4–54) days	15 (4–79) days	12 (4–108) days
ICU mortality	29%	35%	43%
Hospital mortality	35%	41%	44%
1 year mortality	49%	50%	49%

γ$P = 0.06$, *$P <0.05$, **$P <0.01$ and ***$P <0.005$ in comparison with the oral decontamination group.

approach to prevent colonization at this site was a very effective method of infection prevention, and larger multi-centred studies will test whether such an approach has an impact on outcomes such as length of hospital stay and mortality.

A randomized clinical trial of intermittent sub-glottic secretion drainage in patients receiving mechanical ventilation.

Smulders K, van der Hoeven H, Weers-Pothoff I, Vandenbroucke-Grauls C. *Chest* 2002; **121**(3): 858–62.

B A C K G R O U N D . This randomized controlled study from the Netherlands investigated the effect of sub-glottic secretions drainage on the incidence of VAP in patients receiving mechanical ventilation. One hundred and fifty patients with an expected duration of mechanical ventilation >72 h were enrolled in the study. Patients were randomly assigned to receive either an endotracheal tube with a dorsal lumen for intermittent sub-glottic secretions drainage (duration 8 seconds and 20-second intervals) or a standard endotracheal tube (routine suction every 4 hours or if there developed an increased airways resistance or audible/visible secretions in the endotracheal tube). The outcome measurements were the incidence of VAP, duration of mechanical ventilation, length of ICU stay, length of hospital stay, and mortality.

I N T E R P R E T A T I O N . Seventy-five patients were randomized to sub-glottic secretion drainage, and 75 patients were randomized to the control group. The two groups were similar at the time of randomization with respect to demographic characteristics and severity of illness. VAP was seen significantly less in the active arm receiving intermittent sub-glottic secretion drainage (*P* = 0.01). There was no significant difference, however, in length of ICU stay or mortality rates (Table 14.2). In summary, intermittent sub-glottic secretion drainage reduced the incidence of VAP in patients receiving mechanical ventilation, although had no impact on the length of stay or mortality rates. Larger studies are needed to determine whether this technique is reproducible and has an

Table 14.2 Outcomes comparing the active arm (intermittent sub-glottic secretion drainage) with the standard arm (routine secretion drainage from endotracheal tube). In the active arm, fewer patients developed VAP but there was no significant difference in length of intensive care unit stay or mortality rates

	Active arm	Standard arm
Number	75	75
Mean age ± SD years	63.7 ± 13.2	62.8 ± 15.6
Per cent developed VAP	4%*	16%
Mean length of ICU stay ± SD	9.3 ± 7.4 days	12.3 ± 3.6 days
Mortality	16%	13.3%

*P <0.05.

impact on outcome variables such as incidence of VAP, length of ICU stay and mortality rates.

Comment

The studies by Bergmans *et al.* and Smulders *et al.* presented interesting strategies to prevent VAP. The studies using oral decontamination and intermittent sub-glottic drainage both reduced the incidence of VAP but did not show improved outcomes such as reduced length of ICU stay or reduced mortality rates. The numbers that developed VAP in each study were small which may explain why there was no impact on length of ICU stay or mortality, despite a reduced incidence of VAP. Further large multi-centred studies with oral decontamination and intermittent sub-glottic drainage are needed to confirm the reduced incidence of VAP and whether this can lead to improved outcomes.

Alveolar and serum procalcitonin: diagnostic and prognostic value in ventilator associated pneumonia.

Duflo F, Debon R, Monneret G, Bienvenu J, Chassard D, Allaouchiche B.
Anesthesiology 2002; **96**(1): 74–91.

B A C K G R O U N D . This French study examined the potential role of serum and alveolar procalcitonin as early markers of VAP and as a prognostic tool. Ninety-six patients with a strong suspicion of VAP were prospectively enrolled and the diagnosis of VAP was based on a positive quantitative culture obtained via a mini-bronchoalveolar lavage of $\geq 10^3$ colony-forming units/ml (cfu/ml). Blood and alveolar samples were collected for procalcitonin measurement and analysed for diagnostic and prognostic evaluation on days 0, 3 and 6. Sensitivity, specificity, positive likelihood ratio and receiver-operating characteristic curves were analysed to define ideal cut-off values and approach the decision analysis. Antibiotics were started following the Gram stain results from the bronchoalveolar lavage.

I N T E R P R E T A T I O N . Serum procalcitonin was significantly increased in the VAP group compared with the non-VAP group at days 0 and 3 but not significantly different at day 6 (Table 14.3). A serum procalcitonin concentration >3.9 ng/ml (best cut-off value) was considered positive for the VAP diagnosis with a sensitivity of 41% and a specificity of 100%. The mean (95% CI) serum procalcitonin was significantly increased ($P <0.02$) in the non-survivors compared with the survivors for the VAP group: 16.5 ng/ml (95% CI 8.1–24.9) in patients that died and 2.9 ng/ml (1.2–4.7) for patients that survived. The best cut-off value for serum procalcitonin of the non-survivors in the VAP group was 2.6 ng/ml with a sensitivity of 74%, specificity of 75% and a positive likelihood ratio of 2.96. Regarding VAP diagnosis and prognosis, no significant differences were found for alveolar procalcitonin in all groups. In summary this small study suggests that serum procalcitonin may be a useful tool in the early diagnosis of ventilator associated pneumonia and may be a helpful marker of prognosis. Further multi-centre studies evaluating the use of procalcitonin are awaited.

Table 14.3 The mean serum procalcitonin concentrations were elevated in the VAP group at days 0 and 3. There was no significant difference at day 6 (data not shown)

	VAP group	Non-VAP group
Number	44	52
Mean age (95% CI) years	53 (48.4–56.4)	48 (44–52)
Mean serum procalcitonin concentrations (ng/ml) (95% CI) Day 0	11.5 (5.9–17.0)*	1.5 (1.1–1.9)
Mean serum procalcitonin concentrations (ng/ml) (95% CI) Day 3	7.5 (6.3–8.7)*	1.25 (1.03–1.47)

*$P < 0.02$.

Comment

The study highlighted that serum procalcitonin may be a useful clinical marker to aid in the diagnosis of VAP and may have prognostic significance. Procalcitonin is normally produced in the C cells of the thyroid gland and is the precursor of calcitonin. Normally all procalcitonin is cleaved and none is released in the bloodstream and, therefore, procalcitonin levels are usually undetectable (<0.1 ng/ml). During severe infections, however, procalcitonin levels may increase to >100 ng/ml and it is probably produced by extra-thyroid tissues. In view of its high specificity, it may turn out to be a useful routine clinical test in cases suspected of VAP, but this single-centred study needs confirmation from larger multi-centre studies.

Clinical importance of delays in the initiation of appropriate antibiotic treatment for ventilator associated pneumonia.

Iregui M, Ward S, Sherman G, Fraser VJ, Kollef MH. *Chest* 2002; **122**(1): 262–8.

BACKGROUND. This US study investigated the influence of initially delayed appropriate antibiotic treatment on the outcome of 107 patients receiving mechanical ventilation and antibiotic treatment for VAP.

INTERPRETATION. All 107 patients (mean age ± SD was 56.6 ± 16.8 years) eventually received treatment with an antibiotic regimen that was shown *in vitro* to be active against the bacterial pathogens isolated from their respiratory secretions. Antibiotic treatment was standardized so patients received the combination treatment with Vancomycin and at least one of the following antibiotics (Ciprofloxacin, Imipenum,

Table 14.4 Risk factors associated with increased hospital mortality by logistic regression analysis

Risk factor	OR (95% CI)	P value
Antibiotic administration >24 hours	7.68 (4.5–13.09)	<0.001
Presence of malignancy	3.20 (1.79–5.71)	0.04
Apache score	1.13 (1.09–1.18)	0.001

Cefepime or Piperacillin-Tazobactam) to cover MRSA and *Pseudomonas aeruginosa*. A total of 30.8% received antibiotic treatment that was delayed for ≥24 h after initially meeting diagnostic criteria for VAP, and this was mainly due to a delay in writing the antibiotic orders (75.8%). A total of 18.2% were accounted for by the presence of a bacterial species resistant to the initially prescribed antibiotic regimen. The mean time ± SD interval from initially meeting the diagnostic criteria for VAP until the administration of antibiotic treatment was 28.6 ± 5.8 hours among patients who had delayed antibiotic therapy, compared with 12.5 ± 4.2 hours for all other patients ($P <0.001$). The mortality was 69.7% for the delayed antibiotic group compared with 28.4% for the group receiving antibiotics within 24 hours ($P <0.01$). Overall 41.1% with VAP died during their hospitalization. Increasing APACHE scores, the presence of malignancy and the administration of delayed antibiotic therapy were identified as risk factors independently associated with increased hospital mortality by logistic regression analysis (Table 14.4).

Comments

In summary this single-centre US study emphasizes the importance of prompt antibacterial therapy in patients with VAP and that a delay ≥24 hours is associated with an increased hospital mortality. The development of antibiotic protocols will likely improve the early initiation of appropriate antibiotic therapy. These protocols will likely be driven locally by pathogens normally identified, sensitivities, cost and availability of antibiotics. There is a danger, however, of indiscriminately using potent antibiotics in both high dependency units and ICUs which will encourage drug resistance. Thus, targeting antibiotic therapy is encouraged where possible.

The final section is on bronchiectasis and discusses both the pathogenesis and treatment strategies.

15

Bronchiectasis

Many patients with bronchiectasis are chronically colonized with bacteria, when apparently clinically stable, and suffer from recurrent bacterial chest infections. The first two studies investigated bacterial colonization in patients with clinically stable bronchiectasis and investigated the risk factors, the microbiological pattern and its influence on airways inflammation.

The mainstay of treatment in bronchiectasis is regular chest physiotherapy, yearly influenza vaccination, and prompt antibiotic treatment for infective exacerbations. Antibiotics are routinely recommended for infective exacerbations, and long-term antibiotics are considered for patients with frequent infective exacerbations to try and reduce the exacerbation frequency. Long-term antibiotics are used routinely in patients with cystic fibrosis chronically colonized with *Pseudomonas aeruginosa* to reduce the frequency of exacerbations and hopefully attenuate the decline in FEV_1 (forced expiratory volume in one second). It is not known, however, whether there should be a similar approach in patients with bronchiectasis chronically colonized with *Pseudomonas aeruginosa*. The study by Couch was a randomized placebo controlled study and examined the impact of 4 weeks' treatment with nebulized Tobramycin solution.

The papers following evaluate the role of surgical intervention. Surgery is normally considered in patients with bronchiectasis with localized disease and recurrent infective exacerbations or life-threatening haemoptysis. Two retrospective studies are presented on the surgical outcome in patients with bronchiectasis selected for surgical intervention.

As stated previously, regular physiotherapy is recommended and many methods are now available to aid sputum expectoration. The flutter valve, a hand-held pipe-like device causing oscillating positive expiratory pressure within the airways, is a newer method to aid sputum expectoration and the study by Thompson *et al.* compared the flutter valve with the more conventional active cycle breathing technique.

The final study compared the outcome of nurse- and doctor-led clinics. There is an increasing pressure on doctor-led clinics both in primary and secondary care, and a lack of consultation time is commonly complained about. Nurse-led clinics are being promoted in many chronic diseases, such as asthma and diabetes, to try and combat this. The provision of specialized clinics may improve healthcare as protocols are likely to be adhered to, patients may have more time with the nurse practitioner and patient groups can be formed.

Bacterial colonization in patients with bronchiectasis: microbiological pattern and risk factors.
Angrill J, Agusti C, de Celis R, *et al. Thorax* 2002; **57**(1): 15–19.

BACKGROUND. This 2-year prospective Spanish study investigated the risk factors of airway colonization in 77 patients with bronchiectasis whilst in a stable clinical condition.

INTERPRETATION. The demographics for the study group are shown in Table 15.1. The incidence of bronchial colonization with potential pathogenic micro-organisms was 64%. The most frequent organisms isolated were *Haemophilus influenzae* (55%) and *Pseudomonas species* (26%). Resistance to β lactam antibiotics was found in 30% of the patients colonized with *Haemophilus influenzae, Streptococcus pneumoniae*, or *Moraxella catarrhalis*. When the sputum sample was satisfactory, the operative characteristics of the sputum cultures were similar to those obtained with the protective specimen brush taken as a gold standard. Risk factors associated with bronchial colonization in the multivariate analysis were diagnosis of bronchiectasis before the age of 14 years, FEV_1 <80% predicted and the presence of varicose or cystic bronchiectasis (Table 15.2).

Comment
In summary there is a high prevalence of bronchial colonization by potential pathogenic micro-organisms in clinically stable patients with bronchiectasis. Sputum

Table 15.1 Demographics for the study population

	Patients with bronchiectasis
Number	77
Age	58 ± 14 years
Current smokers	6%
FEV_1 (% predicted)	75 ± 23%

Data presented as mean ± SD.

Table 15.2 Risk factors for bronchial colonization

	OR (95% CI)
Age <14 years	3.92 (1.29–11.95)
FEV_1 <80% predicted	3.91 (1.30–11.78)
Cystic or varicose bronchiectasis	4.80 (1.11–21.46)

All P <0.01.

samples obtained from patients with bronchiectasis are usually of good quality with little squamous cell contamination. This study confirmed that sputum culture was a good alternative to the invasive bronchoscopic procedures for evaluation of this colonization assuming an adequate sample. The risk factors for colonization included the early diagnosis of bronchiectasis, the more advanced forms of bronchiectasis (varicose and cystic forms), and the presence of airflow obstruction with an FEV_1 <80% predicted likely, reflecting more advanced bronchiectasis. The study following looks at the impact of bacterial colonization on airways inflammation.

Bronchial inflammation and colonization in patients with clinically stable bronchiectasis.

Angrill J, Agusti C, De Celis R, *et al. Am J Respir Crit Care Med* 2001; **164**(9): 1628–32.

BACKGROUND. This Spanish study evaluated the bronchial inflammatory response and its relationship to bacterial colonization in patients with bronchiectasis. Bronchoalveolar lavage (BAL) was carried out in 49 patients with bronchiectasis in a stable clinical condition and in 9 non-smoking control subjects without respiratory disease (Table 15.3). The BAL was processed for differential cell counts, quantitative bacteriologic cultures, and measurement of inflammatory mediators.

INTERPRETATION. An increase in the number and percentage of neutrophils was found in patients with bronchiectasis compared with control subjects (Table 15.4). The non-colonized bronchiectasis patients had a higher per cent of neutrophils than the control subjects. There was, however, a higher per cent of neutrophils in bronchiectasis patients colonized by micro-organisms with potential pathogenicity (defined as colonization $\geq 10^3$ cfu/ml from BAL) compared with both non-colonized patients with bronchiectasis and controls (Table 15.5). In addition, the higher the bacterial load ($\geq 10^4$ cfu/ml), the more intense was the inflammation. In summary there is neutrophilic inflammation in the airways in patients with bronchiectasis in a stable clinical condition. This is potentiated by the presence of potential pathogenic bacteria, and the higher the bacterial load the more intense the inflammation.

Table 15.3 Demographics for the study group (data presented as mean ± SD). Patients with bronchiectasis had lower mean FEV_1 compared with control subjects

	Patients with bronchiectasis	Control subjects
Number	49	9
Age	57 ± 14 years	58 ± 13 years
Number of current smokers	3	0
FEV_1 (% predicted)	79 ± 21%	103 ± 10%*

*P <0.005.

Table 15.4 Patients with bronchiectasis had increased neutrophilic airways inflammation compared with control subjects. Data presented as median (interquartile range)

	Patients with bronchiectasis	Control subjects	P value
Per cent neutrophils	37 (0–98)	1 (0–4)	0.001
Neutrophils (10^5 cells ml^{-1})	1.92 (0–376)	0.1 (0–0.48)	0.002

Table 15.5 Patients with bronchiectasis that were not colonized had an increased per cent of neutrophils compared to controls. Colonized patients with bronchiectasis had an increased per cent of neutrophils compared with non-colonized patients with bronchiectasis and controls

	Colonized patients with bronchiectasis ($\geq 10^3$ cfu/ml)	Non-colonized patients with bronchiectasis	Controls
Per cent neutrophils	57 (0–98)*+	8 (0–93)*	1 (0–4)

*$P < 0.05$ comparisons with the control group; +$P < 0.05$ comparisons with the non-colonised patients with bronchiectasis.

Comment

This study highlights that neutrophilic inflammation is important in the aetiology of bronchiectasis whilst patients are clinically stable even in the absence of bacterial colonization. This neutrophilic inflammation is potentiated by bacterial coloniz-ation, and this study confirmed that this was positively related to bacterial load (increased neutrophilic airways inflammation with increased bacterial loads). This study did not look at exacerbations, but increased neutrophilic airways inflamma-tion would be expected.

The neutrophil has the potential to cause damage to the airways as the activated neutrophil can release proteolytic enzymes and reactive oxygen species that can damage host defences, and thereby promote bacterial colonization. This in itself can further perpetuate airways inflammation and can lead to a vicious circle of on-going inflammation and bacterial colonization, a feature often present in patients with bronchiectasis.

Treatment with tobramycin solution for inhalation in bronchiectasis patients with *Pseudomonas aeruginosa*.

Couch LA. *Chest* 2001; **120**(3): 114S–17S.

BACKGROUND. The treatment of *Pseudomonas aeruginosa* colonization is common practice in patients with cystic fibrosis. It is not clear whether a similar approach is needed for patients with non-cystic fibrosis bronchiectasis. This US randomized, placebo-controlled, multi-centre trial evaluated the safety and efficacy of 300 mg aerosolized tobramycin solution for inhalation administered twice daily for 4 weeks in 74 bronchiectasis patients colonized with *Pseudomonas aeruginosa* $\geq 10^4$ colony forming units per gram of sputum.

INTERPRETATION. There were 37 patients evenly divided between tobramycin therapy and placebo. Following 4 weeks tobramycin therapy, there was a mean reduction in sputum *Pseudomonas aeruginosa* density, and 2 weeks following the end of therapy *Pseudomonas aeruginosa* was eradicated in 35% of patients (Table 15.6). In the placebo arm there was no effect on sputum *Pseudomonas aeruginosa* density and there was no eradication of *Pseudomonas aeruginosa*. There was no significant effect on FEV_1 (per cent predicted) in either arm of the study (Table 15.6). A higher percentage (62%) of tobramycin treated patients were judged by a physician as having an improved general health status compared with 38% of placebo treated patients, although this failed to reach statistical significance ($P = 0.06$). In the tobramycin treatment arm, however, 92% clinically improved if *Pseudomonas aeruginosa* was eradicated as compared with 46% in the rest of the tobramycin treated group ($P = 0.01$). Eight per cent withdrew from the tobramycin treated group whereas there were no withdrawals from the placebo group ($P = 0.2$); the main withdrawals were related to increased wheeze, breathlessness and chest tightness.

Table 15.6 Outcomes comparing the treatment arm (4 weeks nebulized tobramycin) with the placebo arm

End of treatment	Treatment arm	Placebo arm
Mean change in sputum *Pseudomonas aeruginosa* density ($\log_{10}$ colony forming units/g sputum)	−4.5	+0.02*
Per cent *Pseudomonas aeruginosa* eradicated at 6 weeks (2 weeks after treatment ended)	35%	0*
Improvement as assessed by physician	62%	38%
Change in FEV_1 (% predicted)	−2.3%	+1.5%
Withdrawal with adverse effects	8%	0%

*$P < 0.001$.

Comment

This small study showed that aerosolized tobramycin 300 mg twice daily for 4 weeks reduced the bacterial load and eradicated *Pseudomonas aeruginosa* in 35% patients at least in the short term, which led to a clinical improvement as judged by the treating physician. Eight per cent were unable to tolerate the aerosolized tobramycin and had to be withdrawn from the study, which relates to the bronchospasm caused by the aerosolized tobramycin.

Patients colonized with *Pseudomonas aeruginosa* often have recurrent exacerbations, and enter a vicious circle of inflammation and bacterial colonization. The eradication of *Pseudomonas aeruginosa* would be expected, in theory, to lead to clinical improvements if patients could remain eradicated from *Pseudomonas aeruginosa*. This may have an impact on reducing exacerbations, reducing lung function decline and improving health status, but longer-term studies are needed to investigate this.

Surgery for bronchiectasis.
Prieto D, Bernardo J, Matos MJ, Eugenio L, Antunes M. *Eur J Cardiothorac Surg* 2001; **20**(1): 19–23.

B A C K G R O U N D . This study evaluated the role of surgery in patients with bronchiectasis in Portugal. Between 1988 and 1999, the authors had operated on 119 patients with bronchiectasis, 71 female and 48 male, with a mean age of 42.2 years (range 11–77 years).

I N T E R P R E T A T I O N . The main indications for surgery and the surgery performed are shown in Table 15.7. There was no operative mortality and peri-operative morbidity occurred in 12.6%, including temporary broncho-pleural fistulae in 5.8% and post-operative haemorrhage and atrial arrhythmias in 3.4% each. After a mean follow-up of 4.5 years, 67% of this group were asymptomatic, 29% had meaningful clinical improvement, while only 4% maintained or worsened prior symptoms. There were no differences in the spirometry, comparing pre- and post-operative data, with a 2-year minimum interval. The mean VC was 91 and 89% and the FEV_1 was 83 and 81% of expected, respectively before and after $\geq$2 years following surgery ($P > 0.05$).

Surgical treatment in bronchiectasis: analysis of 166 patients.
Kutlay H, Cangir AK, Enon S, *et al. Eur J Cardiothorac Surg* 2002; **21**(4): 634–7.

B A C K G R O U N D . This study reviewed the morbidity and mortality rates and outcome of surgical treatment for bronchiectasis. Between 1990 and 2000, 166 patients (92 female and 74 male patients) underwent pulmonary resection for bronchiectasis. The mean age was 34.1 years (range 7–70 years).

Table 15.7 The outcomes of surgery for bronchiectasis are summarized for the last 2 studies

	Prieto *et al.*	Kutlay *et al.*
Number	119	166
Country	Portugal	Turkey
Mean age	42.2 years	34.1 years
Main indications for surgery		
Failure with medical therapy	55%	95%
Haemoptysis	26%	3%
Main operations		
Lobectomy	62%	72%
Pneumonectomy	7.4%	8%
Segmentectomy	10%	13%
Operative mortality	0	1.8%
Operative morbidity	13%	10.8%
Mean follow up	4.5 years	4.2 years
Clinical status post surgery		
1. Asymptomatic	67%	75%
2. Improvement	29%	21%
3. No change or worse	4%	4%

INTERPRETATION. The main indications for surgery and the surgery performed are shown in Table 15.7. The operative mortality and morbidity were seen in 1.8% and 10.8% patients respectively. Follow-up was complete in 148 patients with a mean of 4.2 years. Overall, 75% of patients were asymptomatic after surgical treatment, symptoms were improved in 21%, and unchanged or worse in 4%. The outcome from these two studies indicates that surgery is relatively 'safe' and many patients can have good long-term functional improvement.

Comment

The precise role for surgical intervention is unclear but surgery may be useful in the management of patients with localized disease that have recurrent exacerbations or life-threatening haemoptysis. Randomized controlled studies are needed to compare conventional therapy and surgery, although data from these non-randomized controlled studies suggests a good outcome from surgery in the majority of patients that either failed medical therapy or have had major haemoptysis.

Randomized crossover study of the Flutter device and the active cycle of breathing technique in non-cystic fibrosis bronchiectasis.

Thompson CS, Harrison S, Ashley J, Day K, Smith DL. *Thorax* 2002; **57**(5): 446–8.

B A C K G R O U N D . **Airway clearance techniques are an important part of the routine care of patients with bronchiectasis. The use of the Flutter device, a hand-held pipe-like device causing oscillating positive expiratory pressure within the airways, has been proposed as an alternative to the more conventional airway clearance techniques. This was a randomized crossover UK study performed in 17 stable patients with non-cystic fibrosis bronchiectasis at home, in which 4 weeks of daily active cycle of breathing technique (ACBT) were compared with 4 weeks of daily physiotherapy with the Flutter device.**

I N T E R P R E T A T I O N . There was no significant difference between the two physiotherapy techniques in the daily sputum weights, daily duration of physiotherapy (Table 15.8), peak expiratory flow rate, breathlessness (Borg score) or health status (Chronic Respiratory Disease Questionnaire). Subjectively (11/17) patients preferred the Flutter to ACBT for routine use, three preferred ACBT and three had no preference. In summary the daily use of the Flutter device in the home is as effective as ACBT in patients with non-cystic fibrosis bronchiectasis, and has a high level of patient acceptability.

Comment

This study compared physiotherapy techniques and the Flutter valve offers a useful alternative to conventional physiotherapy techniques (the ACBT in this study), and from this study has a high patient acceptability. There were no short-term differences between physiotherapy techniques, but if the Flutter valve truly has higher patient acceptability, this may improve compliance with ongoing physiotherapy, which ultimately may affect the prognosis. Longer-term studies are needed.

Table 15.8 There were no significant differences in the daily duration of physiotherapy and sputum volume comparing the Flutter valve and ACBT

	Flutter	ACBT
Daily sputum volume Median (interquartile range)	23.4 g (16.8–36.2)	26.6 g (15.0–45.2)
Duration of physiotherapy Mean ± SD daily	25.9 ± 6 11.7 minutes	29.5 ± 17.0 minutes

A randomized controlled crossover trial of nurse practitioner versus doctor led outpatient care in a bronchiectasis clinic.

Sharples LD, Edmunds J, Bilton D, *et al. Thorax* 2002; **57**(8): 661–6.

BACKGROUND. This UK randomized controlled crossover trial was used to compare nurse-led care with doctor-led care in a bronchiectasis outpatient clinic. Eighty patients were recruited and randomized to receive 1 year of nurse-led care and 1 year of doctor-led care in random order. Patients were followed up for 2 years to ensure patient safety and acceptability and to assess differences in lung function. Outcome measures were FEV$_1$, 12-minute walk test, health related quality of life, and resource use.

INTERPRETATION. The demographics are shown in Table 15.9. There were no significant differences in FEV$_1$, other clinical or health related quality of life measures comparing nurse- and doctor-led care. Nurse-led care, however, resulted in a significantly increased resource use compared with doctor-led care (mean difference £1497, 95% CI £688–2674, $P <0.001$), a large part of which resulted from the number and duration of hospital admissions and antibiotic use. The mean difference in resource use was greater in the first year (£2625) than in the second year (£411). In the bronchiectasis outpatient clinic, nurse-led care is as safe and effective as doctor-led care, but may use more resources.

Comment

The final study examined the efficacy of a nurse-led bronchiectasis clinic. In other areas, the development of nurse-led clinics has helped in the management of chronic diseases such as asthma, diabetes and lung cancer. This randomized controlled trial showed very similar outcomes with a nurse- or doctor-led service which is reassuring and will hopefully lead to more nurse-led clinics, as long as there is appropriate clinical back-up (training and supervision) from medical staff, ongoing audit and evaluation of the service. There was an increased cost with nurse-led clinics but the costs were reduced on the second year of the study, so there may have been a learning effect. Some of the potential benefits include easing the burden on doctor-led

Table 15.9 There were no significant differences between either group with bronchiectasis (data presented as mean ± SD)

	Doctor care then nursing care	Nursing care then doctor care
Number	41	39
Mean age	53.1 ± 13.8 years	63.7 ± 10.3 years
Mean FEV$_1$ (% predicted)	70.3 ± 17.5	70.4 ± 23.4

clinics both in primary and secondary care, increasing the use of protocol driven clinics, increasing consultation times for patients, and the formation of patient groups.

Overall section conclusion

The fifty papers selected from 2001 and 2002 to make up the infection section for *Year in Respiratory Medicine 2003* have made important contributions in building evidence-based practice to help in both the investigation and management of patients with tuberculosis, community acquired pneumonia, ventilator associated pneumonia and patients with bronchiectasis.

There has been concern about the tuberculin skin test which can be influenced by environmental mycobacteria, high mycobacterial load, concomitant infections, prior BCG vaccination and immunosuppression, in particular HIV infection, and is prone to errors both in the placement and in the reading of results. In view of this there has been recent interest in measuring interferon gamma from blood using purified protein derivative as the antigen or more specific antigens, such as early secretory antigenic target (ESAT-6), which is restricted to Mycobacterium tuberculosis complex, Mycobacterium kansassi, marinum, flavescens, and szulgai. ESAT-6 is, therefore, absent from all strains of Mycobacterium bovis BCG and the majority of environmental bacteria. The chosen papers showed ESAT-6 is less influenced by prior BCG vaccination and environmental mycobacteria. This increased specificity is an improvement over the tuberculin skin test and will help in the diagnosis of latent tuberculosis infection. There are many strategies for the treatment of latent tuberculosis infection and there has been increased interest in the shorter 2-month regimen with Rifampicin and Pyrazinamide as opposed to the conventional 6-month Isoniazid regimen. The shortened regimen, however, had increased hepatotoxicity. If this regimen is used it is advised that there is monitoring of the liver function tests.

To improve the eradication of tuberculosis there has been a drive for the implementation of directly observed therapy. The study by Walley *et al.* and the Cochrane review, however, have shown that directly observed therapy does not improve completion rates or alter outcome.

There has been interest in whether the addition of a single dose of Mycobacterium vaccae to conventional tuberculosis treatment would improve cure rates. The studies by Mwinga *et al.* and the Cochrane review have shown that the addition of a single dose of Mycobacterium vaccae confers no additional benefit to standard tuberculosis treatment, which is independent of the patient's HIV status. There has also been recent interest in the once-weekly Rifapentine and Isoniazid regimen for treatment in the continuation phase of tuberculosis. This regimen was as efficacious as the standard twice-weekly directly observed therapy regimen with Rifampicin and Isoniazid, and without an increased side-effect profile, in patients with uncomplicated tuberculosis.

Multi-drug resistant tuberculosis (MDRTB) is a global problem but there is widespread variance throughout the world. The study by Tahaoglu *et al.* revealed that there can be an approximate 75% cure in MDRTB patients (if HIV negative) if they can be treated with at least 3 susceptible drugs for 18 months following conversion to negative tuberculosis cultures. The factors associated with a poor outcome are increasing age, being immunocompromised, and the inability to be treated with at least 3 susceptible drugs. Surgery can be a useful adjunct to medical therapy in patients with MDRTB that have localized disease, adequate cardio-pulmonary reserve, and failure with medical therapy. Studies highlight the importance of treatment before surgery and to continue therapy for around 18 months post-surgery. This approach led to recurrence rates of MDRTB <7%.

The current treatment of Mycobacteria other than tuberculosis with Rifampicin and Ethambutol ± Isoniazid has disappointing 5-year cure rates. We await with interest the further British Thoracic Society trial with treatment with Rifampicin and Ethambutol and either Ciprofloxacin or Clarithromycin and/or Mycobacterium vaccae.

The next section moves on to community acquired pneumonia. Community acquired pneumonia is common with incidence rates between 5–11 per 1000 adult population. Important aspects from the British and American Thoracic Societies are discussed, in particular the epidemiology, the placement of patients and the recommended antibiotic regimens. There is an increased incidence of community acquired pneumonia in the elderly. The study by Kaplan *et al.* revealed there was an increased mortality rate with increasing age, patients admitted from nursing homes, patients with comorbid illness, patients that required admission to intensive care or required mechanical ventilation, male patients and patients that develop acute organ dysfunction.

Although *Streptococcus pneumonia* remains the main aetiological pathogen, Gram-negative bacteria can be implicated in up to 11% of cases. Risk factors include aspiration, prior hospitalization or antibiotic therapy within the preceding 30 days, and bronchiectasis. There was an increased mortality rate in patients with a Gram-negative aetiology.

Although the role of nasal intermittent positive pressure ventilation (NIV) is well established in chronic obstructive pulmonary disease patients with hypercapnic respiratory failure, its role in pneumonia has not been established. In addition, whether continuous positive airways pressure (CPAP) or NIV should be used has not been clarified. The study by Hilbert *et al.* found that NIV reduced the need for mechanical ventilation and improved mortality rates in immunosuppressed patients with pulmonary infiltrates, fever and acute respiratory failure. Further specific randomized controlled studies are needed to assess the role of pressure support ventilation in patients with severe community acquired pneumonia (in non-immunosuppressed patients). In addition, further studies are needed to decide whether CPAP or NIV should be the method used in patients with pneumonia.

The guidelines issued by the British and American Thoracic Societies define severe pneumonia but only a small percentage of patients that meet the diagnostic criteria for severe pneumonia subsequently require mechanical ventilation. Patients that require admission to an intensive care unit subsequently have a longer hospital stay, have an increased mortality rate, incur greater costs, and have a greater need if surviving discharge to require nursing or other institutional care.

The final study in this section by Halm *et al.* highlighted the importance of patients being medically stable at discharge, and as expected patients that have instabilities at discharge have higher rates of hospital readmission and a greater mortality rate.

The penultimate section covers ventilator associated pneumonia which affects 8–28% of patients. Both oral decontamination and regular sub-glottic secretion drainage have been shown to reduce the incidence of ventilator associated pneumonia, but being small studies they failed to have an impact on intensive care unit stay or mortality. There need to be larger multi-centre studies to confirm the reduced incidence of ventilator associated pneumonia and to see if this has an impact on outcomes such as length of stay and mortality rates.

The diagnosis of ventilator associated pneumonia may be helped by the measurement of serum procalcitonin. This measurement has low sensitivity but high specificity and may be a useful adjunct to conventional methods for the diagnosis of ventilator associated pneumonia. In addition serum procalcitonin may have prognostic value (higher serum concentrations had a poorer prognosis). Further studies are awaited.

The final study in this section by Iregui *et al.* highlighted the importance of appropriate and early antibiotic therapy showing that patients with delayed treatment had an increased mortality rate.

The last section was on bronchiectasis. The studies by Angrill *et al.* highlighted that 64% of patients are colonized with potential pathogenic bacteria whilst clinically stable and this stimulates neutrophilic airways inflammation. In addition the greater the bacterial load the more intense the inflammation. The use of long-term nebulized antibiotics is now used routinely in patients with cystic fibrosis chronically colonized with *Pseudomonas aeruginosa* but it is not known whether there should be a similar approach in patients with bronchiectasis. The study by Couch revealed that 4 weeks of Tobramycin therapy managed to eradicate *Pseudomonas aeruginosa* in 35% of patients. Long-term studies are required to see if this has an effect on exacerbation frequency and rate of decline in lung function.

The studies by Prieto *et al.* and Kutlay *et al.* showed that surgery can be successful in patients with bronchiectasis with localized disease in patients that have recurrent exacerbations and life-threatening haemoptysis.

Finally, the study by Sharples *et al.* provided the evidence that nurse-led clinics for patients with bronchiectasis were feasible and gave similar outcomes to doctor-led clinics. Training, supervision and audit would be important components to the continuing success of these clinics.

The fifty articles selected have made important contributions in building evidence-based practice to help in both the investigation and management of patients with respiratory infection.

Part IV

Lung cancer

16

Early detection and prevention of lung cancer

Screening for lung cancer

Introduction

Lung cancer is the most common cancer in terms of incidence (1 040 000 new cases per year, 12.8% of the world total) and mortality (921 000 deaths, 17.8% of the world total). Five-year survival as measured by the SEER (surveillance, epidemiology and end results) programme in the USA is 14% with a figure of approximately 8% recorded in Europe. Currently more than three-quarters of patients with lung cancer have locally advanced or metastatic disease (Stages III and IV) at diagnosis with only the remaining 22% with possibly curable disease (Stage I and II). Five-year survival in early stage disease treated by resection is good (approximately 70% for Stage I). The prognosis for lung cancer has improved slightly in the last 30–40 years. This has been due to refined surgical and oncological techniques and, to some degree, to stage migration with improved staging procedures. This compares poorly with other cancers in which mortality has declined by 25% in the same time-period, primarily due to improvements in medical care, screening, diagnosis and treatment.

Lung cancer is closely related to smoking but as half of the new cases of lung cancer occur in ex-smokers the benefits of a mass smoking cessation programme are limited. In most trials, only 10–20% of people will succeed in stopping smoking. Smoking cessation would eventually defeat the disease but there is no sign that smoking habits on a worldwide basis are declining. Indeed, although the incidence of current smoking is being reduced in the Western world these changes are being outstripped by increases in the smoking habits of the developing world.

There is no public health strategy for the early detection of lung cancer despite the fact that screening is accepted in both breast and cervical cancer and recommended in colon and prostate cancer in some countries. However, for 50 years workers have been interested in screening the population for lung cancer. This was in an effort to find early stage cases that may be cured by surgery. Small, uncontrolled studies of chest imaging conducted during the 1950s and 60s did not suggest a reduction in lung cancer mortality from screening. In the 1970s and 80s the National Cancer Institute sponsored three large randomized controlled trials of chest radiography and sputum cytology as lung cancer screening tools |**1–3**|. No decrease in lung cancer mortality was observed, although these studies had a number of shortcomings. Nevertheless, the results have dissuaded mass screening policies over the last 25 years.

Computed tomography (CT) scanning has been used to diagnose lung cancer in symptomatic patients for many years. Recently data have appeared indicating that a low radiation dose spiral CT scan is capable of detecting abnormalities, including those suggestive of early primary lung cancer, in asymptomatic high-risk individuals. Data from the Early Lung Cancer Action Project (ELCAP) was the first to show the ability of low dose spiral CT scan to find early lung cancer |4|. The study enrolled a thousand individuals at elevated risk of lung cancer. CT detected non-calcified nodules in 233 participants (chest X-ray had shown only 68). Twenty-seven malignancies were eventually revealed of which 85% were Stage I. This study has awakened an interest in screening for lung cancer once more.

Screening for lung cancer.
Manser RL, Irving LB, Stone C, *et al.* (*Cochrane Review*). The Cochrane Library, 2002; **4**: Oxford: Update Software.

BACKGROUND. **While population-based screening for lung cancer has not been universally adopted, large numbers of patients have been put into trials of screening for lung cancer. It is not clear whether sputum cytology, chest radiography or newer methods such as CT are effective in reducing mortality.**

INTERPRETATION. This was a Cochrane Review, which selected controlled trials of screening for lung cancer using sputum cytology, chest radiography and chest CT scanning. Literature was searched from 1966–2000. Seven trials were included (6 randomized controlled studies and one non-randomized controlled trial) with 245 610 subjects. Unfortunately, there were no studies with an unscreened control group. In most of the studies, subjects in the control group were offered screening at longer intervals. Recruitment to most trials took place between 1960 and 1980. Methodological problems with the studies were common. Often concealment of randomization was inadequate and statistical analysis was inappropriate. The review showed that frequent screening with chest X-rays was associated with an 11% relative increase in the mortality from lung cancer compared with less frequent screening (RR 1.11, CI 1.00–1.23). The reasons for this were not clear. A non-statistically significant trend was observed for reduction in death from lung cancer when screening with chest X-ray and sputum cytology was compared with chest X-ray alone (RR 0.88, CI 0.74–1.03). Rather disappointingly, although resection rates were consistently higher in screened versus controlled groups this had no significant impact on mortality. There were no controlled studies of CT scanning in the literature at the time of this review.

Comment

This is a useful Cochrane Review, which collated the early trials of lung cancer screening using sputum cytology and chest radiography. The advantage of this review is that it looked at the effect of screening on mortality as reported in the literature. The surprising result was the apparent increase in mortality in the treatment group. The reasons for this are not understood. Results from these trials have led to the abandonment of plain X rays as a screening tool. The recent report by Henschke of screening with low dose spiral CT scanning has been augmented by a further report of the findings on repeat screening. A similar trial has also been reported from the Mayo Clinic. A third, much larger study, over 3 years from a Japanese group has also appeared in the literature.

Early lung cancer action project: initial findings on repeat screening.

Henschke GI, Naidich DP, Yankelevitz DF, *et al. Cancer* 2001; **92**: 153–9.

B A C K G R O U N D . The initial publication of the ELCAP reported the preliminary result of screening of a cohort of 1000 patients. This paper reported on the initial findings of repeat screening of this cohort.

I N T E R P R E T A T I O N . One thousand, one hundred and eighty-four annual repeat screenings were performed on the initial cohort of 1000 patients. A positive result was deemed the detection of a new non-calcified nodule with interim growth. A diagnostic algorithm for investigating abnormalities picked up on the screening test was constructed to try to separate benign from malignant lesions. There were 30 positive screens (2.5%). Two of these patients died from unrelated causes before the diagnostic work-up could be completed. Nodules resolved in another 12. In the remaining 16, half had absence of further growth documented by repeat CT scanning, leaving 8 with a growing nodule. All 8 were biopsied and cancer was found in 7 (6 non-small cell, 1 small cell). Of the non-small cell tumours, 5 were Stage Ia and one was Stage IIIa. The small cell lesion was of limited extent. The median size of the nodules found was 8 mm. In another 2 subjects symptoms prompted an interim diagnosis of endobronchial disease (Stage IIb non-small cell lung cancer [NSCLC] and one limited disease small cell). These two were obviously not picked up by annual screening.

Comment

Unlike the original publication, false-positive screening test results were uncommon. These were also usually manageable without biopsy. It appeared that screening annually would allow for earlier diagnosis of more curable tumours. What is uncertain is whether this approach will improve life expectancy in patients about to develop lung cancer. The paper also did not address the problem whether screening would be cost effective. The authors anticipated that screening an individual would cost less than $50 000, which they felt was acceptable. Obviously this figure would have to be extrapolated to all those at risk of lung cancer in their age group.

Screening for lung cancer with low dose spiral computed tomography.

Swensen SJ, Jett JR, Sloan JA, *et al. Am J Respir Crit Care Med* 2002; **165**: 508–13.

BACKGROUND. Much interest in screening for lung cancer with low dose CT was aroused by the original ELCAP report. This publication describes a similar study in a different part of the United States.

INTERPRETATION. One thousand five hundred and twenty individuals were enrolled into the study over a one-year period. They were aged >50 and had to have at least 20 pack-years smoking history. Individuals were recruited from television and newspaper adverts. All subjects recruited to the study had an initial prevalence scan and then 3 annual incidence scans. Annual sputum cytology was also performed. Two thousand, two hundred and forty-four scans were performed in the initial population of 1520 patients. Uncalcified lung nodules were found in 1000 participants (66% of the study population). Only 25 subjects were actually found to have lung cancer after extensive investigations. This represented 1.7% of participants and only 1.1% of abnormal nodules detected. Of these 25, 22 were non-small cell and 3 small cell. Twenty-two of the 25 were picked up on the prevalence scan and 3 on the annual incidence scan. Fifty-seven per cent of the non-small cell tumours were Stage Ia. Seven patients went on to have benign disease resected as this was the only method of making a diagnosis.

Comment

The authors have shown it is possible to perform screening in a large population of patients but as with other studies, there was no evidence that early detection would translate into a lowering of mortality. There was an extremely high false positive rate and it would be anticipated that much anxiety would be raised by these falsely positive scans. This low specificity should render this screening method as prohibitively expensive. Once again, the authors call for a randomized controlled trial to assess whether screening for lung cancer with low dose spiral CT scan is both effective in prolonging survival and is cost-effective.

Results of three-year mass screening programme for lung cancer using mobile low dose spiral computed tomography scanner.

Sone S, Li F, Yang ZG, *et al. Br J Cancer* 2001; **84**: 25–32.

BACKGROUND. The first reports of using low dose CT scanning as a screening tool have appeared from North America. Is lung cancer screening feasible in other parts of the world?

INTERPRETATION. This was a large project evaluating the usefulness of annual screening by spiral CT in the Japanese population. Five thousand, four hundred and eighty-three subjects were recruited to the trial. Their ages ranged from 40–74. Forty-six per cent were women. Interestingly, 54% of the cohort had never smoked with 94% of the female population being life-long non-smokers. Twenty per cent of the male participants had never smoked. After their initial CT scan in 1996, the cohort was scanned annually in 1997 and 1998. Thirteen thousand, seven hundred and eighty-six scans had been performed at the time of the report. On the initial screening scan 279 (5.1%) nodules were found. Twenty-two (8% of nodules found) turned out to have lung cancer. In the subsequent annual screening scan of 1997 subjects remaining in the trial, 173 (3.9% of 4425) had abnormalities of which 25 (14%) had lung cancer. The following year the cohort had fallen to 3878 and 136 (3.5%) had abnormalities on their scans. Nine (7%) of these had lung cancer. The authors calculated that the sensitivity and specificity for CT scanning in the initial scan was 55% and 95%. This rose to 83% and 97% in the subsequent annual scan. Eighty-eight per cent of the lung cancers found were Stage Ia and were treated surgically.

Comment

The power of the study is limited by the fact that there are small numbers of cases of lung cancer compared with other screening programmes. This is the largest cohort of patients screened by CT scanning but unfortunately the selection process allowed a high percentage of patients who were at very low risk of lung cancer to be included. The fact that more than half the patients in the study had never smoked is almost certainly the explanation for this. In addition, patients were younger (average age 63 years) and a high proportion (64%) was female. The strength of the study lies in the completeness of the data and follow-up. As with other screening studies, the majority of lung cancers found were at early stage. The following paper looked at the relationship between the size of the primary tumour and stage, as clearly this has major implications for lung cancer screening.

Stage distribution in patients with a small (<3 cm) primary non-small cell lung cancer: implications for lung cancer screening.

Hayneman LE, Herndon JE, Goodman PC, Patz EF. *Cancer* 2001; **92**: 3051–5.

BACKGROUND. There has been much interest in using low dose CT scanning to detect lung cancer. For this screening to work it is assumed that smaller primary tumours are detected at an earlier stage than larger tumours. This study looked at the stage distribution of small primary NSCLC.

INTERPRETATION. This was a retrospective study looking at 620 patients with pathologically proven NSCLC <3 cm in diameter over a 20-year period. All tumours had been resected and their pathology and imaging was reviewed retrospectively to confirm the size of the primary tumour and the stage of disease at presentation. No statistical relation between stage distribution and the size of the primary lesion was found. This suggested that the detection of small tumours using screening CT might not result in a shift to an earlier stage distribution. Five hundred and sixteen patients (83%) with these small tumours were Stage I but 47 patients (8%) had Stage IV disease with a primary tumour <3 cm in diameter. The mean tumour size in Stage I was 1.93 cm and those in Stage IV 1.99 cm. This suggested that size had very little to do with the biology of the tumour.

Comment

This study cast doubt about the likelihood that screening for lung cancer using CT scanning which picks up small primary tumours could shift the stage distribution of patients. However, the patients included in the study had been referred to a tertiary centre and may be a biased population not accurately reflecting those in a screened population. Once again, the importance of a trial looking to show a change in mortality was stressed.

Screening of 'at risk' populations

The results of the CT screening trials have been encouraging with good pick-up rates in prevalence scans but so far rather disappointing results with repeat screening. This has led some workers to look at screening populations who are at higher risk of lung cancer. The earlier CT studies use cohorts of smokers in middle adult life. Occupational asbestos exposure is known to be a risk factor for lung cancer. A report has recently appeared looking at the potential benefits of screening a population of workers who have been exposed to asbestos.

Computed tomography screening for lung cancer in asbestos-exposed workers.
Tiitola M, Kivisaari L, Huuskonen MS, *et al. Lung Cancer* 2002; **35**: 17–22.

BACKGROUND. The benefits of screening a population of high-risk subjects is not known. This study looked at CT screening for lung cancer of asbestos-exposed workers with known occupational disease.

INTERPRETATION. Finnish physicians enrolled 602 patients (11 women) into the trial. There were 85 cases of asbestosis and 601 of bilateral pleural plaques. Smoking was not an inclusion criterion for the patients with asbestosis. Mean age was 63 years (range 38–81). Mean exposure to asbestos was 26 years. Average smoking history was 24 pack years. All were construction workers. Subjects were interviewed using a standardized questionnaire and were imaged with low dose spiral CT scans and chest radiography. The screening detected 111 patients with non-calcified nodules greater than 0.5 cm in diameter. Sixty-six of them were referred for further hospital examination. Five lung cancers were found (106 false-positive scans). Three cases were potentially operable. There was one false-negative FNA biopsy. After 3 years of follow-up two new lung cancers were reported with no evidence of tumour in the retrospective analysis of the screening by CT scan. The study did not generate enough data for a proper evaluation of the cost-effectiveness of screening this type of population. The results of screening in this study are summarized in Fig. 16.1.

Comment

Once again, CT scanning was capable of finding early lung cancers in a group with considerable asbestos-related pleural and lung pathology. It is perhaps surprising that the false-positive rate was not even higher than the previously reported American studies. Of the study population, 18.4% had abnormal scans compared with 23% in the ELCAP study and more than 60% in the Mayo Clinic project. The patients in this study were younger than in the American trials although it could be argued had a higher risk of lung cancer because of their occupational exposure to asbestos. In addition, the patients screened in the Finnish study had lower smoking

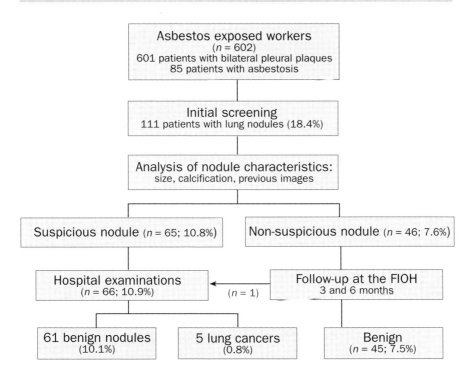

Fig. 16.1 CT screening for lung cancer. Source: Tiitola *et al.* (2002).

histories in terms of total pack years. Further results from repeat screening from this group are awaited.

The lung cancer screening trials reported above gave detection rates at baseline screening which ranged from 0.5–2.7%. This large variability in lung cancer detection almost certainly reflects the differing lung cancer risk between the populations screened. Patients included in these trials had variable smoking histories. Some of the trials even included non-smokers. There is also a wide age range of patients included in the studies. Obviously, to make spiral CT scanning cost-effective in reducing lung cancer mortality it would be rational to scan a population at higher risk. The National Cancer Institute and the American Cancer Society have sponsored a series of international meetings to refine the selection criteria for participation in lung cancer screening trials with spiral CT.

Lung cancer screening by spiral CT. What is the optimal target population for screening trials?

Van Klaveren RJ, de Koning HJ, Mulshine J, Hirsch FR. *Lung Cancer* 2002; **38**: 243–52.

B A C K G R O U N D . **Is it possible to optimize the efficiency of lung cancer screening by spiral CT by targeting a specific population?**

I N T E R P R E T A T I O N . This group from Holland and the United States provide recommendations for the selection of the optimal target population for lung cancer screening trials with spiral CT scanning based on an analysis of risk factors and high-risk populations. The variables considered were smoking history, age, fitness for surgery, history of previous cancer, body weight and previous pneumonectomy. The authors reviewed the literature and found a close link between age and smoking habit. The incidence of lung cancer in a cohort of men aged between 45 and 49 years who smoked 20 cigarettes per day is 83/100 000 of the population. This rises to 1372/100 000 in the cohort of men of similar smoking habit who are aged between 70 and 74 years. The recommendation from this study was that the trial should include subjects with a smoking history of at least 30 years and an average consumption of at least 20 cigarettes per day. The risk of lung cancer falls after smoking cessation and it was decided that ex-smokers who had quit more than 5 years ago should be excluded from the trials. The selection criteria for participation in lung cancer screening trials was summarized in Table 16.1.

Comment

This review will allow future trials to be performed using groups of patients who are at the highest risk of lung cancer. This should improve the effectiveness of population screening of lung cancer with spiral CT scans. Lung cancer screening is a complex issue. The ultimate goal is to reduce lung cancer mortality and none of the trials performed so far have addressed this. If a benefit is there then it will

Table 16.1 Selection criteria for participation in lung cancer screening trials with spiral CT

Selection criteria

(Ex)-smokers who smoked on average ≥20 cigarettes a day for ≥30 years
Ex-smokers who quit <5 years
Men ≤70 years and women ≤75 years
A functional capacity which corresponds with: ≥4 MET (ACC/AHA), and/or the ability to climb
    ≥2 flight of stairs (36 steps) without rest
No previous pneumonectomy
Prior cancer is allowed if curatively treated ≥5 years ago without recurrence
No previous history of breast cancer, melanoma or hypernephroma
Weight <140 kg
Able to lie flat
Able to hold breath for 20 s
No chest CT scan within 1 year before enrolment
Able to sign the consent form
Long-term follow-up is feasible
Willing to undergo curative therapy if lung cancer is detected

Source: Van Klaveren *et al.* (2002).

undoubtedly come with costs both financial and otherwise. Cancer screening uses substantial health care resources and false-positive tests result in unnecessary anxiety as well as unnecessary and sometimes risky further procedures. We need to know whether the benefit of screening outweighs the harm and yet this benefit cannot be quantified and needs to be known before mass screening programmes are established.

Prevention of lung cancer

Introduction

Lung cancer is caused by cigarette smoking. Theories of carcinogenesis have been put forward and postulate that exposure to carcinogenic factors in cigarette smoke result in diffuse tissue damage in the bronchial epithelium. It is thought that cancer develops in a stepwise fashion with an accumulation of molecular alterations progressing through pre-invasive steps to invasive malignant disease. This pathway includes the development of cellular atypia, squamous metaplasia, dysplasia and carcinoma *in situ*. Suppressing one or more of the pre-invasive steps may impede the development of cancer. This has been attempted in the past in lung cancer using both natural and synthetic agents. The results of these chemoprevention studies, however, have been disappointing. The whole topic of the chemoprevention of lung cancer has been well reviewed in the two following papers.

Cigarette smoking and lung cancer: chemical mechanisms and approaches to prevention.

Hecht SS. *Lancet Oncology* 2002; **3**: 461–9.

BACKGROUND. What are the mechanisms by which cigarette smoking causes lung cancer and can this lead to the development of chemopreventative techniques?

INTERPRETATION. This is a comprehensive review of the chemical mechanisms involved in the development of lung cancer. Particular attention is paid to specific carcinogens in cigarette smoke which react with DNA resulting in DNA adducts that cause the genetic changes known in human lung cancer. The authors show the evidence for nicotine derived nitrosoaminoketone as being one of the most important carcinogenic compounds in tobacco smoke. Three important areas are discussed in relation to prevention: first, the variability of uptake of tobacco carcinogens by human lung tissue, with susceptibility to DNA damage being different in individuals with different smoke exposure; second, the differences in the metabolic activation and detoxification of carcinogens and third, a review of chemoprevention techniques in smokers and ex-smokers.

Comment

This review shows clearly that the chemical mechanisms for lung cancer induction are well understood. The results of chemoprevention of tobacco-related cancer in pre-clinical studies have been impressive. The challenge ahead is to demonstrate efficacy in humans.

Lung cancer chemoprevention: an integrated approach.

Lippman SM, Spitz MR. *J Clin Oncol* 2001; **19**: 74s–82s.

BACKGROUND. Is lung cancer chemoprevention a realistic strategy?

INTERPRETATION. This article reviews the history of chemoprevention for lung cancer. The results of definitive randomized controlled lung cancer chemoprevention trials are reviewed. These have taken place in three settings: primary prevention in healthy high-risk smokers, secondary prevention in patients known to have pre-malignant lesions and thirdly tertiary prevention of a second primary tumour in patients already treated for lung cancer. The results of these trials are summarized in the Table 16.2. All these trials have produced negative primary end-point results. In some trials there appear to be a harmful effect of the chemopreventive agent given in the hope of protecting the subject from the development of malignancy. The review looks to the future direction of lung cancer chemoprevention. This involves the development of new molecular targets in the highest risk subgroups of smokers and former smokers.

Table 16.2 Randomized lung cancer chemoprevention trials

Setting	Phase	No. of patients	Agents	Primary end-point
Primary	III			
Smokers		29 133	BC/vitamin E*	Harm/neutral
Smokers/asbestos		18 314	BC + retinal	Harm
Secondary	II			
Metaplasia		150	Etretinate	Neutral
Metaplasia		87	Isotretinain	Neutral
Metaplasia		68	Fenretinide	Neutral
Sputum atypia		73	Vitamin B_{12} + folic acid	Neutral
Sputum atypia		755	BC + retinal	Neutral
Tertiary	III (SPT)			
NSCLC		307	RP	Neutral
NSCLC + HNC		2592	NAC/RP*	Neutral/neutral
NSCLC		1166	Isotretinain	Neutral

BC, beta-carotene; SPT, second primary tumour; NSCLC, non-small-cell lung cancer; HNC, head and neck cancer; NAC, N-acetylcysteine; RP, retinyl palmitate.
* 2 × 2 factorial design.

Source: Lippman *et al.* (2001).

Comment

The results of lung cancer chemoprevention are disappointing. A point of interest is the apparent increase in risk of lung cancer in some of the studies. In the Caret study |5|, prevention of lung cancer was attempted with beta-carotene plus retinol (Vitamin A) in a placebo-controlled fashion in 18 314 asbestos workers and smokers. The trial was terminated when it became clear that there was a significant (28%) increase in lung cancer incidence occurring in patients taking active treatment, with a total increase in mortality of 17%. The significance of this increase was related to an increase in current smokers taking active treatment. It has been postulated that carcinogenesis was actually enhanced when high tissue concentrations of beta-carotene interacted with oxidative tobacco smoke. A similar result was seen in the trial of isotretinoin published in 2001.

Randomized phase III intergroup trial of Isotretinoin to prevent second primary tumours in Stage I non-small cell lung cancer.

Lippman SM, Lee JJ, Karp DD, *et al. J Natl Cancer Inst* 2001; **93**: 605–18.

BACKGROUND. Patients who have been cured of lung cancer are at increased risk of a second lung tumour compared with the normal population. This study investigated

whether treatment with Isotretinoin could prevent secondary primary tumours in this population.

INTERPRETATION. This was a randomized phase III trial of 1166 Stage I NSCLC patients who had been treated by surgery. Patients were recruited to the trial between 6 weeks and 3 years from resection. No patient had prior radiotherapy or chemotherapy. Subjects were randomized to treatment with placebo or to the retinoid Isotretinoin 30 mg daily for 3 years. The primary end-point of the study was the time to development of a second primary tumour and the secondary end-points were the time to recurrence of their original tumour or death. The median follow-up of patients was 3.5 years. There was no difference between Isotretinoin or placebo in all end-points. The hazard ratio of the development of a second primary tumour for the treated group compared with placebo was 1.08 (95% confidence interval: 0.78–1.49), for recurrence of tumour was 0.99 (0.76–1.29) and for overall mortality was 1.07 (0.84–1.35). Smoking was a much more important predictor of recurrence, mortality and the development of a second primary than treatment with isotretinoin. The hazard ratio if the subject was a current smoker increased to 3.11 (1–9.7) for recurrence and 4.39 (1.11–17.294) for mortality in the treatment group. Mucocutaneous toxicity and non-compliance was a problem with the treatment group in this study (40% in the treatment arm and 25% in the placebo arm withdrawing from the study in 3 years).

Comment

This trial produced a negative result for the use of a retinoid in protecting patients with resected lung cancer developing second tumours or from delaying recurrence or improving overall mortality. Significant toxicity of the treatment was seen and this led to high levels of non-compliance.

Perhaps more worrying is an apparent effect of increased recurrence and mortality when patients in the treatment group continued to smoke.

Chemoprevention of lung cancer is still an attractive concept. More is now known about the mechanisms by which tumours appear in the lungs of smokers. Newer protective agents are required and these will only be produced with an increased understanding of the underlying carcinogenesis of lung cancer.

References

1. Flehinger BJ, Melamed MR, Zaman MB, *et al.* Early lung cancer detection: results of the initial (prevalence) radiologic and cytologic screening in the Memorial Sloan-Kettering Study. *Am Rev Respir Dis* 1984; **130**: 555–60.
2. Frost JK, Ball WC, Levin ML, *et al.* Early lung cancer detection: results of the initial (prevalence) radiologic and cytologic screening in the John's Hopkins Study. *Am Rev Respir Dis* 984; **130**: 549–54.

3. Fontana RS, Sanderson DR, Taylor WF, *et al*. Early lung cancer detection: results of the initial (prevalence) radiologic and cytologic screening in the Mayo Clinic Study. *Am Rev Resp Dis* 1984; **130**: 561–70.

4. Henschke CI, McCauley DI, Yankelevitz DF, *et al*. Early lung cancer action project: overall design and findings from baseline screening. *Lancet* 1999; **354**: 99–105.

5. Omenn GS, Goodman GE, Thornquist MD, *et al*. Effects of a combinaion of beta carotene and vitamin A on lung cancer and cardiovascular disease. *N Engl J Med* 1996; **334**: 1150–5.

17

Diagnosis and staging of lung cancer

Diagnosis and staging

Introduction

In general, making the diagnosis of lung cancer is not particularly difficult. Most patients present with new respiratory symptoms and the diagnosis is suspected when a chest radiograph is performed. It is known that up to 95% of patients with lung cancer have an abnormal chest X-ray. The next important step is obtaining a histological diagnosis. This is done either at bronchoscopy or by performing a transthoracic biopsy of the lung. In other patients, a histological diagnosis is achieved by sampling metastatic disease in mediastinal lymph nodes or in sites of a distant metastasis. Once a histological diagnosis is confirmed, it is important to stage the patient accurately. This is vital in selecting appropriate management and for giving an estimate of prognosis. Currently patients are staged using standard chest radiography and computed tomography (CT) scanning. Other specific scans of bone, brain, liver and adrenals may also establish the extent of disease. There have been a number of recent advances in the diagnostic and staging procedures performed in lung cancer. Perhaps the most significant development has been the introduction of positron emission tomography (PET) scanning.

PET scanning

PET scanning is based on the principle that cancer cells have a higher rate of glycolysis and an increased cellular uptake of glucose than non-cancer cells. A labelled tracer, 18 fluorodeoxyglucose (FDG) is taken up into cells, metabolically trapped and accumulates. [18]FDG is a positron emitter and, therefore, can be measured using a scanner. PET, therefore, provides evidence of metabolic activity in tumour cells.

The place of PET scanning in the evaluation of lung cancer is being formulated. Two important reviews have appeared in the year 2001. The first is a meta-analysis and the second a systematic review.

Accuracy of positron emission tomography for diagnosis of pulmonary nodules and mass lesions. A meta-analysis.

Gould MK, McLean CC, Kushner WG, *et al. JAMA* 2001; **285**: 914–24.

BACKGROUND. Controversy exists over the management of solitary pulmonary nodules. CT scanning is useful especially if calcification can be demonstrated suggesting a benign aetiology. A decision whether nodules should be biopsied, resected or followed-up, however, has to be made. There has been much interest in the use of PET scanning to see whether the sensitivity and specificity of CT scanning could be improved. This is a meta-analysis to estimate the diagnostic accuracy of PET scanning for nodules and mass lesions.

INTERPRETATION. Standard meta-analysis techniques were used to find studies concerning PET scanning published between 1966 and 2000. Reports in all languages were considered. Studies with greater than 10 patients were included if there were at least 5 malignant diagnoses and the sensitivity and specificity for malignancy were calculated. Of the 727 potentially relevant studies of PET scanning in lung cancer, only 40 were eligible. These involved 1474 patients with a median prevalence of malignancy of 72%. The sensitivity of PET scanning was calculated at 96.8% (range 83–100%) and the specificity at 77.8% (52–100%). Only 8 patients had nodules less than 1 cm in diameter. Of these, 3 patients had false-negative results. In lesions bigger than 1 cm diagnostic accuracy did not depend on the size of the lesion ($P = 0.43$). Both qualitative and semi-quantitative methods of reporting the scans were used. FDG imaging with a modified gamma camera was considered and three studies that compared PET with FDG imaging with gamma camera were included. There were no differences between these techniques in terms of sensitivity and specificity but the numbers were extremely small.

Comment

This is a useful study looking at the current literature on the diagnostic accuracy of PET scanning. It should be concluded that it is an accurate non-invasive imaging test for the evaluation of solidary pulmonary nodules and masses. The technique is not, however, particularly sensitive or specific in small nodules (<1 cm). Its high cost, however, may prevent its routine use in many parts of the world.

Positron emission tomography in the diagnosis and staging of lung cancer: a systematic, quantitative review.

Fischer BM, Mortensen J, Hojgaard L. *Lancet Oncology* 2001; **2**(11): 659–66.

BACKGROUND. How useful a diagnostic tool is positron emission tomography in terms of sensitivity, specificity and accuracy in the diagnostic evaluation of small cell lung cancer (SCLC)?

INTERPRETATION. A systematic literature search was carried out using Medline, Embase databases and the Cochrane Controlled Trials Register. Fifty-five original works on the diagnostic performance of PET in the investigation of non-small cell lung cancer (NSCLC) were identified. For the diagnosis of NSCLC the mean sensitivity and specificity were 96% and 78% for dedicated PET and 92% and 86% for gamma camera PET. In the mediastinal staging of NSCLC the corresponding results were 83% and 96% for dedicated PET and 81% and 95% for gamma camera PET.

Comment

These results are similar to the previous review showing that PET scanning in lung cancer has a high sensitivity and specificity when compared with CT scanning. Information is now required on just where PET scanning should be placed in the diagnostic work-up of patients. For instance, how important is it to confirm positive findings in PET scanning? An important study looking at this appeared in the literature in 2001.

Mediastinal lymph node sampling following positron emission tomography with fluorodeoxyglucose imaging in lung cancer staging.

Gupta NC, Tamim WJ, Graeber GG, Bishop HA, Hobbs GR. *Chest* 2001; **120**(2): 521–7.

BACKGROUND. What is the predictive accuracy of PET scanning in detecting metastatic intrathoracic lymph node involvement in patients with NSCLC?

INTERPRETATION. Seventy-seven patients with suspected or proven NSCLC underwent CT and PET-FDG scanning. The results of these scans were correlated with the histological findings of hilar and mediastinal lymph node sampling using mediastinoscopy, open biopsy, thoracotomy and thoracotomy with resection. Patients were then classified into resectable and unresectable depending initially on PET results correlated to histological findings. The sensitivity, specificity and accuracy of CT scanning was 68%, 61% and 63%. PET scanning gave much better results (87%, 91% and 82%). The change of management with routine sampling following PET was seen in five of six patients with false-positive findings but none in four patients with false-negative findings. False-negative results did not change management in these patients.

Comment

This study suggests that the addition of PET scanning to conventional CT scanning might save unnecessary sampling procedures and thoracotomy in patients with lung cancer.

Can PET scanning save futile thoracotomies?

Despite widely published guidelines for the assessment of patients for resection, a significant number (up to 50%) of patients undergoing potentially curative surgery for suspected NSCLC, end up having recurrence of disease or peri-operative morbidity and mortality. It is known that PET scanning is more accurate than conventional staging in the diagnosis of NSCLC. There has been no evidence in the literature, however, that PET scanning could lead to better selection of patients for surgery. An important trial was reported in 2002 addressing this issue.

Effectiveness of positron emission tomography in the preoperative assessment of patients with suspected non-small cell lung cancer: the PLUS multi-centre randomized trial.

Van Tinteren H, Hoekstra OS, Smit EF, *et al. Lancet* 2002; **359**: 1388–93.

BACKGROUND. Can PET scanning lead to a reduction in the number of futile thoracotomies for patients with potentially resectable NSCLC?

INTERPRETATION. This was a randomized controlled trial reported from the Netherlands. One hundred and eighty-eight patients from nine hospitals were randomly allocated to either conventional work-up (CW) or conventional work-up and PET scanning (CW + PET) prior to surgical assessment. Patients were followed up for one year post-operatively. The primary end-point of the study was the rate of futile thoracotomies in each group. A futile thoracotomy was defined as an operation on a patient who had benign disease, an open and closed case, pathological N2 disease, or post-operative relapse or death within 12 months of randomization. Analysis was by intention to treat. Ninety-six patients were randomized to the CW group and 92 to the CW + PET. Two patients in the CW + PET group did not undergo PET scanning. Eighteen patients in the CW group and 32 in the CW + PET group did not go on to have a thoracotomy after mediastinoscopy. In the CW group 39 (41%) patients had a futile thoracotomy compared with 19 (21%) in the CW + PET group. This gave a relative reduction in futile thoracotomies of 51% (95% CI 32–80, $P = 0.003$).

Comment

This study showed for the first time that pre-operative PET scanning could have an influence on treatment decisions and outcomes. The rate of futile thoracotomies in the CW group would appear to be high (41%) compared with many centres. However, PET scanning saved many futile operations. It is likely that PET scanning, therefore, will improve the results of surgery by allowing surgeons to operate on more patients with potentially curable disease.

PET scanning in small cell lung cancer

Small cell lung cancer accounts for about 25% of all cases of lung cancer diagnosed annually. Most patients have metastatic disease at presentation and the staging of this disease is usually divided into 'limited' (where the disease is confined to one hemithorax) or 'extensive' where tumour has spread outside the ipsilateral thorax. The standard approach to staging includes CT scanning, brain or magnetic resonance imaging (MRI) scanning, bone marrow biopsy or a bone scan and liver ultrasound. PET scanning has been shown to be more accurate and sensitive than CT scanning in staging mediastinal disease in NSCLC. Data is only now appearing concerning the usefulness of PET scanning in staging patients with small cell histology.

Whole body FDG-PET for the evaluation and staging of small cell lung cancer: a preliminary study.
Chin R, McCain TW, Miller AA, *et al. Lung Cancer* 2002; **37**: 1–6.

BACKGROUND. Does PET scanning have any additional advantage over standard staging tests in patients with SCLC?

INTERPRETATION. This prospective study performed in the United States involved 18 patients with SCLC who underwent total body FDG-PET in addition to conventional staging procedures. The agreement between PET and conventional scanning in identifying metastatic disease and, therefore, correctly staging disease was assessed. Overall FDG-PET agreed with conventional staging examinations in 15 out of 18 (83%) patients. Eight had extensive and seven limited disease. PET scanning showed disease that was more extensive in two of the three patients where there was disagreement between the two staging methods.

Comment

This was a small prospective study looking at the usefulness of PET scanning as a single test to stage SCLC. The results indicate that PET scanning could find disease that was missed by other scans and suggested that this procedure may be able to replace the combination of current imaging modalities. This would be extremely helpful for the patient in that a single attendance for a scan would be all that was required for accurate staging. The exception for this would be patients with brain metastasis. No patient in this study had brain metastasis but PET scanning is not as useful as MRI in this situation as glucose uptake in the brain is extremely high.

FDG-PET imaging for the staging and follow-up of small cell lung cancer.

Schumaker T, Brink I, Mix M, *et al. Eur J Nucl Med* 2001; **28**: 483–8.

BACKGROUND. Does PET scanning have any additional advantage over standard staging tests in patients with SCLC?

INTERPRETATION. Thirty patients were included in this study, which compared PET scanning with the currently recommended staging procedures. Thirty-six PET scans were performed. In 24 patients, the scan was done as a primary staging of the disease, in four at follow-up after treatment and in two patients both as primary staging and as follow-up. Identical results for PET scanning and conventional investigations were seen in 23 of 36 patients. Six had limited disease, 12 extensive disease, and in five no disease was found (follow-up scans). In seven patients, PET scanning upstaged patients to extensive disease. There were discordant results in five patients with respect to disease in lung, bone, liver and adrenal glands but this did not affect the overall staging. Table 17.1 summarizes concordance and discordance of PET with conventional scanning. PET scanning was found to be more sensitive for the detection of mediastinal and hilar lymph nodes and bone metastases.

Comment

The results of this study are similar to the previous trial. Once again, PET scanning found disease not seen by conventional methods. The numbers, however, were small. Before PET scanning can replace conventional investigations in SCLC, comparative studies with pathological confirmation are required before the accuracy and cost-effectiveness can be fully evaluated. In addition, where FDG-PET and conventional scanning differ, survival data may indicate which staging protocol most optimally determines prognosis and, therefore, can guide treatment.

Table 17.1 Summary of FDG-PET results and rate of concordance and discordance with respect to the sum of conventional examinations

	Concordant with other examinations	Discordant with other examinations
Patients (*n* = 30)	17 (57%)	13 (43%)
Investigations (*n* = 36)	23 (64%)	13 (36%)
Tumour localizations (*n* = 77)	60 (78%)	17 (22%)
		PET confirmed: 11
		PET disproved: 3
		Unknown: 3

Source: Schumaker *et al.* (2001).

Safety of transthoracic needle biopsy

Transthoracic needle biopsy of lung lesions is traditionally performed as an outpatient procedure. The most common major complication is pneumothorax. The incidence of post-lung biopsy pneumothorax in the literature varies between 5 and 57% with between 1.6 and 17% requiring chest tube insertion. It has been estimated that most pneumothoraces occur within 30 minutes of the biopsy. In a large retrospective study of 673 procedures |1| the optimum time for performing a post-biopsy chest radiograph was assessed. Eighty-eight per cent of pneumothoraces were detected immediately but the authors recommended both 1- and 4-hour post-biopsy radiographs. This obviously involves the patient having to stay in the hospital for a significant time, which may be difficult in a busy X-ray department. The following study assessed whether it was possible to discharge patients within 30 minutes if there was no immediate pneumothorax.

Transthoracic needle biopsy of the lung: results of early discharge in 506 out-patients.
Dennie CJ, Matzinger FR, Marriner JR, Maziak DE. *Radiology* 2001; **219**: 247–51.

BACKGROUND. This was a study determining the safety of early discharge (30 minutes) after transthoracic needle biopsy of the lung.

INTERPRETATION. This was a prospective study of 506 consecutive lung biopsies. Four hundred and forty patients underwent FNA only and 66 patients also had a core biopsy. Patients were discharged after a 30-minute post-biopsy chest film if there was no pneumothorax. Patients who had an asymptomatic pneumothorax were kept for a further 30 minutes and were followed up one day and/or one week after biopsy to identify late complications. Patients with symptomatic or enlarging pneumothorax were treated with an 8F pigtail catheter and a Heimlich valve as an outpatient and followed up 24 hours later for chest tube removal. The pneumothorax rate in the study was 22.9%. Eight-one of these 116 patients had asymptomatic pneumothoraces and only 33 (6.5%) had a pigtail catheter inserted. Seven patients developed a pneumothorax after discharge and two patients (0.4%) had to undergo large-bore chest tube insertion. There were no deaths or major complications.

Comment

This study suggested that an observation period of 30 minutes after lung biopsy might be sufficient for patients without a pneumothorax. The authors constructed a post-biopsy treatment algorithm (Fig. 17.1).

One of the limitations of the study was there was no control group in which a more traditional 1- or 4-hour post-biopsy film was taken. The authors concluded,

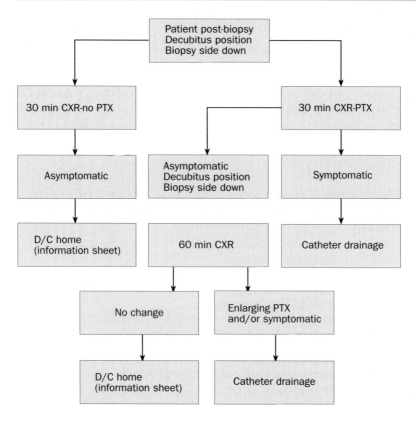

Fig. 17.1 Flow chart shows the proposed patient treatment algorithm after lung biopsy. CXR = chest radiograph, D/C = discharged, PTX = pneumothorax. Source: Dennie *et al.* (2001).

however, that discharge 30 minutes after lung biopsy in the absence of a pneumothorax is a safe approach.

Endoscopic ultrasound in the staging of lung cancer

CT scanning remains the mainstay of imaging the mediastinum but has limited sensitivity and specificity for detecting nodal involvement. Large benign reactive nodes are frequently present in patients with a lung primary and conversely micrometastasis may exist in normal-sized lymph nodes. The finding of enlarged nodes on the CT scan, usually leads to mediastinoscopy or mediastinotomy to obtain histological proof of involvement. These procedures are invasive and have a small but significant morbidity. Endoscopic ultrasound (EUS) is a new technique by which a modified endoscope with ultrasound transducer on its tip allows unparalleled views of structures adjacent to the gut lumen. Scanning from the oesophagus, therefore, gives excellent views of the subcarinal space and the posterior mediastinum. This is an area where mediastinoscopy may be difficult. There have been studies in recent years reporting on the use of EUS in the staging of the mediastinum in lung cancer. The great advantage of this procedure over CT scanning is that it is possible to sample the lymph nodes by fine needle aspirate, thus allowing differentiation of benign from malignant nodes.

Evaluation of mediastinal lymphadenopathy with endoscopic, ultrasound-guided fine needle aspiration biopsy.

Wiersema MJ, Vazquez-Sequeiros, Wiersema LM. *Radiology* 2001; **219**: 252–7.

BACKGROUND. How safe and accurate is endoscopic ultrasound-guided fine needle aspiration (FNA) biopsy of mediastinal lymph nodes.

INTERPRETATION. Eighty-six patients with mediastinal lymphadenopathy were examined by EUS. In 29, the patients were known to have NSCLC and the EUS was part of the staging procedure. In the remaining 57, it was performed to obtain a primary diagnosis. Final diagnosis was based on clinical follow-up and/or surgical results. In 82 patients in whom a final diagnosis was available (35 benign, 47 malignant) a sensitivity, specificity, accuracy, negative and positive predicted value of endoscopic ultrasound FNA in distinguishing benign from malignant nodes was 96, 100, 98, 94 and 100%

Table 17.2 Comparison of endoscopic US-guided FNAB results with surgical pathologic, cytologic, or extended clinical follow-up results in patients with mediastinal lymphadenopathy

Endoscopic US-guided FNAB*	Final diagnosis	
	Benign	Malignant
Benign	33	2
Inconclusive	2	0
Malignant	0	45
Total	35	47

Note data are numbers of patients.
* For endoscopic US-guided FNAB, the sensitivity was 96% (45/47; 95% CI: 85%, 99%); specificity. 100% (95% CI: 89%, 100%); accuracy, 98% (78/80; 95% CI: 91%, 100%); negative predictive value, 94% (33/35; 95% CI: 81%, 99%); positive predictive value, 100% (95% CI: 92%, 100%); and inconclusive test result rate, 2% (2/82; 95% CI: 0, 9%).

Source: Wiersema *et al.* (2001).

respectively. Ultrasound-guided FNA had superior accuracy compared with endoscopic ultrasound alone and CT alone (both 79%). The results of endoscopic ultrasound-guided FNA prompted a change to non-surgical management in 80% of the 82% who underwent the procedure. One minor complication (fever post-procedure) was encountered. This resolved with oral antibiotics.

Comment

Endoscopic ultrasound and FNA would appear to be accurate and safe for the evaluation of mediastinal nodes in the staging of NSCLC. It may be useful in establishing a primary diagnosis (Table 17.2).

 Endoscopic ultrasound-guided biopsy of mediastinal lesions has a major impact on patient management.
Larsen SS, Krasnik M, Vilmann P, *et al. Thorax* 2002; **57**(2): 98–103.

BACKGROUND. **Does endoscopic ultrasound-guided biopsy of the mediastinum change patient management in lung cancer?**

INTERPRETATION. Over a 6-year period 84 patients underwent EUS FNA. In all, CT scanning had shown a lesion in the mediastinum suspicious of malignancy. The history of each patient up to referral was reviewed by a Board of Thoracic Specialists to decide the further course if EUS FNA had not been available. This diagnostic strategy was compared with the actual clinical course after EUS FNA. EUS FNA had a sensitivity in this study of 92%, a specificity of 100% and an accuracy of 94%. In 18 of 37 patients (49%) thoracotomy/thoracoscopy was avoided as a result of EUS FNA and in 28 of 41 (68%) mediastinoscopy was avoided. A final diagnosis on EUS FNA of SCLC was made in eight patients resulting in a referral for chemotherapy, and in another three patients with benign disease specific treatment was initiated for sarcoidosis, abscess and benign tumour of the oesophagus. The accuracy of EUS FNA is summarized in Table 17.3.

Table 17.3 Comparison of EUS FNA results with final diagnoses obtained by thoracotomy, mediastinoscopy, or clinical follow-up in all patients (*n* = 84) suspected of mediastinal malignancy

Final diagnosis	EUS FNA		
	Malignant	Benign	Total
Malignant	54	5	59
Inconclusive	0	5	5
Benign	0	20	20
Total	54	30	84

Source: Larsen *et al.* (2002).

Comment

This is another study showing the benefits of EUS FNA in a specific group of patients with suspected mediastinal involvement with lung cancer. The one drawback of this study was the use of a Board of Thoracic Specialist to review the patients' histories. There was a possibility of bias, as the study authors themselves formed the Panel assessing the impact of the test in question. Although the authors do not report this, it is likely that the procedure is cost effective as it saves a significant number of procedures.

EUS FNA should have a central role in the investigation of patients with mediastinal masses and in the staging of those with potentially resectable lung cancer. Comparative studies with PET scanning are needed before its place in the management of lung cancer is established. It certainly has the potential of saving a significant number of invasive procedures.

Reference

1. Perlmuth LM, Brann SD, Newman GE, *et al.* Timing of chest film follow-up after transthoracic needle aspiration biopsy. *Am J Roentgenol* 1986; **162**: 389–91.

18

Treatment of lung cancer

Introduction

Survival from lung cancer has not changed dramatically over the last two or three decades. The vast majority of patients present with advanced disease and are treated with palliative intent. Five-year survival has been reported from Europe and North America at around 6–15%. In most registry-based series, three-quarters of patients do not survive a year. Prolonged survival is related to surgical resection and radical radiotherapy. Multi-modality therapy for small cell lung cancer (SCLC) is also associated with a very small proportion of patients gaining significant improvement in life expectancy.

There have been a number of advances in lung cancer management over the last few years. This chapter deals with a number of these areas. Advances in surgical management include the better selection of patients for surgery, the value of systematic lymph node dissection and the place of pre-operative chemotherapy. Other issues include the management of a solitary metastasis in a patient with resectable disease and the use of surgical sealant for preventing air leaks.

Chemotherapy is now accepted treatment in the management of non-small cell lesions. This chapter will cover a number of different areas concerning dosage, scheduling and new agents in this area. In addition, the place of radiotherapy for both palliative and curative treatment will be covered.

Chemotherapy remains the treatment of choice for patients with small cell lesions. This condition is also sensitive to radiotherapy and the effectiveness of dual modality therapy has been accepted. What is unclear is how these treatments should be timed for optimal benefit. Other areas covered in the section on SCLC, include prophylactic cranial irradiation and the management of superior vena caval (SVC) obstruction.

The final section deals with two important topics. The first is the search for newer treatments for the management of patients with non-small cell lung cancer (NSCLC) and the second is some interesting work concerning how lung cancer patients who have received therapy should be followed-up.

Surgery

Selection of patients for surgery

Operative and survival rates for lung cancer appear to be higher in the United States and mainland Europe than in the United Kingdom. The reasons for this are not clear but possibly include the fact that patients may present later with more advanced disease in the United Kingdom, that they may have more co-morbidity and be less fit for surgery or that there is a general nihilistic approach amongst clinicians referring patients to surgeons. These factors may all lead to a lower resection rate. In order to address this problem the British Thoracic Society and the Society of Cardiothoracic Surgeons of Great Britain and Ireland formed a Working Party to write formal guidelines on the selection of patients with lung cancer for surgery. These were published in 2001 in Thorax.

Guidelines on the selection of patients with lung cancer for surgery.

British Thoracic Society and Society of Cardiothoracic Surgeons of Great Britain and Ireland Working Party. *Thorax* 2001; **56**: 89–108.

BACKGROUND. **Guidelines may be useful to improve the accuracy of the selection process for physicians, surgeons and oncologists who manage potentially operable patients.**

INTERPRETATION. The joint BTS/SCTS Working Party selected two major areas for concern as follows:

1 Fitness for surgery	2 Operability
a Age	a Diagnosis and staging
b Pulmonary function	b Adjuvant therapy
c Cardiovascular fitness	c Operations available
d Nutrition and performance status	d Locally advanced disease
e Small cell lung cancer	

The literature on these topics was examined in a systematic way, the evidence was considered and recommendations were based on the evidence graded according to the SIGN system. Altogether 53 recommendations were made covering the above areas. Of these recommendations, only four were at level A requiring at least one randomized controlled trial, 28 were at Grade B which requires well conducted clinical studies but no randomized trials, and 21 were at Grade C where there was absence of directly applicable studies of good quality. A useful algorithm showing assessment of fitness for surgery in terms of lung function was presented within the Guidelines.

Comment

These guidelines are thorough and cover all the contentious areas for patients undergoing thoracic surgery for lung cancer. Assessing patients' fitness for surgery is carefully considered and the guidelines allow clinicians to fit patients into high risk, average risk and low risk categories depending on both simple and complicated pulmonary function tests. The Guidelines are clearly evidence-based and are accompanied by an extensive literature review (182 references). They should provide an invaluable tool to the thoracic surgeons involved in the resection of lung cancer as well as to the clinicians who are referring lung cancer patients for resection.

The value of systematic lymph node dissection

The management of mediastinal lymph nodes during major pulmonary resection varies throughout the world. Surgical management ranges over a spectrum that extends from random sampling of suspicious nodes through systematic dissection of each mediastinal node station to radical block dissection of all mediastinal nodes and lymphatic vessels. The optimal approach remains the subject of debate. There is no doubt that the value of accurately determining node status cannot be over-emphasized. Without reliable staging, there can be no basis for comparison of results and ultimately no ability to compare treatment strategies. What is not known is whether systematic nodal dissection in resectable lung cancer has an impact on survival. Exponents of block dissection point to excellent long-term survival results with early stage disease and attribute this to the removal of lymph nodes. Others argue that this apparent enhanced survival results from an effect of staging whereby patients have simply been more accurately allocated to the relevant group. In the last year, two studies have appeared in the literature addressing the place of mediastinal lymph node dissection in patients with resectable disease. The first was a retrospective analysis and the second a randomized trial.

Should mediastinal nodal dissection be routinely undertaken in patients with peripheral small-sized (2 cm or less) lung cancer? Retrospective analysis of 225 patients.

Watanabe S, Oda M, Go T, et al. Eur J Cardio-Thoracic Surg 2001; 20: 1007–11.

BACKGROUND. Is systematic nodal dissection useful when resecting small peripheral lung cancers?

INTERPRETATION. This was a retrospective analysis performed from a surgical centre in Japan. Two hundred and twenty-five patients were included over a 25-year period. This represented 13.1% of resections. These subjects had a small (2 cm or less) peripheral tumour and they had undergone lobectomy and systematic nodal dissection. The vast majority (75.6%) had adenocarcinoma histology. Of these 170 patients, 38 (22.4%) showed hilar or mediastinal lymph node metastases. No metastases were encountered in all of the squamous cell carcinomas or in the small (less than 1 cm) adenocarcinomas and small cell lesions. The authors concluded that mediastinal nodal dissection was unnecessary in patients with peripheral small tumours fulfilling the following criteria:

1. squamous cell carcinoma less than 2 cm;

2. adenocarcinoma less than 1 cm;

3. localized bronchoalveolar cell carcinoma;

4. small cell carcinoma less than 1 cm.

The above criteria were satisfied by 28.4% of the 225 patients included in this study.

Comment

This study would suggest there is a subgroup of patients who could potentially benefit from systematic nodal dissection. The study, however, was retrospective and unrandomized.

A randomized trial of systemic nodal dissection in resectable non-small cell lung cancer.
Wu Y, Huang Z, Wang S, *et al. Lung Cancer* 2002; **36**: 1–6.

BACKGROUND. The usefulness of systematic nodal dissection in prolonging long-term survival and preventing local recurrence is still a matter of controversy in the surgical treatment of NSCLC.

INTERPRETATION. This was a randomized trial from China comparing systematic nodal dissection (SND) and mediastinal lymph node sampling (MLS) in resectable NSCLC. Five hundred and thirty-two patients were enrolled into the study, 268 were randomized to lung resection combined with SND and 264 were treated with lung resection combined with MLS. Patients with Stages I to IIIa were included. After surgical restaging only 471 cases were eligible for follow-up. Median survival was 59 months in the group given SND and 34 months in the MLS group. This was highly significant. Survival at each stage was increased by SND: Stage I five-year survival 82.16 versus 57.49%, Stage II 50.42 versus 34.05%, Stage IIIa 26.98 versus 6.18%. In a multivariate analysis, other factors shown to influence survival were tumour stage, size and the number of lymph node metastases (Table 18.1).

Comment

This trial seems to show major survival advantage for lymph node dissection. One possible confounding phenomenon, however, is that SND resulted in a significant stage migration. There were more Stage I (42 versus 24%) and fewer Stage IIIa cases (28 versus 48%) in patients undergoing lymph node sampling only. This suggests

Table 18.1 Characteristics of 471 eligible patients

	SND (*n* = 240)	MLS (*n* = 231)
Gender		
Male (%)	182 (76)	184 (80)
Female (%)	58 (24)	47 (20)
Age		
Range (years)	20–70	26–70
Median (years)	57.0	57.0
Pathology		
Squamous cell carcinoma (%)	93 (39)	89 (38)
Adenocarcinoma (%)	109 (45)	103 (45)
Other (%)	38 (16)	39 (17)
Stage (1997, UICC)		
I (%)	58 (24)	98 (42)
II (%)	67 (28)	69 (30)
IIIA (%)	115 (48)	64 (28)

SND, systematic nodal dissection; MLS, mediastinal lymph nodal sampling.

Source: Wu *et al.* (2002).

that MLS is less accurate in staging the disease and that stage migration may have influenced survival in this trial within stage subgroups. However, the survival advantage to the whole group randomized to surgery and SND was impressive, and it must be assumed that overall stage was similar in the two groups. No other differences were seen in the characteristics of the patients included in the study.

In addition, only scanty details of morbidity for the different surgical procedures were presented. The authors claim that SND is a safe procedure and should be the standard operation in NSCLC. Opponents of complete mediastinal lymph node dissection may draw different conclusions from the study.

Pre-operative chemotherapy

Results of surgical resection for lung cancer are closely related to the stage of disease at operation. The concept of 'down-staging' a patient who has advanced stage disease to an operable stage has generated much interest over the years. One concern of thoracic surgeons is that pre-operative treatment with cytotoxic drugs will delay 'effective' surgical resections and the use of these agents will increase operative morbidity and mortality. Pre-operative chemotherapy in more than 30 phase II trials has proved to be feasible at the expense of mild post-operative morbidity or mortality. In the last decade, three small, randomized trials have suggested impressive survival advantage for patients with Stage IIIa disease [1–3].

One of these studies [3] was initially criticized because of poor survival in the surgery alone group but the advantage of chemotherapy appeared to continue many years after the trial was completed. It is known that chemotherapy produces results that are more impressive if the tumour burden is small and, therefore, it is surprising perhaps that pre-operative chemotherapy has not been tried in better stage patients previously. It is likely this was due to worries from thoracic surgeons that patients who had operable (and, therefore, potentially curable) disease could not afford to wait while having chemotherapy and not only would their disease perhaps become inoperable but that the toxicity of chemotherapy would make thoracic resection more hazardous. A large trial examining the place of pre-operative chemotherapy in early stage NSCLC was published in 2002.

Pre-operative chemotherapy followed by surgery compared with primary surgery in resectable Stage I (except T_1N_0) II and IIIa non-small cell lung cancer.
Depierre A, Milleron B, Moro-Sibilot D, *et al. J Clin Oncol* 2001; **20**: 247–53.

B ACKGROUND . **This study was designed to evaluate whether pre-operative chemotherapy could improve survival in early stage NSCLC patients.**

I NTERPRETATION . This French randomized trial compared pre-operative chemotherapy to primary surgery in patients with early stage NSCLC. Chemotherapy consisted of two cycles of mitomycin, ifosfamide and cisplatin with two additional post-operative cycles for responding patients. In both arms of the study patients with T3 disease or N2 disease post-operatively received thoracic radiotherapy. Three hundred and fifty-five patients were randomized. Overall response to pre-operative chemotherapy was 64%. There were two pre-operative toxic deaths. Post-operative mortality was 6.7% in the chemotherapy arm and 4.5% in the primary surgery group. Median survival was 37 months (95% CI 26.7–48.3) for those patients getting pre-operative chemotherapy and 26 months (95% CI 19.8–33.6) for the primary surgery group ($P = 0.15$). Survival difference between arms increased from 3.8% at one year to 8.6% at 4 years. The benefit of pre-operative chemotherapy was most marked in patients with N0 and N1 disease. Disease-free survival time was significantly longer in the chemotherapy arm ($P = 0.033$) (Fig. 18.1).

Comment

Although impressive differences in median, 3 and 4-year survival, were observed between the groups, they were not statistically significant except for patients with Stage I and II disease. Patients who had T1N0 Stage Ia disease were not included in the trial. The lack of efficacy of pre-operative chemotherapy in Stage IIIa disease conflicts with the results of three previously published phase III trials. This lack of effect may be due to the efficacy of chemotherapy being poor in bulkier disease with drugs being more active on micrometastasis and not on local or regional lymphatic spread. This trial, which involved large numbers of patients, would seem to cast

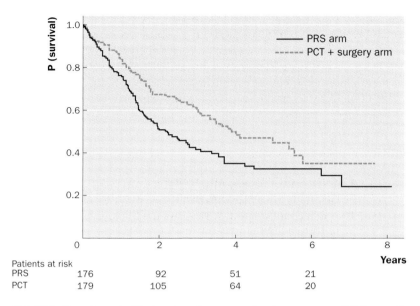

Patients at risk
PRS	176	92	51	21
PCT	179	105	64	20

Fig. 18.1 Overall survival by treatment arm: arm A, primary surgery (PRS); arm B, pre-operative chemotherapy (PCT) + surgery. Source: Depierre *et al.* (2001).

some doubt on the validity of earlier smaller studies in patients with more advanced disease. Results of ongoing trials including the MRC (LU22) trial in the UK and in Europe are eagerly awaited and hopefully, will allow the correct positioning of multimodality therapy in potentially operable patients.

Who should perform resections for lung cancer?

The influence of hospital volume on survival after resection for lung cancer.
Bach PB, Cramer LD, Schrag D, *et al. N Engl J Med* 2001; **345**: 181–8.

BACKGROUND. **It is known that there is wide variation in post-operative morbidity and mortality for many different surgical procedures depending upon the centre performing the operation. This study looked at the influence of volume of cases on survival after resection for lung cancer in a group of hospitals in the USA.**

INTERPRETATION. Information was extracted from the SSER database for lung cancer resections performed in 76 different hospitals in the United States for the period 1985–1996. The study involved 2118 patients. Survival and frequency of post-operative complications were the main end-points of the study. These results were then correlated with the annual workload of the hospital. Thirty-four of the 76 hospitals performed between one and three resections per year, 16 undertook 20–66 and two hospitals operated on between 67 and 100 cases per year. Five-year survival after surgery was 33% in the group of hospitals performing the least surgery and 44% in the two busiest hospitals. This was a significant difference ($P < 0.001$). There were no differences in lengths of stay. Post-operative complications were twice as high in the low volume hospital group (44 versus 20%). Teaching hospitals fared the same as non-teaching hospitals.

Comment

This study would appear to show that hospitals performing high numbers of operations had better outcomes in terms of 5-year survival and post-operative complications. Unfortunately, the study did not include data concerning case mix or co-morbidity. This is likely to have an effect on outcomes. There was also no data on adjuvant treatments performed which may have had an impact on survival. The authors concluded that it was possible to target variations in surgical care but did not conclude that the number of centres performing surgery should be reduced in order to keep workloads high. The evidence was that the already high volume hospitals could not cope with further work.

Surgical management of a synchronous solitary metastasis

The finding of a single metastatic lesion outwith the thorax makes patients with NSCLC inoperable and at Stage IV. Standard treatment in these patients would be chemotherapy. Retrospective studies, however, suggest that a small number of patients with solitary M1 disease may benefit from resection of both the primary and metastatic site of disease. The majority of experience in this area comes from the resection of a single brain metastasis followed by treatment of the primary tumour by thoracotomy |**4**|.

This form of management is controversial, however. Further reports concerning the management of isolated M1 disease have recently appeared in the literature. The first gives the long-term results of a combined resection policy and the second looks at the place of chemotherapy in this scenario.

Prolonged survival after extracranial metastasectomy from synchronous resectable lung cancer.

Ambrogi V, Tonini G, Mineo TC, *et al. Annals of Surg Oncol* 2001; **8**: 663–6.

B A C K G R O U N D . Is prolonged survival possible after combined resection of primary lung cancer and a solitary metastasis?

I N T E R P R E T A T I O N . This study was a retrospective analysis of a small group of NSCLC patients who were treated by resection of the primary tumour and surgical management of a synchronous solitary extracranial metastasis. These patients were accrued over a 7-year period. Nine patients were described. The single metastatic site was adrenal in five, cutaneous in two, axillary lymph node in one and kidney in one. The criteria for operating included a locally resectable primary tumour, non-small cell histology, no pre-operative evidence of N2 disease and complete resection of the proven metastasis. Resection was achieved in all patients, the primary tumour being treated by lobectomy. No mortality or major morbidity was reported. Five-year survival rate in this small group was 55.6% with five patients surviving more than 5 years. The 2 patients who were found to have N2 disease at surgery did not have prolonged survival.

Comment

This is a small series of patients but suggests that if carefully selected it may be possible to get prolonged survival in patients who have easily resectable primary disease and a single solitary extracranial metastasis that is amenable to surgery. The following study looks at the place of chemotherapy in these patients.

A phase II trial of chemotherapy and surgery for non-small lung cancer patients with a synchronous solitary metastasis.
Downey RJ, Ng KK, Kris MG, *et al. Lung Cancer* 2002; **38**: 193–7.

BACKGROUND. Is the combining of surgery and chemotherapy in solitary M1 disease feasible and of benefit to the patients?

INTERPRETATION. This was a prospective trial in patients with solitary synchronous M1 NSCLC with or without N2 disease. Treatment consisted of three cycles of mitomycin, vinblastine and cisplatin (MVP) chemotherapy followed by resection of all disease sites and then two cycles of VP therapy. Solitary brain metastases were to be resected before chemotherapy. Twenty-three patients were recruited over a 7-year period. Median age was 55 years. N2 involvement was seen in 12. M1 sites were brain (14), adrenal (3), bone (3), spleen (1), lung (1) and colon (1). Twelve patients completed all three cycles of induction chemotherapy and eight underwent resection. Five further patients were resected without completing induction chemotherapy. Eight patients completed post-operative chemotherapy. Median survival was 11 months only. Two patients survived 5 years without disease.

Comment

The results of this study are quite different to those observed in the surgery only trial. This was almost certainly due to the fact that patients with worse prognosis (known N2 disease) were included. The number of patients with this solitary M1 disease who qualified for the combined treatment was small. The induction chemotherapy was poorly tolerated and when compared to the historical experience of surgery alone overall survival was poor. These studies highlight the fact that surgical treatment of solitary M1 disease is still controversial, that in a small proportion of patients prolonged survival is possible and that the selection of patients for this form of treatment is crucial. Chemotherapy would seem to add little to surgery alone.

Management of post-operative air leaks

Surgical sealant for preventing air leaks after pulmonary resections in patients with lung cancer.
Rami R, Mateu M. *Cochrane Review*. The Cochrane Library, 2002;
4: Oxford: Update Software.

BACKGROUND. **Surgical sealants of different types have been developed to prevent or reduce post-operative air leaks. This systematic review was undertaken to evaluate the evidence of the effectiveness of this strategy.**

INTERPRETATION. Standard electronic medical databases, Medline, Embase and Cancerlit were searched to identify published trials concerning surgical sealant. Randomized controlled clinical trials were included, in which standard closure techniques plus a sealant were compared with the same intervention with no use of sealant in patients undergoing elective lung cancer resection. Two hundred and thirty-two patients from four trials were included in the review. In two trials, there were no differences between treatment and control patients in terms of reduction of duration of air leaks, chest tube drainage, hospital stay or complications. In the other two trials, post-operative air leaks were significantly reduced in the treatment groups but there were no differences in hospital stay, complications, chest tube drainage or cost.

Comment

A variety of surgical sealants has been used in thoracic surgery to prevent air leaks and to treat bronchopleural fistulae. The effectiveness of such sealants has not been fully established in patients with lung cancer undergoing lung resection. This review concluded that some sealants may have some beneficial effect in reducing post-operative air leaks but since the evidence was not uniform, the systematic use of surgical sealants in clinical practice could not be recommended by the review. The studies included in the review contained patients with other diseases than lung cancer and the heterogeneity of the underlying diseases of the patients may be responsible for some of the discrepancies in the results reported. In the trials where there were positive results, post-operative air leaks were reduced from 66 to 39% in the treatment group. Rather surprisingly, this did not translate into significant differences in hospital stay or other complications. Significantly, there were no significant cost savings from the use of sealants.

Chemotherapy for non-small cell lung cancer

Introduction

Chemotherapy has become accepted treatment for NSCLC. This follows the meta-analysis published in 1995 showing that the addition of chemotherapy to all other treatment modalities, including best supportive care, gave a significant survival advantage |6|. A number of important studies have appeared in the last year concerning various aspects of chemotherapy in NSCLC. The first looked at the new generation of drugs that have appeared. The second concerned a comparison of platinum-based and non-platinum-based regimens. The next study looked at the question of duration of chemotherapy in patients with advanced disease and finally a study from the same group looked at the effectiveness of outpatient chemotherapy in Stage IIIb and IV patients.

Clinical and cost-effectiveness of paclitaxel, docetaxel, gemcitabine and vinorelbine in non-small cell lung cancer: a systematic review.

Clegg A, Scott DA, Hewitson P, *et al. Thorax* 2002; **57**: 20–8.

BACKGROUND. There is now cautious optimism that chemotherapy can improve symptom relief, quality of life and survival in NSCLC. A new generation of drugs have appeared. This review summarizes the cost-effectiveness of four new drugs used in NSCLC.

INTERPRETATION. Eleven electronic databases were searched for studies involving paclitaxil, docetaxel, gemcitabine and vinorelbine in NSCLC. Clinical effectiveness was assessed using the outcomes of survival, quality of life and adverse effect. Cost-effectiveness was assessed by developing a costing model and presenting the results as incremental cost per life year saved and compared this with the cost of best supportive care. Survival gains due to chemotherapy were within the range of 2–4 months, quality of life usually improved and the drugs were described as 'reasonably' cost-effective. Incremental cost per life year saved versus best supportive care ranged from £4091 for single agent vindesine up to £17 546 for docetaxel given as second line treatment.

Comment

This review was published from the data generated by the National Institute of Clinical Excellence (NICE) in their review of chemotherapy for NSCLC. There is an argument that drug costs may be cheaper than reported since the patients studied were involved in clinical trials. In patients treated off protocol, chemotherapy may well be stopped earlier if less effective and costs thereby reduced. Most patients included in these studies had advanced disease (most Stage IV). It is possible that the benefits of chemotherapy were somewhat exaggerated because survival in untreated patients is so poor (in the region of approximately 5 months). Also, the quality of life data in most of these studies was extremely variable and since survival was only being increased by a couple of months then the indication for drug treatment in these patients was one of palliation and the cost-effectiveness in terms of improvement in quality of life was difficult to measure.

Platinum-based and non-platinum-based chemotherapy in advanced non-small cell lung cancer: a randomized multi-centre trial.

Georgoulias V, Papadakis E, Alexopoulous A, *et al. Lancet* 2001; **357**: 1478–84.

BACKGROUND. The first active regimens in NSCLC contain platinum. This study compared platinum-based and non-platinum-based chemotherapy in advanced NSCLC.

INTERPRETATION. This was a multi-centre study from a Greek group. They compared a regimen containing platinum (cisplatin and docetaxel) with chemotherapy without platinum (gemcitabine and docetaxel). Four hundred and forty-one patients were randomized to the two treatments. All patients had received no chemotherapy previously, and were Stage IIIb or IV NSCLC. All patients received human granulocyte colony stimulating factor in an attempt to protect their marrow. Objective response rate were similar in the two groups (32.4% platinum-based, 30.2% non-platinum-based). There was no difference in the median duration of response (7 months in both groups), time to tumour progression (8 versus 9 months) or overall survival (10 versus 9.5 months). One and two year survival rates were virtually identical at around 20 and 4%. The gemcitabine plus docetaxel regimen had a much better toxicity profile than the platinum-based regimen.

Comment

This is a large randomized study in advanced disease patients. The two regimens showed equivalent potency. One interesting finding from the study was that non-adenocarcinoma histology had a higher response rate with the platinum-containing regimen (40 versus 23%). In virtually all studies of NSCLC patients, no distinction is made between different histological types of the disease. This study provides some evidence that patients with different histologies may respond differently to certain regimens and that perhaps chemotherapy should be tailored to histological subtypes within the NSCLC population.

Duration of chemotherapy in advanced non-small cell lung cancer: a randomized trial of three versus six courses of mitomycin, vinblastine and cisplatin.

Smith IE, O'Brien MER, Talbot DC, *et al. J Clin Oncol* 2001; **19**: 1336–43.

BACKGROUND. There are no published data on the optimal duration of chemotherapy for advanced NSCLC. Six cycles are usually recommended. This is a multi-centre, randomized trial comparing different durations of treatment with chemotherapy in NSCLC.

INTERPRETATION. Three hundred and eight patients were included in the study. All had Stage IIIb or IV NSCLC and a performance status 0–2. All patients were treated with standard MVP (mitomycin, vindesine, platinum) chemotherapy in cycles every 21 days. Patients were randomized to either three or six cycles of treatment. Quality of life, response, toxicity and duration of symptom relief were the primary end-points of the study. One hundred and fifty-five patients were randomized to receive three courses of chemotherapy. Those receiving only three treatments were less likely to get complete resolution of symptoms (5 vs 14%) compared with the 153 patients who were given six treatments. Median survival in both groups was around 6.5 months. One-year survival in both groups was also similar (22 vs 25%). Duration of symptom-relief was identical in the two groups (4.5 months), quality of life was much better in the group receiving three treatments with significant reduction in fatigue ($P = 0.03$) and a definite trend in a reduction in nausea and vomiting ($P = 0.06$).

Comment

This is a well-designed study looking specifically at the benefits of receiving three or six cycles with chemotherapy in NSCLC. There appeared to be no evidence for any benefit in terms of survival or quality of life in receiving six courses of treatment. Survival in both groups was poor as only patients with advanced disease were included. Since this is palliative chemotherapy, it would seem reasonable to recommend that patients receive only three cycles of therapy. However, they are less likely to get complete resolution of their symptoms.

Mitomycin C, vinblastine and carboplatin: effective outpatient chemotherapy for advanced non-small carcinoma of the lung.

Gregory RK, Smith IE, Norton A, *et al. Clin Oncol* 2001; **13**: 483–7.

BACKGROUND. Chemotherapy for NSCLC can be fairly toxic and usually requires in-patient therapy. This study looks at an outpatient chemotherapy regimen for NSCLC.

INTERPRETATION. Forty-three patients with Stage IIIb and IV NSCLC were enrolled into a study of outpatient chemotherapy. Six patients with IIIa disease who were unfit for radical treatment were also included. Since there was no platinum in the regimen, it was possible to give treatment as an outpatient as no hydration pre-chemotherapy was required. Performance status was 1 in 15, 2 in 22 and six patients had a performance status of three. The median number of courses given was three (range 1–6). Thirteen out of 43 (30%) had an objective response to the treatment with three having a complete response. Twenty-six out of 43 (60%) had a symptomatic improvement on treatment. The symptoms that responded were malaise, pain, cough, breathlessness, haemoptysis and anorexia. Only 5 out of 43 patients had a worsening of symptoms whilst on treatment. Median survival in the group was 7 months.

Comment

Comparing this regimen with MVP toxicity was similar although there was more thrombocytopenia. Survival was virtually identical. The carboplatin, however, made the regimen more expensive but with no in-patient stay, the regimen was overall much cheaper to administer. Although it should be stressed that this was not a randomized study, it was possible to show that in a group of patients with poor performance status with advanced disease, reasonable benefit from out-patient chemotherapy could be obtained.

Radiotherapy in non-small cell lung cancer

Historically radiotherapy has always played a central part in the management of patients with NSCLC. In general, patients are treated with two different strategies. High dose radical radiotherapy is given to patients to prolong survival and in a small proportion of patients provide a cure. This is especially important for patients who are considered not sufficiently fit for surgery due to co-morbidity or in patients who have inoperable disease of more advanced stage. The vast majority of patients receiving radiotherapy for NSCLC, however, are being treated with palliative intent. A number of different regimens of palliative radiotherapy in NSCLC exist and there is no obvious gold standard treatment. Important variables in palliative radiotherapy regimens include the dose and fractionation of treatment given and whether the patient should be given immediate treatment at diagnosis when symptoms may be few or whether it is more rational to wait until symptoms develop before administering palliative radiotherapy. Trials looking at these variables have appeared in the last year.

Immediate versus delayed palliative thoracic radiotherapy in patients with unresectable locally advanced non-small cell lung cancer and minimal thoracic symptoms: a randomized controlled trial.

Falk SJ, Girling DJ, White RJ, *et al.*, on behalf of the MRC Lung Cancer Working Party. *Br Med J* 2002; **325**: 465–8.

BACKGROUND. Should palliative radiotherapy be given immediately to asymptomatic patients with incurable lung cancer or 'as needed' to treat symptoms as they emerge?

INTERPRETATION. This was a multi-centre randomized controlled trial carried out in 23 centres in the United Kingdom, Ireland and South Africa. Two hundred and thirty previously untreated patients with minimal thoracic symptoms were randomized to receive either immediate palliative radiotherapy or delayed treatment when symptoms arose. All patients were given supportive therapy as needed. A number of different regimens of palliative radiotherapy were given although 90% received 17 Gy in two fractions or 10 Gy as a single dose. Forty-two per cent of patients in the delayed group eventually received radiotherapy and 56% died without receiving any treatment. The primary end-point of the study was patients being symptom-free at 6 months with secondary end-points being quality of life, adverse events and survival. There was no difference between the two groups in terms of the primary end-point with 28% of patients receiving immediate palliative radiotherapy being symptom-free at 6 months compared with 26% of the delayed group. There was no evidence of any difference between the groups in activity, anxiety and depression or psychological distress when measured with standard quality of life instruments. Adverse events were more common in the immediate treatment group. There was no survival advantage for immediate palliative radiotherapy. Median survival in this group was 8.3 months compared with 7.9 months in the other group, with 1-year survival 31% in the immediate treatment group compared with 29% in the delayed group.

Comment

The need for this trial arose because of differing practices in administering palliative radiotherapy. Most respiratory physicians believe that there is no point in giving radiotherapy if the patient does not have symptoms. Their belief is that toxicity from radiotherapy would actually impair a patient's quality of life. Radiation oncologists have believed that patients should be treated when they are well and that this would prevent symptoms occurring, rather than waiting for the patient to experience sometimes distressing symptoms, and perhaps not be fit enough for palliative treatment. The results of the study would suggest that there is no difference in symptom control using these two regimens with the group being treated immediately experiencing more adverse events. Perhaps not surprisingly no survival advantage materialized from this palliative treatment. The study has been criticized by some radiation oncologists who felt that the palliative regimens were 'old fashioned'. There is now a belief that palliative radiotherapy can actually offer some survival advantage if given to fit patients. Some evidence for this emerged from the following study.

Randomized phase III trial of single versus fractionated thoracic radiation in the palliation of patients with lung cancer.
Bezjak A, Dixon P, Brundage M, *et al. Int J Rad Oncol Biol Phys* 2002; **54**: 719–28.

BACKGROUND. The exact schedule for palliative radiotherapy in NSCLC has not been established. This study compared two well used regimens.

INTERPRETATION. This was a multi-institutional phase III randomized study comparing 10 Gy in a single fraction of radiotherapy with 20 Gy in five fractions for the palliation of thoracic symptoms in lung cancer. The primary end-point was palliation of symptoms at one month post-radiotherapy. Patient completed daily diary cards were used as an evaluation tool. Secondary end-points included quality of life, toxicity and survival. Two hundred and thirty patients were randomized in the study. At one month, no difference was found in symptom control between the two arms as judged by daily diary scores. There was a suggestion, however, that patients receiving fractionated radiotherapy (20 Gy) had a greater improvement in certain areas such as quality of life, pain and ability to carry out normal activities. No significant difference was found in treatment-related toxicity. Patients who received five fractions survived, on average, two months longer than patients receiving one fraction ($P = 0.03$).

Comment

This study was conducted in Canada where single fractions of radiotherapy have not been accepted as an effective palliative regimen. Work from the United Kingdom Medical Research Council had shown that 30 Gy in 10 fractions was equivalent to 17 Gy in two fractions and subsequently that 17 Gy in two fractions was equivalent to 10 Gy in one fraction |5,6|. The Canadian study showed that the two treatment strategies provided a similar degree of palliation in terms of thoracic symptoms. However, there were differences in survival between the two study arms of clinically relevant magnitude. Patients receiving five fractions had a median survival of six months (95% CI 4.9–7.9) while those given single fraction treatment survived for a median of 4.2 months (95% CI 3.7–5.4, $P = 0.03$). This difference was not seen in poor performance status patients (Fig. 18.2).

Small cell lung cancer

Introduction

Chemotherapy is the treatment of choice for SCLC and dual modality therapy confers significant survival advantage. In this section the timing of radiotherapy

(a)

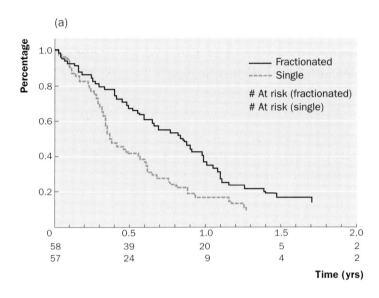

(b)

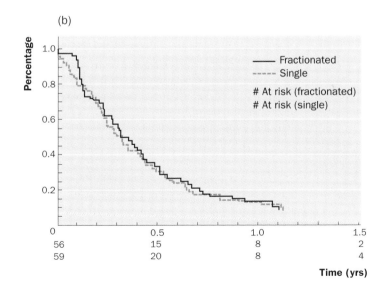

Fig. 18.2 Survival in good performance status (0–1) graph (a), or poor performance status (2–3) graph (b). Source: Bezjak *et al.* (2002).

and chemotherapy, the different regimens used in small cell patients and the effectiveness of prophylactic cranial irradiation will be covered. The final paper is a Cochrane Review looking at the management of superior vena caval obstruction. This is an important complication of patients with both small cell and non-small lesions.

Timing of radiotherapy and chemotherapy

In general, SCLC is acutely sensitive to both chemotherapy and radiotherapy although in the vast majority of patients the disease eventually relapses and causes death. There have been many randomized studies addressing the issue of the timing of radiotherapy when given in high doses with chemotherapy in the initial stage of management. An area of interest has been whether treatment with radiotherapy and chemotherapy should be given concurrently or sequentially. Two trials have demonstrated a statistically significant advantage to early concurrent therapy; three revealed no advantage to earlier radiotherapy and a study published this year shows a strong trend towards a better outcome with early concurrent therapy.

Phase III study of concurrent versus sequential thoracic radiotherapy in combination with cisplatin and etoposide for limited stage small cell lung cancer: results of the Japan Clinical Oncology Group Study 9104.

Takada M, Fukuoka M, Kwahara M, et al. J Clin Oncol 2002; **20**: 3054–60.

BACKGROUND. This study was designed to evaluate the optimal timing for thoracic radiotherapy in patients undergoing chemotherapy for limited disease SCLC.

INTERPRETATION. This was a randomized phase III study performed by the Lung Cancer Study Group of the Japan Clinical Oncology Group. Two hundred and thirty-one patients with limited disease SCLC were enrolled into the trial. All patients received four cycles of cisplatin plus etoposide chemotherapy. Patients were randomized to receive either sequential or concurrent radiotherapy with this chemotherapy. Radiotherapy consisted of 45 Gy over three weeks (1.5 Gy twice daily). Patients in the sequential treatment arm received their chemotherapy treatment every 3 weeks whilst those in the concurrent arm were treated every 4 weeks. Radiotherapy was begun on day two of the first cycle of radiotherapy in the concurrent arm and after the fourth cycle in the sequential arm. Concurrent radiotherapy yielded better survival than sequential radiotherapy although this difference was not statistically significant ($P = 0.097$). The median survival time was 19.7 months in the sequential arm versus 27.2 months in the concurrent arm (Fig. 18.3). The 2, 3 and 5 year survival rates for patient who received sequential radiotherapy were 35.1, 20.2 and 18.3% respectively, opposed to 54.4, 29.8 and 23.7% respectively, for the patients receiving concurrent radiotherapy. Haematological toxicity was more severe in the concurrent arm. Severe oesophagitis was infrequently seen in both arms, occurring in 9% of patients treated concurrently and 4% in the sequential treatment group.

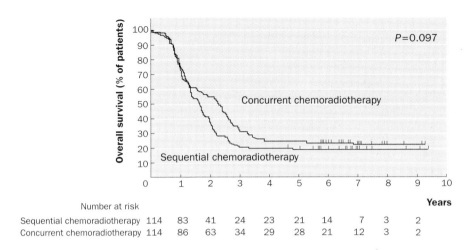

Fig. 18.3 Overall survival of patients with LS-SCLC who were assigned to treatment with sequential chemoradiotherapy of concurrent chemoradiotherapy.
Source: Takada *et al.* (2002).

Comment

The study suggests that cisplatin plus etoposide and concurrent radiotherapy is more effective in the treatment of limited disease SCLC than cisplastin plus etoposide and sequential radiotherapy. The rates of severe oesophageal toxicity were modest compared with other studies looking at concurrent chemotherapy and radiotherapy. In one previous trial |7| a 27% toxicity rate was seen with accelerated radiation and chemotherapy. The use of 4-weekly chemotherapy intervals might explain the modest rate in the above study. However, this may also have resulted in a clinically significant decrease in chemotherapy dose intensity perhaps explaining the failure of the study to achieve statistical significance. Interestingly, the study also showed that early concurrent therapy seemed to reduce the risk of brain metastases as the first failure. An important finding from this trial is that the outcome in both arms was significantly better than expected. The trial design anticipated an increase in median survival from 12–18 months. The actual results showed an increase from 19.7–27.2 months. This difference was not statistically significant due, in part, to the sample size of 231 patients. The trial was thus underpowered to detect a clinically relevant difference in survival based on the timing of radiotherapy. This reaffirmed the importance of large randomized clinical trials in oncology.

Chemotherapy regimens in small cell lung cancer

Many studies have shown that although chemotherapy is active in SCLC few patients achieve long-term survival. There are hundreds of trials in the literature of many different regimens. A gold standard treatment has not been identified, though a number of regimens are more popular than other ones. A national survey of chemotherapy regimens used to treat SCLC has recently been carried out in the United Kingdom.

A national survey of the chemotherapy regimens used to treat small cell lung cancer in the United Kingdom.

Sambrook RJ, Girling DJ. *Br J Cancer* 2001; **84**: 1447–52.

BACKGROUND. It is known that different regimens are used for the management of SCLC. This survey looked at chemotherapy practice in the United Kingdom.

INTERPRETATION. This was an MRC study looking at chemotherapy regimens in SCLC. One thousand two hundred and fourteen questionnaires were sent to clinicians who were thought to be treating SCLC patients with chemotherapy (clinical oncologists, medical oncologists, respiratory physicians and general physicians). One thousand and seventy questionnaires were returned giving a response rate of 88%. Thirty-six per cent of patients were treated by clinical oncologists, 30% by medical oncologists, 27% by respiratory physicians and 7% by others. Overall, 34 different regimens were reported. One hundred and fifty-one combinations of dose and schedule were used. The three regimens most widely used in good prognosis patients were ACE (doxorubicin, cyclophosphamide and etoposide), CAV (cyclophosphamide, doxorubicin and vincristine) and PE (platinum and etoposide). The main reasons given for the choice of regimen included cost, quality of life considerations, patients convenience and routine local practice. Few clinicians based their choice of regimens on the results of clinical trials.

Comment

This study revealed a surprising variation in the routine management of SCLC patients in the United Kingdom. It would be difficult to extrapolate these results to other parts of the world where cost considerations may be different. The message to be taken from the study is that no standard chemotherapy for SCLC exists and it may be difficult to compare results between clinicians in routine practice if different regimens are being used.

Prophylactic cranial irradiation in small cell lung cancer

Cranial irradiation for preventing brain metastases of small cell lung cancer in patients in complete remission.
Prophylactic Cranial Irradiation Overview Collaborative Group. *Cochrane Review*. The Cochrane Library, 2002; **4**: Oxford: Update Software.

BACKGROUND. It is known that prophylactic cranial irradiation (PCI) significantly reduces the rate of brain metastases in patients with SCLC who respond to chemotherapy. Individual randomized trials conducted on patients in complete remission have been unable to clarify whether this treatment improves survival. This systematic review addresses this question.

INTERPRETATION. Electronic databases were searched for randomized trials comparing prophylactic cranial irradiation with no PCI in patients with NSCLC in complete remission. Seven trials with a total of 987 participants were included. The relative risk of death in the treatment group compared with the control group was 0.84 (95% CI 0.73–0.97, $P = 0.01$). This effect corresponds to a 5.4% increase in the 3-year survival (20.7% in the treatment group versus 15.3% in the control group). PCI also increased disease-free survival (RR 0.75, 95% CI 0.65–0.86, $P = 0.01$) and decreased the risk of brain metastases (RR 0.46, 95% CI 0.38–0.57, $P = 0.001$). There did not appear to be a relationship between dose of irradiation and the risk of brain metastases though a trend appeared to exist.

Comment

It has long been known that the risk of brain metastases can be virtually halved by prophylactic cranial irradiation in patients with SCLC who go into complete remission with standard chemotherapy. This review shows that there is a significant improvement in survival with this treatment and an extension of the disease-free survival. There is a suggestion that there may be potentially greater benefit on brain metastases rate if PCI is given earlier or at a higher dose although further clinical trials specifically looking at these two points are required.

Management of SVC obstruction

Steroids, radiotherapy, chemotherapy and stents for superior vena caval obstruction in carcinoma of the bronchus.
Rowell NP, Gleeson FV. *Cochrane Review*. The Cochrane Library, 2002; **4**: Oxford: Update Software.

BACKGROUND. Superior vena caval obstruction (SVCO) affects a minority of patients with lung cancer. Treatment options include radiotherapy, chemotherapy, steroids and

an insertion of an expandable metal stent. This review defines more clearly the relative merits of the different treatment modalities in this unpleasant complication of lung cancer.

INTERPRETATION. This Cochrane review searched a number of different databases for both randomized and non-randomized trials in which patients with carcinoma of the bronchus and a diagnosis of SVCO had been treated with any combination of steroids, chemotherapy, radiotherapy or insertion of an expandable metal stent. Three randomized and 98 non-randomized studies were found of which two and 44 respectively met the inclusion criteria of the review. The one randomized study that compared radiotherapy and chemotherapy against radiotherapy alone was excluded as not all patients had a diagnosis of lung cancer. No studies were found reporting the effectiveness of steroid therapy. There were 22 radiotherapy/chemotherapy studies and 23 stent studies that formed the basis of review. In SCLC, chemotherapy and or radiotherapy relieved SVCO in 77%. In NSCLC 60% had relief of SVCO following chemotherapy and/or radiotherapy. Insertion of an SVC stent relieved SVCO in 95% of patients. The relapse rates for SCLC, NSCLC and stenting were 17, 19 and 11% respectively. Recanalization was frequently achieved with stenting resulting in long-term patency in 92%. Morbidity following stent insertion was greater if thrombolytics were administered.

Comment

Chemotherapy and radiotherapy was, therefore, effective in relieving SVCO in a high proportion of patients with SVCO. Stent insertion, however, appears to provide relief in a higher proportion and more rapidly. There is no evidence for the use of steroid therapy in this condition.

New therapies for lung cancer

While cytotoxic chemotherapy is accepted as the treatment of choice for the vast majority of patients with SCLC, it has been only in the last decade that this form of treatment has become accepted for patients with NSCLC. Modest benefits in survival, reduction in symptoms and improving quality of life have been reported when compared with best supportive care |8,9|.

Chemotherapy for advanced NSCLC remains controversial as the introduction of newer cytotoxic agents has resulted in only minor improvements in survival. Trials reported recently of newer chemotherapy regimens have shown results only slightly superior to historical controls and it seems clear that our investment in cytotoxic chemotherapy for NSCLC has reached the point of diminishing returns. Novel treatment modalities are needed and there are currently a number of agents emerging from advances made in the understanding of the biology of the disease. A number of molecular and biological targets for NSCLC have been identified and it is likely that these will form the bases of more sophisticated biological therapies. These therapies have recently been reviewed.

Targeted therapy in non-small cell lung cancer.
Giaccone G. *Lung Cancer* 2002; **38**(Suppl 2): S29–32.

BACKGROUND. New agents are urgently required to improve outcomes in patients with NSCLC. This article reviews these developments.

Comment

This short paper outlines different treatment strategies that focus on cell signalling and other biological pathways involved in the development of tumours. This approach is different from standard cytotoxic chemotherapy in that the focus of treatment is to inhibit specific biological pathways in a cytostatic way rather than attacking tumour proliferation, which is how most cytotoxic drugs work. Examples of the biological agents considered are outlined in Table 18.2.

Two of the newer therapies that have reached clinical trials and have caused much interest include the epidermal growth factor receptor (EGFR) inhibitor IRESSA and a new anti-folate compound Pemetrexed.

Epidermal growth factor receptor inhibition

Tyrosine kinases are proteins involved in normal cell growth and malignant transformation. Since first discovered more than 20 years ago numerous different families of tyrosine kinases have been identified many of which are involved with transmembrane receptors that act to transduce extracellular signals to intracellular

Table 18.2 Examples of biologic agents with potential use in NSCLC

Signal transduction/cell cycle inhibitors	Farnesyl transferase inhibitors Antisense oligonucleotides to protein kinase C Flavopiridol Retinoids UCN-101
Angiogenesis inhibitors	Anti-VEGF antibody VEGF receptor inhibitors (SU5416, SU6668, ZD6474) Matrix metalloproteinase inhibitors (Prinomostat, marimastat) Endostatin/angiostatin TNP-470
EGFR inhibitors	Anti-EGFR antibodies (trastuzumab, cetuximab) EGFR tyrosine kinase inhibitors (ZD1839, OS1774, PK1166, C11033)

Source: Giaccone (2002).

responses. Increased tyrosine kinase activity is a hallmark of neoplastic cells and correlates well with the degree of malignant transformation. Of all the tyrosine kinases much is now known about the EGFR subfamily. Stimulation of the EGFR promotes tumour growth by increasing cell proliferation, motility, adhesion and invasive capacity. EGFR expression is associated with metastases, advanced disease, resistance to chemotherapy and radiotherapy and a poor prognosis |10|. EGF signalling can be blocked by small molecule EGFR tyrosine kinase inhibitors. The most exciting results have been seen with an oral preparation ZD 1839 (IRESSA) on which phase I and II studies have been reported.

Selective oral epidermal growth factor receptor tyrosine kinase inhibitor ZD 1839 is generally well-tolerated and has activity in non-small cell lung cancer and other solid tumours: results of a phase I trial.

Herbst RS, Maddow A-M, Rothenberg ML, *et al. J Clin Oncol* 2002; **20**: 3815–25.

BACKGROUND. This was a phase I dose escalation, tolerability trial of oral ZD 1839.

INTERPRETATION. Seventy-one patients were given ZD 1839 at seven different dose levels. Most had NSCLC ($n = 39$) or head and neck cancer ($n = 18$). Sixty-eight of the 71 had received prior chemotherapy. The primary dose-limiting toxicities were diarrhoea and an acne-like follicular rash. Pharmacokinetic analysis showed that steady-state kinetics occurred by day seven. Initial tumour activity was manifested by prolonged stable disease though one patient had a partial response. Anti-tumour activity was observed at all doses.

Comment

This study shows that this oral drug is reasonably well tolerated. It is not surprising perhaps that as EGFRs are found on squamous epithelium that the majority of adverse events should occur in the skin and GI tract (Fig. 18.4).

Total EGFR levels were not changed after therapy but there was a trend towards reduction in activated EGFR. Significant decreases in proliferation markers such as mitogen-activated protein kinase were seen and although this was a phase I study, anti-tumour activity was observed. A significant number of patients remained clinically stable for up to 30 months on treatment. These patients had failed standard cytotoxic chemotherapy. Two Phase II trials of ZD 1839 appeared in abstract form in 2002.

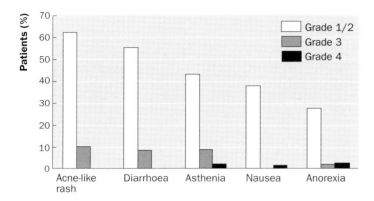

Fig. 18.4 Five most common adverse events (occurring in >30% of the population) over all dose levels. Source: Herbst *et al.* (2002).

Final results from a phase II trial of ZD 1839 ('IRESSA') for patients with advanced non-small cell lung cancer (IDEAL I).

Fukuoka M, Yano S, Giaccone G, *et al. Proc ASCO* 2002; **21**: 1188 Abstract.

A phase II trial of ZD 1839 ('IRESSA') in advanced non-small cell lung cancer (NSCLC) patients who had failed platinum—and docetaxel-based regimens (IDEAL 2).

Kris MG, Natale RB, Herbst RS, *et al. Proc ASCO* 2002; **21**: 1166 Abstract.

B ACKGROUND . **These two phase II trials reported on response rates and safety of ZD 1839, a new agent in NSCLC.**

I NTERPRETATION . IDEAL 1 reported on 210 previously treated patients with locally advanced or metastatic NSCLC. Patients were randomized to 250 or 500 mg per day of oral ZD1839. There were no differences between the two doses in response rates, progression-free survival and overall survival. Adverse events were mild and similar to that seen in phase I studies. Fewer patients experienced these effects on the 250 mg per day dose. Response rates of 18.4 and 19% with overall survival of 7.6 and 8 months were seen in the two dose regimens. IDEAL 2 was a similar study in heavily pre-treated patients (41% had failed two, 33% had failed three and 25% had failed four or more previous regimens). Response rates were 11.8 and 8.8% for the two dose regimens with symptom response rates of 43 and 35%. Median survival for both groups was in the region of 6 months. Similar levels of adverse events were seen.

Comment

These phase II trials in heavily pre-treated patients with NSCLC confirmed the phase I trial results of IRESSA suggesting that the drug was well tolerated and had activity against the tumours. Two, phase III studies comparing IRESSA in combination with standard cytotoxic chemotherapy against chemotherapy alone were reported in abstract form in the same year. These studies were performed in patients who had not previously been treated.

A phase III clinical trial of ZD1839 ('IRESSA') in combination with gemcitabine and cisplatin in chemotherapy-naïve patients with advanced non-small cell lung cancer (INTACT I).

Giaccone G, Johnston DH, Manegold C, *et al. Ann Oncol* 2002; **13**(Suppl 5): 2 Abstract 40.

ZD1839 ('IRESSA') in combination with paclitaxel and carboplatin in chemotherapy-naïve patients with advanced non-small cell lung cancer: results from a Phase III clinical trial (INTACT 2)

Johnston DH, Herbst R, Gianccone G, et al. *Ann Oncol* 2002; **13**(Suppl 5): 127 Abstract 4680.

BACKGROUND. These two phase III studies compare IRESSA in combination with standard chemotherapy with chemotherapy alone in patients with NSCLC who had not been previously treated.

INTERPRETATION. INTACT I was a randomized double-blind placebo-controlled multi-centre trial. Chemotherapy naïve patients with phase III or IV disease and performance status 0 were randomized to chemotherapy (6 cycles gemcitabine plus cisplatin plus placebo or chemotherapy plus 250 mg per day of IRESSA or chemotherapy plus 500 mg per day of IRESSA). The primary end-point was overall survival although secondary end-points included progression-free survival, symptom improvement, quality of life and safety. One thousand and ninety-three patients were recruited from 165 sites worldwide. There were no statistically significant differences in overall survival, progression-free survival and time to worsening of symptoms in the three arms. The toxicity profile of IRESSA combined with chemotherapy was similar to chemotherapy alone with the exception of dose-dependent diarrhoea and skin rashes. INTACT 2 was a similar study enrolling 1037 patients from 200 sites worldwide but predominantly in the USA. The chemotherapy used was carboplatin and paclitaxel every 3 weeks for six cycles. Patients were continued on IRESSA or placebo until diseases progression. Overall survival was similar (8.7–9.9 months) in the three arms.

Comment

IRESSA in combination with two-agent chemotherapy for advanced NSCLC did not improve treatment outcomes. These results were disappointing in view of the favourable phase I and II results. The trials have shown that the addition of IRESSA to standard chemotherapy was unhelpful but the trials did not include an IRESSA monotherapy arm. Clearly since IRESSA is not a standard cytotoxic agent, it may be important to evaluate the drug in a different way. Its place in the treatment of advanced NSCLC remains to be found but perhaps its role may be in keeping patients in remission post-chemotherapy rather than being given concurrently with cytotoxic drugs. Further studies looking at this promising agent are awaited.

Pemetrexed (ALIMTA)

In the past anti-folates have only had a minor role in the treatment of lung cancer with perhaps methotrexate being the most widely used agent. Pemetrexed (ALIMTA) is a new antimetabolite that inhibits a number of enzymes involved in DNA synthesis [11].

Pre-clinical studies have shown activity against a wide variety of tumours including lung cancer. A phase I trial showed peak serum concentrations considerably above the IC_{50} for pre-clinical cytotoxicity. Partial responses were reported in 11% of evaluable patients. Grade IV leucopenia developed in 25%.

Phase II studies have been performed in Canada and in Australia and South Africa. In the Canadian study, 33 previously untreated patients were given ALIMTA 600 mg/m^2 intravenously every 3 weeks. Dose reduction was required because of mucositus, vomiting and myalgia. Seven partial responses were seen out of 30 evaluable patients. Median survival was 9.2 months. Twenty-seven per cent of patients had significant neutropenia and skin rash. The response rate in the other study was 16% of 57 evaluable patients. Median survival was 7.2 months. Forty-two per cent had significant neutropenia and 31% a Grade III/IV skin rash. A trial of ALIMTA in combination with cisplatin has been reported.

Phase II trial of pemetrexed sodium, (multi-targeted antifolate) and cisplatin as first line therapy in patients with advanced non-small cell lung carcinoma.
Shepherd FA, Dancey J, Arnold A, *et al. Cancer* 2001; **92**: 595–600.

BACKGROUND. Pemetrexed is a new anti-folate with activity in NSCLC. This is a phase II trial of the drug in combination with cisplatin.

INTERPRETATION. Thirty-one patients were enrolled into the study over a year. Pemetrexed 500 mg/m^2 was given intravenously with cisplatin 75 mg/m^2. Median age was 60 years. Twenty-six patients had Stage IV disease with five patients having Stage IIIb. There were 29 patients evaluable for response. Thirteen had partial responses with an overall response rate of 43% (95% CI 26–64%). Median duration of response was 6.1 months and the median survival was 8.9 months. The response rate of 46% in the 24 Stage IV patients was remarkable. The regimen appeared reasonably tolerated. Grade III/IV granulocytopenia was seen in seven patients, Grade III/IV anaemia in six patients and Grade III nausea and vomiting in two patients.

Comment

The combination of pemetrexed with cisplatin resulted in higher response rates than those seen with single agent therapy. This, of course, was not a randomized trial. The toxicity profile was encouraging. Results from a German study using a similar regimen gave an overall response rate of 39% in 36 chemotherapy-naïve patients. Median survival was 10.9 months. A much higher proportion, however, had significant granulocytopenia (59%). Results of ongoing studies of pemetrexed with other cytotoxic agents are awaited. There are theoretical reasons to hope that this drug may be particularly valuable in patients who have been pre-treated as it acts at targets other than those of drugs used in first line therapy.

Follow-up

Patients with lung cancer have an extremely poor prognosis with 80% dying within a year. Patients undergoing treatment, however, do require follow-up, though long-term survival in non-surgical patients is unusual. Currently most patients with cancer are routinely seen for regular follow-up appointments in outpatient clinics. There is little evidence that this routine follow-up actually provides an environment conducive to supporting patients and that perhaps patients do not get enough time to raise concerns. Most clinics are run by busy doctors who may fail to detect patient's emotional distress. In the last few years experienced nurse practitioners with a specialist interest in lung cancer have appeared. In the last year, two papers have been published looking at different methods of following up lung cancer patients. The first investigates an open access arrangement where routine appointments were not given but patients could be seen at any time and in the second study the use of lung cancer nurses to manage follow-up compared to routine medical follow-up was evaluated in a randomized trial.

Open access follow-up for lung cancer: patient and staff satisfaction.

Ardlard JW, Joseph J, Brammer CV, Gerrard GE. *Clin Oncol* 2001; **13**: 404–8.

B A C K G R O U N D . To evaluate an open access follow-up clinical for lung cancer in terms of patient and staff satisfaction.

I N T E R P R E T A T I O N . This study was undertaken in a District General Hospital that ran a weekly oncology clinic. After consultation with local general practitioners, an open-access lung cancer clinic was set up. Over a 2-year period, 160 new patients were included. Median survival was 5 months with 18% alive at 1 year. Thirty-eight patients underwent radical therapy or were too unwell to consider any treatment, leaving 122 patients undergoing palliative treatment or having no symptoms. These patients were seen routinely six week post-therapy. Forty-seven, however, died in this time-span leaving 75 patients eligible for the study. Ten patients considered this follow-up unsuitable or declined open access follow-up leaving 65 patients within the study. Forty-four of these actually used the service, 28 were only seen on one occasion with 6 patients being seen on three or more occasions. There were 66 clinic visits altogether which is fewer than if all patients had been given a routine 3 month follow-up. In 90% of cases, the reason for the clinic visit was a symptom of tumour progression. Questionnaires were sent to patients, carers and staff and a high level of satisfaction was seen. Local general practitioners welcomed the service.

Comment

This is not a randomized trial but results would suggest that open access follow-up is certainly possible and popular with patients and staff respectively. The clinic was apparently more efficient than if routine follow-up had been arranged and almost certainly saved money. Levels of anxiety from patients post-therapy were not recorded but in general, high levels of satisfaction were obtained from patients. There was a high drop out rate from the study with only 65 patients included from the original 160 patients recruited.

Nurse-led follow-up and conventional medical follow-up in management of patients with lung cancer: a randomized trial.

Moore S, Corner J, Haviland J, *et al. BMJ* 2002; **325**: 1145.

B A C K G R O U N D . This study assessed the effectiveness of a nurse-led follow-up clinic in the management of patients with lung cancer.

I N T E R P R E T A T I O N . This was a randomized controlled trial in a specialist cancer hospital. Two hundred and three patients with lung cancer who had completed their initial treatment and who were expected to survive for at least 3 months were enrolled. Nurse-led follow-up of outpatients was compared with conventional medical follow-up. The main outcome measures were quality of life, patient satisfaction, general practitioner satisfaction, survival, resource use and cost. Seventy-five per cent of eligible patients consented to participate. Patients followed up by nurses had less severe breathlessness at 3 months and better scores for emotional functioning at 12 months. No significant differences in general practitioner overall satisfaction was seen between the two groups and there was no difference in survival. Nurses tended to record progression of symptoms sooner than doctors did. Patients followed up by nurses were much more likely to die at home rather than in hospital and attended fewer consultations with a hospital doctor, had fewer X-rays and more radiotherapy. Nurse-led follow-up appeared to be cost-effective.

Comment

Follow-up of patients with lung cancer by clinical nurse specialists appears to be safe, acceptable and cost effective. At no time in the study did patients wish to revert to conventional medical follow-up. Forty per cent of patients who received nurse-led follow-up died at home compared with 23% of patients who received conventional medical follow-up. It is known that 50% or more of UK patients with terminal cancer express a preference to die at home.

These interesting developments in the methods by which patients are followed-up need to be rolled out into larger programmes to assess whether they are acceptable and cost-effective.

References

1. Roth JA, Fossella F, Komaki R, Ryan MB, Putnam JB Jr, Lee JS, Dhingra H, De Caro L, Chasen M, McGavran M, et al. A randomized trial comparing peri-operative chemotherapy and surgery with surgery alone in resectable stage III a non-small cell lung cancer. J Natl Cancer Inst 1994; **86**: 673–80.

2. Pass HI, Pogrebniak HW, Steinberg SM, Mulshine J, Minna J. Randomized trial of neoadjuvant therapy for lung cancer: interim analysis. Ann Thoracic Surg 1992; **53**: 992–8.

3. Rosell R, Gomez-Codina J, Camps C, Maestre J, Padille J, Canto A, Mate JL, Li S, Roig J, Olazabal A, et al. A randomized trial comparing pre-operative chemotherapy plus surgery with surgery alone in patients with non-small cell lung cancer. N Engl J Med 1994; **330**: 153–8.

4. Wronski M, Arbit E, Burt M, Galicich JH. Survival after surgical treatment of brain metastases from lung cancer: a follow-up study of 231 patients treated between 1976 and 1991. J Neurosurg 1995; **83**: 605–16.

  5. MRC Lung Cancer Working Party. Report to the MRC inoperable non-small cell lung cancer (NSCLC): A Medical Research Council randomized trial of palliative radiotherapy with two fractions or ten fractions. *Br J Cancer* 1991; **63**: 265–70.

  6. MRC Lung Cancer Working Party. A Medical Research Council (MRC) randomized trial of palliative radiotherapy with two fractions or a single fraction in patients with inoperable non-small cell lung cancer (NSCLC) and poor performance status. *Br J Cancer* 1992; **65**: 934–41.

  7. Turrisi AT IIIrd, Kim K, Blum R, Sause WT, Livingston RB, Komaki R, Wagner H, Aisners S, Johnson DH. Twice-daily compared with once daily thoracic radiotherapy in limited small cell lung cancer treated concurrently with cisplatin and etoposide. *N Engl J Med* 1999; **340**: 265–71.

  8. Non-small Cell Lung Cancer Collaborative Group. Chemotherapy in non-small-cell lung cancer, a meta-analysis using updated data on individual patients from 52 randomized clinical trials. *BMJ* 1995; **311**: 899–909.

  9. Marino P, Pampallona S, Preatoni A, Cantoni A, Invernizzi F. Chemotherapy v supportive care in advanced non-small cell lung cancer: results of a meta-analysis of the literature. *Chest* 1994; **106**: 861–5.

  10. Woodburn JR. The epidermal growth factor receptor and its inhibition in cancer. *Pharmacol Ther* 1999; **82**: 241–50.

  11. Postmus PE. Activity of pemetrexed (Alimta), a new antifolate, against non-small cell lung cancer. *Lung Cancer* 2002; **38**(Suppl 2): S3–7.

List of abbreviations

α_1AT	alpha$_1$-antitrypsin
ACBT	active cycle of breathing technique
ACE	doxorubicin, cyclophosphamide and etoposide
ACQUIP	Ambulatory Care Quality Improvement Project
ACRN	Asthma Clinical Research Network
ADI	AIDS-defining illness
AHR	airway hyper-responsiveness
AIA	aspirin-intolerant asthma
ALT	alanine aminotransferase
AMP	adenosine monophosphate
APACHE	Acute Physiology and Chronic Health Evaluation
ASM	airway smooth muscle
AST	aspartate aminotransferase
ATRA	all-*trans*-retinoic acid
ATS	American Thoracic Society
BAL	bronchoalveolar lavage
BALF	bronchoalveolar lavage fluid
BC	beta-carotene
BCG	Bacillus Calmette-Guerin
BD	bronchodilator
BDI	baseline dyspnoea index
BDP	beclomethasone dipropionate
BMD	bone mineral density
BMI	body mass index
BTS	British Thoracic Society
BUD	budesonide
CAV	cyclophosphamide, doxorubicin and vincristine
CD	cluster of differentiation
CES-D	Centers for Epidemiologic Studies Depression
cfu	colony forming units
CI	confidence interval
CO	carbon monoxide
COPD	chronic obstructive pulmonary disease

CPAP	continuous positive airways pressure
CRDQ	Chronic Respiratory Diseases Questionnaire
CT	computed tomography
CW	conventional work-up
CXR	Chest radiography
DALY	disability adjusted life year
D/C	discharged
DNA	deoxyribonucleic acid
DPD	dry powder device
E	Ethambutol
ECP	eosinophil cationic protein
EGFR	epidermal growth factor receptor
ELCAP	Early Lung Cancer Action Project
eNO	exhaled nitric oxide
ESAT-6	early secretory antigenic target
EUS	endoscopic ultrasound
ev	explained variance
F	formaterol
FDG	fluorodeoxyglucose
FEV$_1$	forced expiratory volume in 1 second
FiO$_2$	fractional concentration of oxygen in inspired air
FLAP	five lipoxygenase activating protein
fMLP	formyl methionyl leucyl phenylalanine
FNA	fine needle aspiration
FP	fluticasone propionate
FRC	functional residual capacity
FVC	forced vital capacity
GC	glucocorticoid
GP	general practitioner
HAART	highly active antiretroviral therapy
HDM	house dust mite
HNC	head and neck cancer
HRCT	high resolution computerized tomography

I	Isoniazid	$PaCO_2$	partial pressure of carbon dioxide in arterial blood
ICS	inhaled corticosteroids		
ICTP	carboxy-terminal cross-linked telopeptide of type I collagen	PaO_2	partial pressure of oxygen in arterial blood
ICU	intensive care unit	PAP	pulmonary artery pressure
IFNγ	Interferon gamma	PC	provocative concentration
IgE	immunoglobulin E	PCI	prophylactic cranial irradiation
IL	interleukin		
IQR	interquartile range	PE	platinum and etoposide
ITU	intensive therapy unit	PEEP	positive end-expiratory pressure
Kco	carbon monoxide		
kPA	kilo Pascales	PEFR	peak expiratory flow rate
LABA	long acting β-2 agonists	PET	positron emission tomography
LHS	Lung Health Study		
LOC	loss of control	PM_{10}	particulate matter of less than 10 _m diameter
LOD	likelihood ratio		
LPS	lipopolysaccharide	PPV	positive predictive value
LTB_4	leukotriene B_4	PTX	pneumothorax
LTBI	latent mycobacterial tuberculosis infection	R	Rifampicin
		ROA	rapid-onset asthma
LVRS	lung-volume reduction surgery	RP	retinyl palmitate
		RR	relative risk
MAC	Mycobacterium avium complex	RV	residual volume
		SaO_2	oxygen saturation in arterial blood
MAS	multi-centre allergy study		
MCD	mucus clearance device	SCLC	small cell lung cancer
MDI	metered dose inhaler	SD	standard deviation
MDRTB	multi-drug resistant tuberculosis	SE	structured educational
		SEER	surveillance, epidemiology and end results
MLS	mediastinal lymph node sampling	SF-36	Short Form 36 Questionnaire
mmHg	mm of mercury	SGRQ	St George's Respiratory Questionnaire
MPO	myeloperoxidase		
MRI	magnetic resonance imaging	SLE	systemic lupus erythematosis
		SND	systemic nodal dissection
MVP	mitomycin, vinblastine and cisplatin	SNP	single nucleotide polymorphism
NAC	N-acetylcysteine	SOA	slow-onset asthma
NETT	National Emphysema Treatment Trial	SPT	second primary tumour
		SVCO	superior vena caval obstruction
NICE	National Institute of Clinical Excellence	TDI	transition dyspnoea index
		Th	T helper
NIV	nasal intermittent positive pressure ventilation	TNFα	tumour necrosis factor alpha
		VA	Veterans Affairs
NMES	neuromuscular electrical stimulation	VAP	ventilator associated pneumonia
NO	nitric oxide		
NPPV	non-invasive positive pressure ventilation	VC	vital capacity
		WHO	World Health Organization
NSCLC	non-small cell lung cancer		
OR	odds ratio		

Index of papers reviewed

Aalbers R, Ayres J, Backer V, Decramer M, Lier PA, Magyar P, Malolepszy J, Ruffin R, Sybrecht GW. Formoterol in patients with chronic obstructive pulmonary disease: a randomized, controlled, 3-month trial. *Eur Respir J* 2002; **19**: 936–43. **140**

Afessa B, Morales IJ, Scanlon PD, Peters SG. Prognostic factors, clinical course, and hospital outcome of patients with chronic obstructive pulmonary disease admitted to an intensive care unit for acute respiratory failure. *Crit Care Med* 2002; **30**: 1610–15. **202**

Ambrogi V, Tonini G, Mineo TC. Prolonged survival after extracranial metastasectomy from synchronous resectable lung cancer. *Annals of Surg Oncol* 2001; 8: 663–6. **318**

American Thoracic Society. Guidelines for the management of adults with community acquired pneumonia. *Am J Respir Crit Care Med* 2001; **163**(7): 1730–54. **245**

Angrill J, Agusti C, de Celis R, Filella X, Rano A, Elena M, De La Bellacasa JP, Xaubet A, Torres A. Bronchial inflammation and colonization in patients with clinically stable bronchiectasis. *Am J Respir Crit Care Med* 2001; **164**(9): 1628–32. **273**

Angrill J, Agusti C, de Celis R, Rano A, Gonzalez J, Sole T, Xaubet A, Rodriguez-Roisin R, Torres A. Bacterial colonization in patients with bronchiectasis: microbiological pattern and risk factors. *Thorax* 2002; **57**(1): 15–19. **272**

Angus DC, Marrie TJ, Obrosky DS, Clermont G, Dremsizov TT, Coley C, Fine MJ, Singer DE, Kapoor WN. Severe community acquired pneumonia: use of intensive care services and evaluation of American and British Thoracic Society Diagnostic criteria. *Am J Respir Crit Care Med* 2002; **166**(5): 717–23. **261**

Arancibia F, Bauer TT, Ewig S, Mensa J, Gonzalez J, Niederman MS, Torres A. Community acquired pneumonia due to Gram-negative bacteria and *Pseudomonas aeruginosa*: incidence, risk, and prognosis. *Arch Intern Med* 2002; **162**(16): 1849–58. **256**

Ardlard JW, Joseph J, Brammer CV, Gerrard GE. Open access follow-up for lung cancer: patient and staff satisfaction. *Clin Oncol* 2001; **13**: 404–8. **339**

Atkinson RW, Anderson HR, Sunyer J, Ayres J, Baccini M, Vonk JM, Boumghar A, Forastiere F, Forsberg B, Touloumi G, Schwartz J, Katsouyanni K. Acute effects of particulate air pollution on respiratory admissions. Results from APHEA 2 Project. *Am J Respir Crit Care Med* 2001; **164**: 1860–6. **93**

Au DH, Curtis JR, Every NR, McDonnell MB, Fihn SD. Association between inhaled β-agonists and the risk of unstable angina and myocardial infarction. *Chest* 2002; **121**: 846–51. **99**

Bach PB, Cramer LD, Schrag D, Downey RJ, Gelfand SE, Begg CB. The influence of hospital volume on survival after resection for lung cancer. *N Engl J Med* 2001; **345**: 181–8. **317**

Basagana X, Sunyer J, Zock JP, Kogevinas M, Urrutia I, Maldonado JA, Almar E, Payo F, Anto JM; Spanish Working Group of the European Community Respiratory

Health Survey. Incidence of asthma and its determinants among adults in Spain. *Am J Respir Crit Care Med* 2001; **164**: 1133–7. **5**

Bellete B, Coberly J, Barnes GL, Ko C, Chaisson RE, Comstock GW, Bishai WR. Evaluation of a whole-blood interferon-gamma release assay for the detection of Mycobacterium tuberculosis infection in 2 study populations. *Clin Infect Dis* 2002; **34**: 1449–56. **212**

Benator D, Bhattacharya M, Bozeman L, Burman W, Cantazaro A, Chaisson R, Gordin F, Horsburgh CR, Horton J, Khan A, Lahart C, Metchock B, Pachucki C, Stanton L, Vernon A, Villarino ME, Wang YC, Weiner M, Weis S; The Tuberculosis Trials Consortium. Rifapentine and Isoniazid once a week versus Rifampicin and Isoniazid twice a week for treatment of drug-susceptible pulmonary tuberculosis in HIV-negative patients: a randomized clinical trial. The Tuberculosis Trials Consortium. *Lancet* 2002; **360**(9332): 528–34. **230**

Bergmans DC, Bonten MJ, Gaillard CA, Paling JC, van der Geest S, van Tiel FH, Beysens AJ, de Leeuw PW, Stobberingh EE. Prevention of ventilator associated pneumonia by oral decontamination: a prospective, randomized, double blind, placebo-controlled study. *Am J Respir Crit Care Med* 2001; **164**(3): 382–8. **265**

Bezjak A, Dixon P, Brundage M, Tu D, Palmer MJ, Blood P, Grafton C, Lochrin C, Leong C, Mulroy L, Smith C, Wright J, Pater JL; Clinical Trials Group of the National Cancer Institute of Canada. Randomized phase III trial of single versus fractionated thoracic radiation in the palliation of patients with lung cancer. *Int J Rad Oncol Biol Phys* 2002; **54**: 719–28. **326**

Bock NN, Sterling TR, Hamilton CD, Pachucki C, Wang YC, Conwell DS, Mosher A, Samuels M, Vernon A; The

Tuberculosis Trials Consortium, Centers for Disease Control and Prevention, Atlanta, Georgia. A prospective, randomized, double blind study of the tolerability of Rifapentine 600, 900, and 1200 mg plus Isoniazid in the continuation phase of tuberculosis treatment. *Am J Respir Crit Care Med* 2002; **165**: 1526–30. **231**

Braun-Fahrländer C, Riedler J, Herz U, Eder W, Waser M, Grize L, Maisch S, Carr D, Gerlach F, Bufe A, Lauener RP, Schierl R, Renz H, Nowak D, von Mutius E; Allergy and Endotoxin Study Team. Environmental exposure to endotoxin and its relation to asthma in school-age children. *N Engl J Med* 2002; **347**: 869–77. **12**

Brightling CE, Bradding P, Syman FA, Holgate ST, Wardlaw AJ, Pavord I. Mast cell infiltration of airway smooth muscle in asthma. *N Engl J Med* 2002; **346**: 1699–705. **53**

British Thoracic Society and Society of Cardiothoracic Surgeons of Great Britain and Ireland Working Party. Guidelines on the selection of patients with lung cancer for surgery. *Thorax* 2001; **56**: 89–108. **312**

Buhl R, Soler M, Matz J, Townley R, O'Brien J, Noga O, Champain K, Fox H, Thirlwell J, Della Cioppa G. Omalizumab provides long-term control in patients with moderate-to-severe asthma. *Eur Respir J* 2002; **20**: 73–8. **78**

Busse W, Corren J, Lanier BQ, McAlary M, Fowler-Taylor A, Cioppa GD, van As A, Gupta N. Omalizumab, anti-IgE recombinant humanized antibody, for the treatment of severe allergic asthma. *J Allergy Clin Immunol* 2001; **108**: 184–90. **76**

Casaburi R, Mahler DA, Jones PW, Wanner A, San PG, ZuWallack RL, Menjoge SS, Serby CW, Witek T. A long-term evaluation of once-daily inhaled tiotropium in chronic obstructive pulmonary disease. *Eur Respir J* 2002; **19**: 217–24. **131**

Shahane A, Zhang J, Reiss TF, Szczeklik A. Improvement of aspirin-intolerant asthma by montelukast, a leukotriene receptor antagonist. *Am J Respir Crit Care Med* 2002; **165**: 9–14. **74**

Dean GL, Edwards SG, Ives NJ, Matthews G, Fox EF, Navaratne L, Fisher M, Taylor GP, Miller R, Taylor CB, de Ruiter A, Pozniak AL. Treatment of tuberculosis in HIV-infected persons in the era of highly active antiretroviral therapy. *AIDS* 2002; **16**(1): 75–83. **228**

de Bruyn G, Garner P. Mycobacterium vaccae immunotherapy for treating tuberculosis. *The Cochrane Library* 2002; **2**: 1–17. **224**

de Marco R, Locatelli F, Cerveri I, Bugiani M, Marinoni A, Giammanco G. Incidence and remission of asthma: a retrospective study on the natural history of asthma. *J Allergy Clin Immunol* 2002; **110**: 228–35. **35**

Dennie CJ, Matzinger FR, Marriner JR, Maziak DE. Transthoracic needle biopsy of the lung: results of early discharge in 506 outpatients. *Radiology* 2001; **219**: 247–51. **305**

Depierre A, Milleron B, Moro-Sibilot D, Chevret S, Quoix E, Lebeau B, Braun D, Breton JL, Lemarie E, Gouva S, Paillot N, Brechot JM, Janicot H, Lebas FX, Terrioux P, Clavier J, Foucher P, Monchatre M, Coetmeur D, Level MC, Leclerc P, Blanchon F, Rodier JM, Thiberville L, Villeneuve A, Westeel V, Chastang C; French Thoracic Cooperative Group. Pre-operative chemotherapy followed by surgery compared with primary surgery in resectable Stage I (except T_1N_0) II and IIIa non-small cell lung cancer. *J Clin Oncol* 2001; **20**: 247–53. **316**

Dimai HP, Domej W, Leb G, Lau K-HW. Bone loss in patients with untreated chronic obstructive pulmonary disease is mediated by an increase in bone resorption associated with hypercapnia. *J Bone Miner Res* 2001; **16**: 2132–41. **115**

Doherty TM, Demissie A, Olobo J, Wolday D, Britton S, Eguale T, Ravn P, Andersen P. Immune responses to the Mycobacterium tuberculosis-specific antigen ESAT-6 signal subclinical infection among contacts of tuberculosis patients. *J Clin Microbiol* 2002; **40**: 704–6. **216**

Donohue JF, van Noord JA, Bateman ED, Langley SJ, Lee A, Witek TJ Jr, Kesten S, Towse L. A 6-month, placebo-controlled study comparing lung function and health status changes in COPD patients treated with tiotropium or salmeterol. *Chest* 2002; **122**: 47–55. **134**

Douglass J, Aroni R, Goeman D, Stewart K, Sawyer S, Thien F. A qualitative study of action plans for asthma. *Br Med J* 2002; **324**: 1003–5. **79**

Downey RJ, Ng KK, Kris MG, Bains MS, Miller VA, Heelan R, Bilsky M, Ginsberg R, Rusch VW. A phase II trial of chemotherapy and surgery for non-small cell lung cancer patients with a synchronous solitary metastasis. *Lung Cancer* 2002; **38**: 193–7. **319**

Drake AJ, Howells RJ, Shield JPH, Prendiville A, Ward PS, Crowne EC. Symptomatic adrenal insufficiency presenting with hypoglycaemia in asthmatic children receiving high dose inhaled fluticasone propionate. *Br Med J* 2002; **324**: 1081–2. **66**

Drobniewski F, Eltringham I, Graham C, Magee JG, Smith EG, Watt B. A national study of clinical and laboratory factors affecting the survival of patients with multiple drug resistant tuberculosis in the UK. *Thorax* 2002; **57**(9): 810–16. **234**

Ducharme FM. Anti-leukotrienes as add-on therapy to inhaled glucocorticoids in patients with asthma: systematic review of current evidence. *Br Med J* 2002; **324**: 1545–8. **75**

gemcitabine and cisplatin in chemotherapy-naïve patients with advanced non-small cell lung cancer (INTACT I). *Ann Oncol* 2002; **13**(Suppl 5): 2 Abstract 40. **336**

Gomersall CD, Joynt GM, Freebairn RC, Lai CKW, Oh TE. Oxygen therapy for hypercapnic patients with chronic obstructive pulmonary disease and acute respiratory failure: a randomized, controlled pilot study. *Crit Care Med* 2002; **30**: 113–16. **193**

Gompertz S, Stockley RA. A randomized, placebo-controlled trial of a leukotriene synthesis inhibitor in patients with COPD. *Chest* 2002; **122**: 289–94. **162**

Gould MK, McLean CC, Kushner WG, Rydzak CE, Owens DK. Accuracy of positron emission tomography for diagnosis of pulmonary nodules and mass lesions. A meta-analysis. *JAMA* 2001; **285**: 914–24. **300**

Green RH, Brightling CE, McKenna S, Hargadon B, Parker D, Bradding P, Wardlaw AJ, Pavord ID. Asthma exacerbations and sputum eosinophil counts: a randomized controlled trial. *Lancet* 2002; **360**: 1715–21. **51**

Gregory RK, Smith IE, Norton A, Ashley S, O'Brien ME. Mitomycin C, vinblastine and carboplatin: effective outpatient chemotherapy for advanced non-small cell carcinoma of the lung (NSCLC). *Clin Oncol* 2001; **13**: 483–7. **323**

Gupta NC, Tamim WJ, Graeber GG, Bishop HA, Hobbs GR. Mediastinal lymph node sampling following positron emission tomography with fluorodeoxyglucose imaging in lung cancer staging. *Chest* 2001; **120**(2): 521–7. **301**

Halm EA, Fine MJ, Kapoor WN, Singer DE, Marrie TJ, Siu AL. Instability on hospital discharge and the risk of adverse outcomes in patients with pneumonia. *Arch Intern Med* 2002; **162**(11): 1278–84. **263**

Hancox RJ, Subbarao P, Kamada D, Watson PM, Hargreave FE, Inman MD. β2-agonist tolerance and exercise-induced bronchospasm. *Am J Respir Crit Care Med* 2002; **165**: 1068–70. **61**

Hattotuwa KL, Gizycki MJ, Ansari TW, Jeffery PK, Barnes NC. The effects of inhaled fluticasone on airway inflammation in chronic obstructive pulmonary disease. A double blind, placebo-controlled biopsy study. *Am J Respir Crit Care Med* 2002; **165**: 1592–6. **127**

Hayneman LE, Herndon JE, Goodman PC, Patz EF. Stage distribution in patients with a small (<3 cm) primary non-small cell lung cancer: Implications for lung cancer screening. *Cancer* 2001; **92**: 3051–5. **289**

Hecht SS. Cigarette smoking and lung cancer: chemical mechanisms and approaches to prevention. *Lancet Oncology* 2002; **3**: 461–9. **294**

Henschke GI, Naidich DP, Yankelevitz DF, McGuinness G, McCauley DI, Smith JP, Libby D, Pasmantier M, Vazquez M, Koizumi J, Flieder D, Altorki N, Miettinen OS. Early lung cancer action project: initial findings on repeat screening. *Cancer* 2001; **92**: 153–9. **287**

Herbst RS, Maddox AM, Rothenberg ML, Small EJ, Rubin EH, Baselga J, Rojo F, Hong WK, Swaisland H, Averbuch SD, Ochs J, LoRusso PM. Selective oral epidermal growth factor receptor tyrosine kinase inhibitor ZD 1839 is generally well-tolerated and has activity in non-small cell lung cancer and other solid tumours: results of a phase I trial. *J Clin Oncol* 2002; **20**: 3815–25. **334**

Hilbert G, Gruson D, Vargas F, Valentino R, Gbikpi-Benissan G, Dupon M, Reiffers J, Cardinaud JP. Non-invasive ventilation in immunosuppressed patients with pulmonary infiltrates, fever, and acute respiratory failure. *N Engl J Med* 2001; **344**(7): 481–7. **259**

Kutlay H, Cangir AK, Enon S, Sahin E, Akal M, Gungor A, Ozdemir N, Kavukcu S. Surgical treatment in bronchiectasis: analysis of 166 patients. *Eur J Cardiothorac Surg* 2002; **21**(4): 634–7. **276**

Lalvani A, Nagvenkar P, Udwadia Z, Pathan AA, Wilkinson KA, Shastri JS, Ewer K, Hill AV, Mehta A, Rodrigues C. Enumeration of T-cells specific for RD1-encoded antigens suggests a high prevalence of latent Mycobacterium tuberculosis infection in healthy urban Indians. *J Infect Dis* 2001; **183**: 469–77. **215**

Lalvani A, Pathan AA, Durkan H, Wilkinson KA, Whelan A, Deeks JJ, Reece WH, Latif M, Pasvol G, Hill AV. Enhanced contact tracing and spatial tracking of Mycobacterium tuberculosis infection by enumeration of antigen-specific T-cells. *Lancet* 2001; **357**: 2017–21. **214**

Lalvani A, Pathan AA, McShane H, Wilkinson RJ, Latif M, Conlon CP, Pasvol G, Hill AV. Rapid detection of Mycobacterium tuberculosis infection by enumeration of antigen-specific T cells. *Am J Respir Crit Care Med* 2001; **163**(4): 824–8. **213**

Larsen SS, Krasnik M, Vilmann P, Jacobsen GK, Pedersen JH, Faurschou P, Folke K. Endoscopic ultrasound-guided biopsy of mediastinal lesions has a major impact on patient management. *Thorax* 2002; **57**(2): 98–103. **308**

Lazarus SC, Boushey HA, Fahy JV, Chinchilli VM, Lemanske RF Jr, Sorkness CA, Kraft M, Fish JE, Peters SP, Craig T, Drazen JM, Ford JG, Israel E, Martin RJ, Mauger EA, Nachman SA, Spahn JD, Szefler SJ; Asthma Clinical Research Network for the National Heart, Lung, and Blood Institute. Long-acting β2-agonist monotherapy vs continued therapy with inhaled corticosteroids in patients with severe asthma: a randomized controlled trial. *JAMA* 2001; **285**: 2583–93. **69**

Lemanske RF, Sorkness CA, Mauger EA, Lazarus SC, Boushey HA, Fahy JV, Drazen JM, Chinchilli VM, Craig T, Fish JE, Ford JG, Israel E, Kraft M, Martin RJ, Nachman SA, Peters SP, Spahn JD, Szefler SJ; Asthma Clinical Research Network for the National Heart, Lung, and Blood Institute. Inhaled corticosteroid reduction and elimination in patients with persistent asthma receiving salmeterol. *JAMA* 2001; **285**: 2594–603. **69**

Leynaert B, Neukirch C, Jarvis D, Chinn S, Burney P, Neukirch F. Does living on a farm during childhood protect against asthma, allergic rhinitis, and atopy in childhood? *Am J Respir Dis Crit Care Med* 2001; **164**: 1829–34. **11**

Lim WS, Macfarlane JT. A prospective comparison of nursing home acquired pneumonia with community acquired pneumonia. *Eur Respir J* 2001; **18**(2): 362–8. **254**

Lim WS, Macfarlane JT, Colthorpe CL. Pneumonia and pregnancy. *Thorax* 2001; **56**: 398–405. **255**

Lippman SM, Lee JJ, Karp DD, Vokes EE, Benner SE, Goodman GE, Khuri FR, Marks R, Winn RJ, Fry W, Graziano SL, Gandara DR, Okawara G, Woodhouse CL, Williams B, Perez C, Kim HW, Lotan R, Roth JA, Hong WK. Randomized phase III intergroup trial of Isotretinoin to prevent second primary tumours in stage I non-small cell lung cancer. *J Natl Cancer Inst* 2001; **93**: 605–18. **295**

Lippman SM, Spitz MR. Lung cancer chemoprevention: an integrated approach. *J Clin Oncol* 2001; **19**: 74s–82s. **294**

Little SA, MacLeod KJ, Chalmers GW, Love JG, McSharry C, Thomson NC. Association of forced expiratory volume with disease duration and sputum neutrophils in chronic asthma. *Am J Med* 2002; **112**: 446–52. **52**

Neder JA, Sword D, Ward SA, Mackay E, Cochrane LM, Clark CJ. Home-based neuromuscular electrical stimulation as a new rehabilitative strategy for severely disabled patients with chronic obstructive pulmonary disease (COPD). *Thorax* 2002; **57**: 333–7. **169**

Nevins ML, Epstein SK. Predictors of outcome for patients with COPD requiring invasive mechanical ventilation. *Chest* 2001; **119**: 1840–9. **199**

Nouira S, Marghli S, Belghith M, Besbes L, Elatrous S, Abroug F. Once daily oral ofloxacin in chronic obstructive pulmonary disease exacerbation requiring mechanical ventilation: a randomized placebo-controlled trial. *Lancet* 2001; **358**: 2020–5. **183**

O'Brien A, Russo-Magno P, Karki A, Hiranniramol S, Hardin M, Kaszuba M, Sherman C, Rounds S. Effects of withdrawal of inhaled steroids in men with severe irreversible airflow obstruction. *Am J Respir Crit Care Med* 2001; **164**: 365–71. **125**

O'Byrne PM, Barnes PJ, Rodriguez-Roisin R, Runnerstrom E, Sandstrom T, Svensson K, Tattersfield A. Low dose inhaled budesonide and formoterol in mild persistent asthma. *Am J Respir Crit Care Med* 2001; **164**: 1392–7. **71**

O'Donnell DE, Forkert L, Webb KA. Evaluation of bronchodilator responses in patients with 'irreversible' emphysema. *Eur Respir J* 2001: **18**: 914–20. **111**

Ojoo JC, Moon T, McGlone S, Martin K, Gardiner ED, Greenstone MA, Morice AH. Patients' and carers' preferences in two models of care for acute exacerbations of COPD: results of a randomized controlled trial. *Thorax* 2002; **57**: 167–9. **177**

Park SK, Lee CM, Heu JP, Song S.D. A retrospective study for the outcome of pulmonary resection in 49 patients with multi-drug resistant tuberculosis. *Int J Tuberc Lung Dis* 2002; **6**(2): 143–9. **239**

Plant PK, Owen JL, Elliott MW. Non-invasive ventilation in acute exacerbations of chronic obstructive pulmonary disease: long-term survival and predictors of in-hospital outcome. *Thorax* 2001; **56**: 708–12. **195**

Platts-Mills T, Vaughan J, Squillace S, Woodfolk J, Sporik R. Sensitization, asthma and a modified Th2 response in children exposed to cat allergen: a population-based cross-sectional study. *Lancet* 2001; **357**: 752–6. **17**

Plaza V, Serrano J, Picado C, Sanchis J. Frequency and clinical characteristics of rapid-onset fatal and near-fatal asthma. *Eur Respir J* 2002; **19**: 846–52. **38**

Pomerantz BJ, Cleveland JC Jr, Olson HK, Pomerantz M. Pulmonary resection for multi-drug resistant tuberculosis. *J Thorac Cardiovasc Surg* 2001; **121**(3): 448–53. **240**

Pneumonia Guidelines Committee of BTS Standards of Care Committee. British Thoracic Society guidelines for the management of community acquired pneumonia in adults. *Thorax* 2001; **56**(Suppl 4): 1–64. **245**

Prescott E, Almdal A, Mikkelsen KL, Tofteng CL, Vestbo J, Lange P. Prognostic value of weight change in chronic obstructive pulmonary disease: results from the Copenhagen City Heart Study. *Eur Respir J* 2002; **20**: 539–44. **97**

Prieto D, Bernardo J, Matos MJ, Eugenio L, Antunes M. Surgery for bronchiectasis. *Eur J Cardiothorac Surg* 2001; **20**(1): 19–23. **276**

Prophylactic Cranial Irradiation Overview Collaborative Group. Cranial irradiation for preventing brain metastases of small cell lung cancer in patients in complete remission. (*Cochrane Review*) The Cochrane Library, 2002; **4**: Oxford: Update Software. **331**

Rami R, Mateu M. Surgical sealant for preventing air leaks after pulmonary

Am J Respir Crit Care Med 2002; **166**: 1062–72. **80**

Schols AMWJ, Wesseling G, Kester ADM, de Vries G, Mostert R, Slangen J, Wouters EF. Dose-dependent increased mortality risk in COPD patients treated with oral glucocorticoids. *Eur Respir J* 2001; **17**: 337–42. **129**

Schumaker T, Brink I, Mix M, Reinhardt M, Herget G, Digel W, Henke M, Moser E, Nitzsche E. FDG-PET imaging for the staging and follow-up of small cell lung cancer. *Eur J Nucl Med* 2001; **28**: 483–8. **304**

Scrivener S, Yemaneberhan H, Zebenigus M, Tilahun D, Girma S, Ali S, McElroy P, Custovic A, Woodcock A, Pritchard D, Venn A, Britton J. Independent effects of intestinal parasite infection and domestic allergen exposure on risk of wheeze in Ethiopia: a nested case-control study. *Lancet* 2002; **358**: 1493–9. **10**

Sears MR, Greene JM, Willan AR, Taylor DR, Flannery EM, Cowan JO, Herbison GP, Poulton R. Long-term relation between breastfeeding and development of atopy and asthma in young adults. *Lancet* 2002; **360**: 901–7. **19**

Sethi S, Evans N, Grant BJB, Murphy TF. New strains of bacteria and exacerbations of chronic obstructive pulmonary disease. *N Engl J Med* 2002; **347**: 465–71. **180**

Shaheen SO, Sterne JAC, Thompson RL, Songhurst CE, Margetts BM, Burney PGJ. Dietary antioxidants and asthma in adults: population based case–control study. *Am J Respir Crit Care* 2001; **164**: 1823–8. **20**

Sharples LD, Edmunds J, Bilton D, Hollingworth W, Caine N, Keogan M, Exley A. A randomized controlled crossover trial of nurse practitioner versus doctor led outpatient care in a bronchiectasis clinic. *Thorax* 2002; **57**(8): 661–6. **279**

Shepherd FA, Dancey J, Arnold A, Neville A, Rusthoven J, Johnson RD, Fisher B, Eisenhauer E. Phase II trial of pemetrexed sodium, (multitargeted antifolate) and cisplatin as first line therapy in patients with advanced non-small cell lung carcinoma. *Cancer* 2001; **92**: 595–600. **337**

Shiraishi Y, Nakajima Y, Takasuna K, Hanaoka T, Katsuragi N, Konno H. Surgery for Mycobacterium avium complex lung disease in the Clarithromycin era. *Eur J Cardiothorac Surg* 2002; **21**(2): 314–18. **242**

Sin DD, Tu JV. Inhaled corticosteroids and the risk of mortality and readmission in elderly patients with chronic obstructive pulmonary disease. *Am J Respir Crit Care Med* 2001; **164**: 580–4. **122**

Smith IE, O'Brien MER, Talbot DC, Nicolson MC, Mansi JL, Hickish TF, Norton A, Ashley S. Duration of chemotherapy in advanced non-small cell lung cancer: A randomized trial of three versus six courses of mitomycin, vinblastine and cisplatin. *J Clin Oncol* 2001; **19**: 1336–43. **323**

Smulders K, van der Hoeven H, Weers-Pothoff I, Van den broucke-Grauls C. A randomized clinical trial of intermittent sub-glottic secretion drainage in patients receiving mechanical ventilation. *Chest* 2002; **121**(3): 858–62. **267**

Soler M, Matz J, Townley R, Buhl R, O'Brien J, Fox H, Thirlwell J, Gupta N, Della Cioppa G. The anti-IgE antibody omalizumab reduces exacerbations and steroid requirement in allergic asthmatics. *Eur Respir J* 2001; **18**: 254–61. **77**

Sone S, Li F, Yang ZG, Honda T, Maruyama Y, Takashima S, Hasegawa M, Kawakami S, Kubo K, Haniuda M, Yamanda T. Results of three-year mass screening programme for lung cancer using

randomized placebo-controlled trial. *Eur Respir J* 2002; **20**: 545–55. **197**

Tiitola M, Kivisaari L, Huuskonen MS, Mattson K, Koskinen H, Lehtola H, Zitting A, Vehmas T. Computed tomography screening for lung cancer in asbestos-exposed workers. *Lung Cancer* 2002; **35**: 17–22. **290**

Turato G, Zuin R, Miniati M, Baraldo S, Rea F, Beghe B, Monti S, Formichi B, Boschetto P, Harari S, Papi A, Maestrelli P, Fabbri LM, Saetta M. Airway inflammation in severe chronic obstructive pulmonary disease. Relationship with lung function and radiologic emphysema. *Am J Respir Crit Care Med* 2002; **165**: 105–10. **107**

Vally H, Taylor ML, Thompson PJ. The prevalence of aspirin-intolerant asthma (AIA) in Australian asthmatic patients. *Thorax* 2002; **57**: 569–74. **6**

Van den Berge M, Kerstjens HA, Meijer RJ, de Reus DM, Koeter GH, Kauffman HF, Postma DS Corticosteroid-induced improvement in the PC_{20} of adenosine $5'$-monophosphate is more closely associated with airway inflammation in asthma than PC_{20} methacholine. *Am J Respir Crit Care Med* 2001; **164**: 1127–32. **46**

Van den Berge M, Meijer RJ, Kerstjens HA, de Reus DM, Koeter GH, Kauffman HF, Postma DS. PC_{20} adenosine $5'$monophosphate is more closely associated with airway inflammation in asthma than PC_{20} methacholine. *Am J Respir Crit Care Med* 2001; **163**: 1546–50. **45**

van den Toorn LM, Overbeek SE, de Johgste JC, Leman K, Hoogsteden HC, Prins J-B. Airway inflammation is present during clinical remission of atopic asthma. *Am J Respir Crit Care Med* 2001; **164**: 2107–13. **57**

Van Eerdwegh P, Little RD, Dupuis J, Del Mastro RG, Falls K, Simon J, Torrey D, Pandit S, McKenny J, Braunschweiger K, Walsh A, Liu Z, Hayward B, Folz C, Manning SP, Bawa A, Saracino L, Thackston M, Benchekroun Y, Capparell N, Wang M, Adair R, Feng Y, Dubois J, FitzGerald MG, Huang H, Gibson R, Allen KM, Pedan A, Danzig MR, Umland SP, Egan RW, Cuss FM, Rorke S, Clough JB, Holloway JW, Holgate ST, Keith TP. Association of the ADAM33 gene with asthma and bronchial hyper-responsiveness. *Nature* 2002; **418**: 426–30. **30**

Van Klaveren RJ, de Koning HJ, Mulshine J, Hirsch FR. Lung cancer screening by spiral CT. What is the optimal target population for screening trials? *Lung Cancer* 2002; **38**: 243–52. **292**

van Manen JG, Bindels PJE, Dekker FW, Ijzermans CJ, van der Zee JS, Schadé E. Risk of depression in patients with chronic obstructive pulmonary disease and its determinants. *Thorax* 2002; **57**: 412–16. **113**

van Tinteren H, Hoekstra OS, Smit EF, van den Bergh JH, Schreurs AJ, Stallaert RA, van Velthoven PC, Comans EF, Diepenhorst FW, Verboom P, van Mourik JC, Postmus PE, Boers M, Teule GJ. Effectiveness of positron emission tomography in the pre-operative assessment of patients with suspected non-small-cell lung cancer: the PLUS multicentre randomized trial. *Lancet* 2002; **359** (9315): 1388–93. **302**

Vekemans J, Lienhardt C, Sillah JS, Wheeler JG, Lahai GP, Doherty MT, Corrah T, Andersen P, McAdam KP, Marchant A. Tuberculosis contacts but not patients have higher gamma interferon responses to ESAT-6 than do community controls in the Gambia. *Infect Immun* 2001; **69**(10): 6554–7. **215**

Volmink J, Garner P. Directly observed therapy for treating tuberculosis. *The Cochrane Library* 2002; **2**: 1–18. **223**

General index

A

ACE (doxorubicin, cyclophosphamide, etoposide) regimen in SCLC 330
action plans for asthma 79, 81
active cycle of breathing technique (ACBT), comparison with flutter valve in bronchiectasis 278
active tuberculosis
    diagnostic role of ESAT-6 212–214, 215–16, 217
    see also tuberculosis
ADAM33 gene, association with asthma 30–1
adenosine monophosphate (AMP) airway hyper-responsiveness 45–8
adrenal insufficiency in high dose inhaled fluticasone propionate therapy 66, 67
air leaks, post-operative 320
air pollution, effects on respiratory admissions 93–5
airborne moulds, effect of sensitization on asthma severity 36, 37
airway hyper-responsiveness (AHR) 35
    demonstration of 45–8
    risk factors for 33–4
    see also asthma
airway inflammation
    in asthma clinical remission 57–8
    in bronchiectasis, impact of bacterial colonization 273–4
    in chronic obstructive pulmonary disease 107–9
        effect of fluticasone 127–8
airway smooth muscle (ASM)
    mast cell infiltration in asthma 53–5
    proliferation in asthma 55–7
airway wall remodelling in asthma 41–3, 57–8
alcohol consumption, effect on chronic obstructive pulmonary disease 95, 96
ALIMTA (pemetrexed) 337–8
allergen avoidance 59–60
allergic rhinitis, protective effect of farm environment 11–12, 15
all-*trans*-retinoic acid (ATRA) therapy 156–7

α_1-antitrypsin deficiency 103–4
α_1-antitrypsin (AT) (α_1 protease inhibitor) therapy 154–6
Ambulatory Care Quality Improvement Project (ACQUIP) 99
ambulatory oxygen, value in COPD 143–5
American Thoracic Society, guidelines for management of community acquired pneumonia 245–52
aminophylline *see* theophylline
anabolic steroids, reversal of COPD-associated weight loss by oxandrolone 167–9
angina risk in beta-2 agonist therapy 99–101
angiogenesis inhibitors 333
antibacterial therapy
    in bronchiectasis 271
    in ventilator associated pneumonia 269–70
        prophylaxis 265–7
anti-cholinergic therapy
    addition of salmeterol 137–9
    see also tiotropium bromide
anti-immunoglobulin E antibody (omalizumab) 76–9
antioxidants, effect on asthma 20, 21
antiretroviral therapy in patients with concomitant HIV and tuberculosis infection 228–30
APHEA 2 Project 93–5
apple consumption, effect on asthma risk 20, 21
asbestos-exposed workers, lung cancer screening 290–1
aspirin-intolerant asthma (AIA) 5
    effect of leukotriene receptor antagonists 74, 75
    prevalence in Australia 6, 7
asthma 3, 84–5
    airway wall remodelling 41–3, 57–8
    cat sensitization 15–18
    clinical course 33–9
    diagnosis 5
        see also asthma: investigations
    effect of housing characteristics 36, 37
    effect of sensitization to airborne moulds 36, 37

KEEPING UP TO DATE IN ONE VOLUME

The Year in Respiratory Medicine 2003

The Year in Respiratory Medicine
appears on a regular basis

To receive more information about the next issue,
or to reserve a copy on publication,
please contact us at the address below:

Clinical Publishing Services Ltd
Oxford Centre for Innovation
Mill Street
Oxford OX2 0JX, UK

T: +44 1865 811116
F: +44 1865 251550
E: info@clinicalpublishing.co.uk
W: www.clinicalpublishing.co.uk

KEEPING UP TO DATE IN ONE SERIES

"The Year in ..."

EXISTING AND FUTURE VOLUMES

The Year in Hypertension 2000   ISBN 0 9537339 0 4
The Year in Rheumatic Disorders 2001   ISBN 0 9537339 1 2
The Year in Neurology 2001   ISBN 0 9537339 5 5
The Year in Gynaecology 2001   ISBN 0 9537339 2 0
The Year in Hypertension 2001   ISBN 0 9537339 4 7
The Year in Diabetes 2001   ISBN 0 9527339 6 3
The Year in Dyslipidaemia 2002   ISBN 0 9537339 3 9
The Year in Interventional Cardiology 2002   ISBN 0 9537339 7 1
The Year in Rheumatic Disorders 2002   ISBN 0 9537339 9 8
The Year in Hypertension 2002   ISBN 1 904392 00 8
The Year in Gynaecology 2002   ISBN 1 904392 01 6
The Year in Allergy 2003   ISBN 1 904392 05 9
The Year in Neurology 2003   ISBN 1 904392 03 2
The Year in Diabetes 2003   ISBN 1 904392 02 4
The Year in Dyslipidaemia 2003   ISBN 1 904392 07 5
The Year in Rheumatic Disorders 2003   ISBN 1 904392 09 1

To receive more information about these books and future volumes,
or to order copies, please contact us at the address below:

Clinical Publishing Services Ltd
Oxford Centre for Innovation
Mill Street
Oxford OX2 0JX, UK

T: +44 1865 811116
F: +44 1865 251550
E: info@clinicalpublishing.co.uk
W: www.clinicalpublishing.co.uk